D1600256

## Index of 'How to... '

# Oxford American Handbook of
# Geriatric Medicine

**Published and Forthcoming Oxford American Handbooks**

Oxford American Handbook of Clinical Medicine
Oxford American Handbook of Anesthesiology
Oxford American Handbook of Clinical Dentistry
Oxford American Handbook of Clinical Diagnosis
Oxford American Handbook of Clinical Pharmacy
Oxford American Handbook of Critical Care
Oxford American Handbook of Emergency Medicine
Oxford American Handbook of Geriatric Medicine
Oxford American Handbook of Nephrology and Hypertension
Oxford American Handbook of Obstetrics and Gynecology
Oxford American Handbook of Oncology
Oxford American Handbook of Otolaryngology
Oxford American Handbook of Pediatrics
Oxford American Handbook of Physical Medicine and Rehabilitation
Oxford American Handbook of Psychiatry
Oxford American Handbook of Pulmonary Medicine
Oxford American Handbook of Rheumatology
Oxford American Handbook of Surgery

# Oxford American Handbook of
# Geriatric Medicine

## Edited by

## Samuel C. Durso

Associate Professor of Medicine
Interim Director
Division of Geriatric Medicine and Gerontology
Johns Hopkins University School of Medicine
Baltimore, Maryland

### with

## Lesley K. Bowker
## James D. Price
## Sarah C. Smith

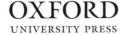

OXFORD
UNIVERSITY PRESS

# OXFORD
UNIVERSITY PRESS

Oxford University Press, Inc. publishes works that further
Oxford University's objective of excellence
in research, scholarship and education.

Oxford  New York

Auckland  Cape Town  Dar es Salaam  Hong Kong  Karachi
Kuala Lumpur  Madrid  Melbourne  Mexico City  Nairobi
New Delhi  Shanghai  Taipei  Toronto

With offices in

Argentina  Austria  Brazil  Chile  Czech Republic  France  Greece
Guatemala  Hungary  Italy  Japan  Poland  Portugal  Singapore
South Korea  Switzerland  Thailand  Turkey  Ukraine  Vietnam

Copyright © 2010 by Oxford University Press, Inc.

Published by Oxford University Press Inc.
198 Madison Avenue, New York, New York 10016

www.oup.com

Library of Congress Cataloging-in-Publication Data

Oxford American handbook of geriatric medicine / edited by Samuel C. Durso ;
with Lesley K. Bowker, James D. Price, Sarah C. Smith.
    p. ; cm. — (Oxford American handbooks)
  Adapted from: Oxford handbook of geriatric medicine / Lesley K. Bowker, James
D. Price, Sarah C. Smith. 2006.
  Includes bibliographical references and index.
  ISBN 978-0-19-537318-9 (flexicover : alk. paper)  1. Geriatrics—Handbooks,
manuals, etc. I. Durso, Samuel C., 1954– II. Bowker, Lesley K. (Leslie Kenyon).
Oxford handbook of geriatric medicine. III. Title: Handbook of geriatric medicine.
IV. Series: Oxford American handbooks.
  [DNLM: 1. Geriatrics—Handbooks.  WT 39 O98 2010]
  RC952.O93 2010
  618.97—dc22

                                                        2009019797

ISBN-13: 978-0-19-537318-9

10  9  8  7  6  5  4  3  2  1

Typeset by Glyph International, Bangalore, India

Printed in China
on acid-free paper

# Preface

Since medical school, I have been a fan of medical handbooks. I like their feel—durable, portable, and readily available. I like the idea they convey, providing expert information boiled down to its essence, yet reliable and proven in the field. A good handbook becomes essential to its user. Its pages become well-thumbed. Its spine acquires a structural memory, opening easily to frequently consulted chapters that correspond to real patient-care experiences at the bedside and office. In creating the *Oxford American Handbook of Geriatric Medicine*, I believe that the publisher and authors have succeeded admirably in creating just such a resource. Collectively, the authors, all colleagues with whom I've worked, have amassed centuries of experience taking care of older adults and thinking about aging. Their expertise comes through clearly.

However, there is something subtler that I have challenged the authors to convey and I hope the reader detects. That is one of tone. The art of geriatric medicine requires competent knowledge and diagnostic skill, certainly, but as much as any specialty, perhaps even more so, it requires a gentle professional temperament, one that is imbued with patience, humility, and wisdom. These are characteristics of the seasoned geriatrician, but are within the grasp of the physician-in-training: patience to listen and be present for the patient; humility to know the limits of scientific and personal knowledge and to respect the patient's self-knowledge; and wisdom to balance competing priorities and see the patient as an individual with unique needs and perspective.

This Handbook is intended to be wedded to these attributes and refreshed by reflection on experience. It is my hope that the physician-in-training will use this resource and follow this path to humane, high-quality medical care of the geriatric patient.

Samuel C. Durso
Baltimore, MD
May 2009

# Acknowledgments

I would like to acknowledge a debt of gratitude to Drs. John Burton, Linda Fried, David Hellmann, and Myron Weisfeldt—all gifted leaders and generous mentors.

I dedicate this book to my wife, Lorna Durso, Ph.D., a superb school psychologist, loving wife and mother, and inspiration for her dedication to her community.

# Contents

# Detailed contents

# List of color plates

# Contributors

**Peter M. Abadir, MD**
Assistant Professor of Medicine,
Division of Geriatric Medicine
and Gerontology
Johns Hopkins University School
of Medicine
Baltimore, Maryland

**Rachel Abuav, MD**
Assistant Professor of
Dermatology
Johns Hopkins University School
of Medicine
Baltimore, Maryland

**Michele Bellantoni, MD**
Associate Professor
Director of Geriatric Medicine
Care Center
Division of Geriatric Medicine and
Gerontology
Johns Hopkins University School
of Medicine
Baltimore, Maryland

**Lisa Boult, MD, MS, MPH**
Assistant Professor
Division of Geriatric Medicine
Johns Hopkins University School
of Medicine
Baltimore, Maryland

**Lynsey Brandt, MD,
PharmD**
Assistant Professor of
Clinical Medicine,
Division of Geriatrics,
University of Pennsylvania
School of Medicine

**Danelle Cayea, MD, MS**
Assistant Professor
Division of Geriatric Medicine
Johns Hopkins University School
of Medicine
Baltimore, Maryland

**Colleen Christmas, MD**
Assistant Professor of
Medicine
Division of Geriatric Medicine
Johns Hopkins University School
of Medicine
Baltimore, Maryland

**Grace Cordts, MD, MPH,
MS, RN**
Clinical Associate
Director of Palliative
Care Service
Johns Hopkins Bayview Medical
Center
Baltimore, Maryland

**Ben Crane, MD, PhD**
Research Fellow in Vestibular
Disease
Department of Otolaryngology
Johns Hopkins University School
of Medicine
Baltimore, Maryland

**Samuel C. Durso, MD, MBA**
Associate Professor of Medicine
Interim Director, Division
of Geriatric Medicine and
Gerontology
Johns Hopkins University School
of Medicine
Baltimore, Maryland

**Cynthia Fields, MD**
Fellow, Geriatric Psychiatry
Johns Hopkins University School
of Medicine
Baltimore, Maryland

**Derek Fine, MD**
Associate Professor of Medicine
Division of Renal Medicine
Johns Hopkins University School
of Medicine
Baltimore, Maryland

**Thomas E. Finucane, MD**

Professor of Medicine
Division of Geriatric Medicine and
Gerontology
Johns Hopkins University School
of Medicine
Baltimore, Maryland

**Rachelle Gajadhar, MD**

Assistant Professor of Medicine
Division of Geriatric Medicine
University of South Carolina
School of Medicine
Columbia,
South Carolina

**F. Michael Gloth, III, MD**

Associate Professor
Division of Geriatric Medicine and
Gerontology
Johns Hopkins University School
of Medicine
Baltimore, Maryland

**William Greenough, III, MD**

Professor of Medicine
Division of Geriatric Medicine
Johns Hopkins University School
of Medicine
Baltimore, Maryland

**Misop Han, MD**

Assistant Professor of Urology
Johns Hopkins University School
of Medicine
Baltimore, Maryland

**Jennifer Hayashi, MD**

Assistant Professor
Director of Elder House Call
Program
Johns Hopkins University School
of Medicine
Baltimore, Maryland

**Franklin Herlong, MD**

Associate Professor of Medicine
Division of Gastroenterology
Johns Hopkins Bayview Medical
Center
Baltimore, Maryland

**Gerald Lazarus, MD**

Professor of Dermatology
Johns Hopkins University School
of Medicine
Baltimore, Maryland

**Shari Ling, MD**

Division of Geriatric Medicine and
Gerontology
Johns Hopkins University School
of Medicine
Research Scientist, National
Institute of Aging
Baltimore, Maryland

**Rafael Llinas, MD**

Associate Professor of
Neurology
Department of Neurology
Johns Hopkins Bayview Medical
Center
Baltimore, Maryland

**Constantine Lyketsos, MD,
MPH**

Chair, Department of
Psychiatry
Johns Hopkins Bayview Medical
Center
Baltimore, Maryland

**Matthew McNabney, MD**

Assistant Professor
Medical Director, Program for
All-Inclusive Care of the Elderly
(PACE)
Director, Fellowship Training
Program
Division of Geriatric Medicine and
Gerontology
Johns Hopkins University School
of Medicine
Baltimore, Maryland

**Richard O'Brien, MD,
Ph.D.**

Chair, Department of
Neurology
Johns Hopkins Bayview Medical
Center
Baltimore, Maryland

**Wilmer Roberts, MD, Ph.D.**
Resident, Department of Urology
Johns Hopkins Hospital
Baltimore, Maryland

**Catherine Schreiber, MD**
Post-Doctoral IRTA Fellow
Longitudinal Research Branch
National Institute on Aging
National Institutes of Health
Baltimore, Maryland

**Gary Shapiro, MD**
Chief of Oncology
Johns Hopkins Bayview Medical Center
Baltimore, Maryland

**Amit Shah, MD**
Assistant Professor of Medicine
University of Texas Southwestern
Dallas, Texas

**Brady Stein, MD**
Fellow, Division of Hematology
Johns Hopkins Hospital
Baltimore, Maryland

**Jeremy Walston, MD**
Professor of Medicine
Co-Director Biology of Frailty
Division of Geriatric Medicine and Gerontology
Johns Hopkins University School of Medicine
Baltimore, Maryland

**Robert Weinberg, MD**
Professor of Ophthalmology
Chief of Ophthalmology
Johns Hopkins Bayview Medical Center
Baltimore, Maryland

**Carlos Weiss, MD, MHS**
Assistant Professor
Division of Geriatric Medicine and Gerontology
Johns Hopkins University School of Medicine
Baltimore, Maryland

**Robert Wise, MD**
Professor of Medicine
Division of Pulmonary Medicine
Johns Hopkins University School of Medicine
Baltimore, Maryland

**James Wright, MD**
Assistant Professor of Urology
Department of Urology
Johns Hopkins Bayview Medical Center
Baltimore, Maryland

**Janet Yellowitz, DMD, MPH**
Associate Professor of Dentistry
University of Maryland School of Dentistry
Baltimore, Maryland

**Jonathan Zennilman, MD, MPH**
Chief of Infectious Disease
Johns Hopkins Bayview Medical Center
Baltimore, Maryland

**Susan Zieman, MD, PhD**
Assistant Professor of Medicine
Division of Cardiology
Johns Hopkins University School of Medicine
Baltimore, Maryland

**Richard Zorowitz, MD**
Chair of Physical Medicine and Rehabilitation
Johns Hopkins Bayview Medical Center
Baltimore, Maryland

# Abbreviations

| | |
|---|---|
| ↓ | decreased |
| ↑ | increased |
| ► | important |
| ►► | don't dawdle |
| A-a | alveolar–arterial |
| AAA | abdominal aortic aneurysm |
| ABG | arterial blood gases |
| ABI | ankle–brachial index |
| ABPI | ankle–brachial pressure index |
| ACD | anemia of chronic disease |
| ACE | angiotensin-converting enzyme; acute care for elders |
| ACS | acute coronary syndrome; American College of Surgeons |
| ACTH | adrenocorticotrophic hormone |
| AD | Alzheimer's disease |
| ADH | antidiuretic hormone |
| ADL | activities of daily living |
| AF | atrial fibrillation |
| AFB | acid-fast bacilli (TB) |
| AICD | automatic implantable cardiac defibrillator |
| AIN | acute interstitial nephritis |
| AL | assisted living |
| ALE | average life expectancy |
| ALP | alkaline phosphatases |
| ALS | advanced life support; amyotrophic lateral sclerosis |
| AMA | American Medical Association |
| AMD | age-related macular degeneration |
| AML | acute myeloid leukemia |
| ANA | antinuclear antibody |
| ANCA | anti-neutrophil cytoplasmic antibody |
| ANUG | acute necrotizing ulcerative gingivitis |
| AOTA | American Occupational Therapy Association |
| ARB | angiotensin receptor blocker |
| ARDS | adult respiratory distress syndrome |
| ARF | acute renal failure |
| ASA | aspirin |
| ATN | acute tubular necrosis |

| AV | atrioventricular |
| --- | --- |
| BCC | basal cell carcinoma |
| bid | two times daily |
| BMI | body mass index |
| BNP | B-type natriuretic peptide |
| BP | blood pressure |
| BPH | benign prostatic hypertrophy |
| BPPV | benign paroxysmal positional vertigo |
| BUN | blood urea nitrogen |
| CABG | coronary artery bypass grafting |
| CAD | coronary artery disease |
| CAM | complementary and alternative medicine |
| CMA | Confusion Assessment Method |
| CBC | complete blood count |
| CBT | cognitive-behavioral therapy |
| CCB | calcium channel blocker |
| CD | *Clostridium difficile*; Crohn's disease |
| CDAD | *Clostridium difficile*–associated diarrhea |
| CDC | Centers for Disease Prevention and Control |
| CDT | clock drawing test |
| CEA | carcinoembryonic antigen; carotid endarterectomy |
| CF | cardiac failure |
| CGA | comprehensive geriatric assessment |
| CHD | coronary heart disease |
| CHF | congestive heart failure |
| ChEI | cholinesterase inhibitor |
| CIDP | chronic inflammatory demyelinating polyradiculoneuropathy |
| CIND | cognitive impairment no dementia |
| CK | creatine kinase |
| CKD | chronic kidney disease |
| CLL | chronic lymphocytic leukemia |
| CMP | complete metabolic profile |
| CMS | Centers for Medicare and Medicaid Services |
| CNS | central nervous system |
| COPD | chronic obstructive pulmonary disease |
| COTA | certified occupational therapist |
| CPR | cardiopulmonary resuscitation |
| CrCl | creatinine clearance |
| CRI | chronic renal insufficiency |

| CRP | C-reactive protein |
| CRRN | Certified Rehabilitation Registered Nurse |
| CSF | cerebrospinal fluid |
| CSS | carotid sinus syndrome |
| CT | computerized tomography |
| CTPA | CT pulmonary angiogram |
| CVD | cardiovascular disease |
| CXR | chest X-ray |
| DAT | dementia of the Alzheimer's type |
| DBP | diastolic blood pressure |
| DEXA | dual X-ray absorptiometry |
| DIC | disseminated intravascular coagulation |
| DIP | desquamative interstitial pneumonia |
| DKA | diabetic ketoacidosis |
| DLB | dementia with Lewy bodies |
| DM | diabetes mellitus |
| DNAR | do not attempt resuscitation |
| DNR | do not resuscitate |
| DOE | dyspnea on exertion |
| DPI | dry-powder inhaler |
| DPOA | durable power of attorney |
| DPOAHC | durable power of attorney for health care |
| DRE | digital rectal examination |
| DSM | *Diagnostic and Statistical Manual of Mental Disorders* |
| DVT | deep vein (venous) thrombosis |
| ECT | electroconvulsive therapy |
| ECG | electrocardiogram |
| ED | emergency department |
| EDD | estimated date of discharge |
| EEG | electroencephalogram |
| EF | ejection fraction |
| ELISA | enzyme-linked immunosorbent assay |
| EMG | electromyogram |
| ENT | ear, nose, throat |
| EORA | elderly-onset rheumatoid arthritis |
| EPS | extrapyramidal side effects |
| ERCP | endoscopic retrograde cholangiopancreatograhpy |
| ESA | erythropoeitic-stimulating agent |
| ESR | erythrocyte sedimentation rate |
| ESRF | end stage renal failure |

| | |
|---|---|
| FBC | full blood count |
| FDA | Food and Drug Administration |
| $FEV_1$ | forced expiratory volume in 1 second |
| FFS | fee for service |
| FNA | fine-needle aspiration |
| FSH | follicle-stimulating hormone |
| FTD | frontotemporal dementia |
| GBM | glomerular basement membrane |
| GCA | giant cell arteritis |
| GCS | Glasgow coma scale |
| GCS-F | granulocyte colony stimulating factor |
| GDS | Genatric Depression Scale |
| GEM | geriatric evaluation and management |
| GERD | gastroesophageal reflux disease |
| GFR | glomerular filtration rate |
| GI | gastrointestinal |
| GN | glomerulonephritis |
| GRECC | geriatric research education and clinical center |
| Hb | hemoglobin |
| $HbA_{1c}$ | glycosylated hemoglobin |
| HCTZ | hydrochlorothiazide |
| HD | hemodialysis |
| HDL | high-density lipoprotein |
| HF | heart failure |
| HHS | hyperosmolar hyperglycemic rate |
| HIV | human immunodeficiency virus |
| HLE | healthy life expectancy |
| HONK | hyperosmolar nonketotic coma |
| HRT | hormone replacement therapy |
| IADL | instrumental activities of daily life |
| IBS | irritable bowel syndrome |
| ICD | implantable cardioverter defibrillator |
| ICU | intensive care unit |
| IDA | iron deficiency anemia |
| IDDM | insulin-dependent diabetes mellitus |
| IFN | interferon |
| IGT | impaired glucose tolerance |
| IHC | immunohistochemistry |
| IHD | ischemic heart disease |
| IM | intramuscular |

| | |
|---|---|
| IP | interphalangeal |
| IPPS | International Prognostic Scoring System; International Prostate Symptom Score |
| IPT | interpersonal therapy |
| ISS | International Staging System |
| IV | intravenous |
| IVC | inferior vena cava |
| IVIG | intravenous immunoglobulin |
| JVP | jugular venous pressure |
| KUB | kidneys, ureter, bladder |
| LACS | lacunar anterior circulation stroke |
| LAD | left axis deviation |
| LBBB | left bundle branch block |
| LDH | lactate dehydrogenase |
| LDL | low-density lipoprotein |
| LFT | liver function tests |
| LH | luteinizing hormone |
| LHRH | luteinizing hormone-releasing hormone |
| LM | lentigo maligna |
| LMN | lower motor neuron |
| LMWH | low-molecular-weight heparin |
| LP | lumbar puncture |
| LST | life-sustaining treatment |
| LTOT | long-term oxygen therapy |
| LUTS | lower urinary tract symptoms |
| LV | left ventricular |
| LVH | left ventricular hypertrophy |
| MAOI | monoamine oxidase inhibitor |
| mcg | microgram(s) |
| MCI | minimal cognitive impairment |
| MCP | metacarpophalangeal |
| MCV | mean cell volume |
| MDI | metered-dose inhaler |
| MDS | minimum data set; myelodysplastic syndrome |
| MGUS | monoclonal gammopathy of undetermined significance |
| MI | myocardial infarction |
| MM | multiple myeloma |
| MMA | methylmalonic acid |
| MMSE | Mini Mental State Examination |
| MRI | magnetic resonance imaging |

| MRSA | methicillin-resistant *Staphylococcus aureus* |
| MSE | mental status examination |
| MSSA | methicillin-sensitive *Staphylococcus aureus* |
| MST | morphine slow release |
| MTP | metatarsophalangeal |
| NG | nasogastric |
| NH | nursing home |
| NIDDM | non-insulin-dependent diabetes mellitus |
| NIH | National Institutes of Health |
| NIV | noninvasive ventilation |
| NMS | neuroleptic malignant syndrome |
| NPH | normal-pressure hydrocephalus |
| NPO | nothing by mouth (nil per os) |
| NSAID | non steroidal anti-inflammatory drug |
| NSIP | nonspecific interstitial pneumonitis |
| NYHA | New York Heart Association |
| OA | osteoarthritis |
| OASIS | Outcome and Assessment Information Set |
| OH | orthostatic hypotension |
| OP | osteoporosis |
| ORT | oral replacement therapy |
| OSA | obstructive sleep apnea |
| OT | occupational therapy (or therapist) |
| OTC | over the counter |
| PA | pulmonary artery |
| PACE | program for all-inclusive care of the elderly |
| $PaCo_2$ | arterial carbon dioxide |
| PACS | partial anterior circulation stroke |
| $PaO_2$ | aterial oxygen |
| PCA | patient-controlled analgesia |
| PCI | percutaneous coronary intervention |
| PCR | polymerase chain reaciton |
| PD | Parkinson's disease; peritoneal dialysis |
| PDD | Parkinson's disease with dementia |
| PE | pulmonary embolism |
| PEC | Physician's Emergency Certificate |
| PEFR | peak expiratory flow rate |
| PEG | percutaneous endoscopic gastrostomy |
| PET | positron emission tomography |
| PHQ-9 | Patient Health Questionnaire (9) |

| PMR | polymyalgia rheumatica |
| PM&R | physical medicine and rehabilitation |
| PO | by mouth (per os) |
| POA | power of attorney |
| POCS | posterior circulation stroke |
| PP | pressure pulse |
| PPI | protein pump inhibitor |
| PPO | preferred provider organization |
| PR | per rectum (anally) |
| PRN | pro re nata (as needed) |
| PSA | prostate-specific antigen |
| PST | problem-solving therapy |
| PT | physiotherapy (or therapist) |
| PTH | parathyroid hormone |
| PVD | peripheral vascular disease |
| qhs | every bedtime |
| qid | four times daily |
| QOL | quality of life |
| RA | rheumatoid arthritis |
| RBBB | right bundle branch block |
| RCT | randomized controlled trial |
| RDW | red cell distribution width |
| RES | reticuloendothelial system |
| RIG | radiographically inserted gastrostomy |
| rt-PA | recombinant tissue plasminogen activator |
| SA | sinoatrial |
| SBP | systolic blood pressure |
| SC | subcutaneously |
| SCC | squamous cell carcinoma |
| SDM | surrogate decision maker |
| SIADH | syndrome of inappropriate ADH secretion |
| SLE | systemic lupus erythematosus |
| SLP | speech–language pathologist |
| SNRI | serotonin–norepinephrine reuptake inhibitor |
| SPECT | single photon emission computed tomography |
| SPF | sun protection factor |
| SR | sustained release |
| SSRI | selective serotonin reuptake inhibitor |
| STD | sexually transmitted disease |
| SVT | supraventricular tachycardia |

| T3 | triiodothyronine |
|---|---|
| T4 | levothyroxine |
| TA | temporal arteritis |
| TAB | temporal artery biopsy |
| TACS | total anterior circulation stroke |
| TB | tuberculosis |
| TBI | toe–brachial index |
| TCA | tricyclic antidepressant |
| TEE | transesophageal echocardiogram |
| TENS | transcutaneous nerve stimulation |
| TFT | thyroid function test |
| TIA | transient ischemic attack |
| tid | three times daily |
| TIV | trivalent inactivated influenza vaccine |
| TNF | tumor necrosis factor |
| TPO | thyroperoxidase |
| TR | transferritin receptor |
| TSH | thyroid-stimulating hormone |
| TURP | transurethral resection of the prostate |
| UA | urinalysis |
| UC | ulcerative colitis |
| U,C+E | urea, creatinine, and electrolytes |
| UFH | unfractionated heparin |
| UIP | usual interstitial pneumonia |
| UMN | upper motor neuron |
| URI | upper respiratory infection |
| USA | unstable angina |
| USPSTF | U.S. Preventive Services Task Force |
| UTI | urinary tract infection |
| VA | Veterans Affairs |
| VaD | vascular dementia |
| VATS | video-assisted thorascopy |
| VBI | vertebrobasilar insufficiency |
| VF | ventricular fibrillation |
| VOR | vestibuo-ocular reflex |
| V/Q | ventilation–perfusion (ratio) |
| VT | ventricular tachycardia |
| WBC | white blood cell |
| WHO | World Health Organization |

# Chapter 1

# Aging

## Jeremy Walston

# The aging person

There are many differences between old and young people. In only some cases are these changes due to true aging, i.e., to changes in characteristics from when the person was young.

## Changes not due to aging

- *Selective survival.* Genetic, psychological, lifestyle, and environmental factors influence survival, thus certain characteristics will be over-represented in older people.
- *Differential challenge.* Systems and services (health, finance, transportation, and retail stores) are often designed and managed in ways that make them more accessible to young people. The greater challenge presented to older people has many effects (e.g., impaired access to health services).
- *Cohort effects.* Societies change, and during the twentieth century change has been rapid. Consequently, both young and old have been exposed to very different physical, social, and cultural environments.

## Changes due to aging

- *Primary aging* is usually due to interactions between genetic (intrinsic, "nature") and environmental (extrinsic, "nurture") factors. Examples include lung cancer in susceptible individuals who smoke, hypertension in susceptible individuals with high salt intake, and diabetes in those with a "thrifty genotype" who adopt a higher-calorie and lower-energy lifestyle. Also, some genes influence more general, cellular aging processes. Only now are specific genetic disease susceptibilities being identified, offering the potential to intervene early and modify risk.
- *Secondary aging* is adaptation to changes of primary aging. These are commonly behavioral, e.g., reduction or cessation of driving as reaction times increase.

## Aging and senescence

Differences between old and young people are thus heterogeneous, and individual effects may be viewed as

- Beneficial (e.g., increased experiential learning, increased peak bone mineral density [reflecting the active youth of older people]),
- Neutral (e.g., graying of hair, pastime preferences), or
- Disadvantageous (e.g., decreased reaction time, development of hypertension).

The bulk of changes, especially those in late middle and older age, are detrimental in meeting pathological and environmental challenges. This loss of adaptability results from homeostatic mechanisms being less prompt, less precise, and less potent than they once were. Thus death rates increase exponentially with age, from a nadir around age 12. In very old age (80–100 years) some tailing-off of the rate of increase is seen, perhaps due to selective survival, but the increase continues nonetheless.

## Further reading

Halter JB, Ouslander JG, Tinetti M, et al. (2009), *Hazzard's Geriatric Medicine and Gerontology*, 6th ed, New York: McGraw-Hill.

# Theories of aging

With few exceptions, all organisms age, manifesting as increased mortality and a finite life span. Theories of aging abound, with over 300 diverse theories existing. Few stand up to careful scrutiny, however, and none has been confirmed as definitely playing a major role. Four examples follow.

## Oxidative damage

Reactive oxygen species fail to be cleared by antioxidative defenses and damage key molecules, including DNA. Damage builds up until key metabolic processes are impaired and cells die.

Despite evidence from in vitro and epidemiological studies supporting beneficial effects of antioxidants (e.g., vitamins C and E), clinical trial results have been disappointing.

## Abnormal control of cell mitosis

For most cell lines, the number of times that cell division can occur is limited (the "Hayflick limit"). Senescent cells may predominate in tissues without significant replicative potential such as cornea and skin. The number of past divisions may be "memorized" by a functional "clock"—DNA repeat sequences (telomeres) shorten until further division ceases.

In other cells, division may continue uncontrolled, resulting in hyperplasia and pathologies as diverse as atherosclerosis and prostatic hyperplasia.

## Protein modification

Changes include oxidation, phophorylation, and glycation (non-enzymatic addition of sugars). Complex glycosylated molecules are the final result of multiple sugar–protein interactions, resulting in a structurally and functionally abnormal protein molecule.

## Wear and tear

There is no doubt that physical damage plays a part in aging of some structures, especially skin, bone, and teeth, but this is far from a universal explanation of aging.

## Aging and evolution

In many cases, theories are consistent with the view that aging is a by-product of genetic selection: favored genes are those that enhance reproductive fitness in earlier life but which may have later detrimental effects. For example, a gene that enhances oxidative phosphorylation may increase a mammal's speed or stamina, while increasing the cumulative burden of oxidative damage that usually manifests much later.

Many genes appear to influence aging. In concert with differential environmental exposures, these result in extreme phenotypic heterogeneity, i.e., people age at different rates and in different ways.

# Demographics: life expectancy

- Life expectancy (average age at death) in the developed world has been rising since accurate records began and continues to rise linearly.
- Life span (maximum possible attainable age) is thought to be around 120 years. It is determined by human biology and has not changed.
- Population aging is not just a minor statistical observation but a dramatic change that is easily observed in only a few generations.
  - In 2006, life expectancy at birth for women born in the United States was 80.4 years, and 75.8 years for men.
  - This contrasts with 49 and 45 years, respectively, at the end of the nineteenth century.
- Although worldwide rises in life expectancy at birth are mainly explained by improvements in perinatal mortality, there is also a clear prolongation of later life in the United States.
  - Between 1981 and 2002, life expectancy at age 50 increased by 4 years for Caucasian and by about 2 years for each gender for non-Caucasian U.S. residents.
  - While projections suggest this trend will continue, it is possible that the modern epidemic of obesity might slow or reverse this.

### Individualized life expectancy estimates

Simple analysis of population statistics reveals that mean male life expectancy is 76 years. However, this is not helpful when counseling an 80-year-old! Table 1.1 demonstrates that as a person gets older their individual life expectancy actually increases. This has relevance in deciding on health-care interventions (see also Chapter 32, Preventive medicine).

**Table 1.1** Predicted life expectancy in United States at various ages by gender and ethnicity

| Age at time of estimate | Median years left to live | | | |
| | Caucasian | | Non-Caucasian | |
| | Male | Female | Male | Female |
| 50 years | 29.1 | 32.9 | 25.3 | 30.2 |
| 60 years | 20.9 | 24.1 | 18.3 | 22.3 |
| 70 years | 13.7 | 16.2 | 12.6 | 15.4 |
| 80 years | 8.1 | 9.7 | 8.2 | 9.7 |

Source: U.S. Department of Commerce, Bureau of Census.

# Demographics: population age structure

### Fertility

*Fertility* is defined as the number of live births per adult female. This rate is currently around 2.1 in the United States, signifying a general stasis in overall population growth. In contrast, during the baby boom years of the 1950s, fertility rates reached almost 3. This bulge in the population pyramid will reach old age in 2010–2030, producing a more rectangular rather then pyramidal future for population structure in the United States. A greater potential economic and caregiving burden will fall to younger members of society.

### Deaths and cause of death

The driver of mortality decline has changed over the twentieth century, from reductions in infant/child mortality to improvements in old-age mortality. The most common cause of death for people aged 50–64 is cancer (lung in men, breast in women). Over the age of 65, circulatory diseases (heart attacks and stroke) are the most common cause of death, followed by lung cancer, Alzheimer's disease, renal failure, and chronic pulmonary diseases.

All these statistics rely on the accuracy of death certification, which is reduced with increasing age when death occurs in the setting of multiple comorbid conditions.

### Population "pyramids"

These demonstrate the age–sex structure of different populations. The shape is determined by fertility and death rates. "Pyramids" from developing nations (and the United States in the past) have a wide base (high fertility but also high death rates, especially in childhood) and triangular tops (very small numbers of older people).

In the developed world the shape has become more squared off (see Fig. 1.1), with some countries having an inverted pyramidal shape—people in their middle years outnumber younger people—as fertility declines below replacement values for prolonged periods.

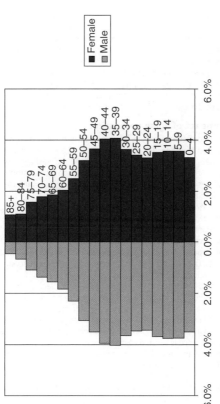

**Fig. 1.1** U.S. age distribution 2000. Source: www.CensusScope.org. Social Science Data Analysis Network of Michigan: www.ssdan.net.

# Demographics: aging and illness

### Healthy life expectancy and prevalence of morbidity

*Healthy life expectancy* (HLE) is that expected to be spent in good or fairly good health. From both an individual and societal perspective it is desirable to have an equivalent or greater rise in healthy life expectancy as in total life expectancy.

"Compression of morbidity," in which illness and disability are squeezed into shorter periods at the end of life, occurs when the rate of disability declines faster than the rate of decline in mortality. Trends in U.S. data since 1982 suggest that compression of morbidity is occurring.

This is most pronounced in individuals with fewer behavioral health risks compared to individuals with more risk factors. Those with fewer behavioral health risks have a quarter of the disability of those with more risk factors and the onset of disability is postponed by 7 to 12 years, which far exceeds the extension of longevity for this group.

### Social impact of aging population

The U.S. population of adults over age 65 is expected to nearly double over the next two decades, increasing from 12% in 2005 to approximately 20% by 2030. The oldest old—those over 80 years of age—will continue to comprise the fastest growing age group. Changes in immigration to the United States (economic migrants are mostly young) will have little effect on the overall shift.

While a large percentage of older adults enter traditional retirement age in good health, more than three quarters have at least one chronic health condition that requires ongoing management. Furthermore, 20% of Medicare beneficiaries have five or more chronic medical conditions. The potential impact of this demographic shift on society's attitudes toward aging adults, the provision of health care, and the overall economy is great. Examples include the following:

- Financing pensions and health services—Social Security in the United States, as in most countries, is financed on a "pay-as-you-go" basis, so will have to be paid for by a smaller workforce. This will mean greater levels of taxation for those in work or a reduction in government pension. Unless private pension investment (from personal savings) improves, there is a risk that many retirees will live in relative poverty.
- Health-care and disability services—the prevalence and degree of disability increases with age. Medicare calculations show that more than a quarter of health-care expenditure is during the last year of a person's life, with half of that occurring during the last 60 days.
- Families are more likely to be supporting older members.
- Retired people comprise a growing market, thus companies and industries that accommodate the needs and wishes of older people will flourish.
- Transport, housing, and infrastructure must be built or adapted.
- Political power of older adults will grow.

### Further reading

http://www.cdc.gov/nchs/fastats/lifexpec.htm
Institute of Medicine (IOM) (2008). *Retooling for an Aging America: Building the Health Care Workforce*. Washington, DC: National Academies Press.

# Illness in older people

One of the paradoxes of medical care of the older person is that the frequency of some presentations (falls, delirium) and of some diagnoses (infection, dehydration) encourages the belief that medical management is straightforward and that investigation and treatment may satisfactorily be inexpensive and low skill (and thus intellectually unrewarding for the staff involved).

However, the objective reality is the reverse. Diagnosis is frequently more challenging, and the therapeutic pathway less clear and more littered with obstacles. However, choose the right path, and the results (both patient-centered and societal [costs of care, etc.]) are substantial.

## Features of illness in older people

- Present atypically and nonspecifically
- Cause greater morbidity and mortality
- May progress much more rapidly—a few hours' delay in diagnosis of a septic syndrome is much more likely to be fatal
- Health, social, and financial sequelae. Failures of treatment may have long-term, wide-ranging effects (e.g., loss of independence requiring institutional care).
- Co-pathology is common. For example, in the older patient with pneumonia and recent atypical chest pain, make sure you exclude myocardial infarction (MI; sepsis precipitates a hyperdynamic, hypercoagulable state, increasing the risk of acute coronary syndromes, and a proportion of atypical pain is cardiac in origin).
- Lack of physiological reserve. If physiological function is "borderline" (in terms of impacting lifestyle or precipitating symptoms), minor deterioration may lead to significant disability. Conversely, apparently minor improvements may disproportionately improve function. For example, identification and correction of several minor disorders may yield dramatic benefits (e.g., stopping medication that causes confusion and removing ear wax that impairs hearing can restore independent function).

## Investigating older people

- *Investigative procedures* may be less well tolerated by older people. Thus the investigative pathway is more complex, with decision-making dependent on clinical presentation, sensitivity and specificity of test, side effects and discomfort of the test, hazards of "blind" treatment or "watchful waiting," and, of course, the wishes of the patient.
- *Consider the significance of positive results.* Fever of unknown cause is a common presentation, and urinalysis a mandatory investigation. But what proportion of healthy, community-dwelling, older women has asymptomatic bacteriuria and a positive dipstick? (A: around 30%, depending on sample characteristics). Therefore, in what proportion of older people presenting with fever and a positive dipstick is urinary tract infection (UTI) the significant pathology? (A: much less than 100%!).

The practical consequence of this is missing fever arising from chest, abdominal, or central nervous system infection that is erroneously attributed to UTI following positive urinalysis.

## Treating disease in older people

- *Benefit may be substantial* from clinical interventions—e.g., thrombolysis for acute coronary syndrome). For example, an older and sicker person with an ejection fraction (EF) of 30% (perhaps, an 80-year-old with heart failure) may derive relatively great benefit from aggressive action that preserves left ventricular function. Note that the important consideration is function, not age.
- *Benefit may be marginal.* Life expectancy and the balance of risks and benefits must be considered in decision-making. For example, avoidance of medication-induced dizziness and falls is more likely to be a priority in a frail 95-year-old than long-term benefit from control of hypertension.
- *Side effects* of therapies are more likely. In coronary care, beta-blockade, aspirin, angiotensin-converting enzyme (ACE) inhibitors, thrombolysis, and heparin may all have significant life- (and quality-of-life-) saving effects in older patients. Studies show that these agents are underused in MI patients of all ages, but much more so in the elderly population. The frequency of side effects (bradycardia and block, profound hypotension, renal impairment, and bleeding) is greater in older people, although a significant net benefit remains.
- *Response to treatment may be less immediate.* Convalescence is slower, and the physician and health-care team may not see the eventual outcome of their work (the patient having been transferred to rehabilitation, for example).

## Further reading

Fried LP, Storer DJ, King DE, Lodder F (1991). Diagnosis of illness in the elderly. *J Am Geriatr Soc* **39**(2):117–123.

# Geriatric care continuum

**Jennifer Hayashi**
**Michele Bellantoni**
**Matthew McNabney**

# Navigating the geriatric care continuum

### The role of physicians and care teams

Geriatricians are trained in the care of older adults and are keenly aware of the complex needs of that population as well as the sites of care along the continuum. Specialty training for geriatricians is done primarily within the care settings described in this chapter. Careful attention by the physician to *care transitions* is critical to successful navigation of this continuum by older adults.

Although geriatricians are specifically trained in the care of older adults, most of the care is provided by generalists (internists and family physicians). Important skills for all physicians who provide care for older adults are the awareness of care options, good communication with patients and their families, and attention to medications.

Physicians often work within care teams when they provide care for older adults. These teams typically consist of professionals from different disciplines To understand the components and value of team-based care, it is important to consider who should be on the team and how team members work together.

Characteristics of cohesive care teams include the following:
- Clear goals with measurable outcomes
- Clinical and administrative systems
- Division of labor
- Training of all team members
- Effective communication

Teams with greater cohesion are associated with better clinical outcome measures and higher patient satisfaction. However, a number of barriers to team formation exist, chiefly related to the challenges of human relationships and personalities.

### Comprehensive geriatric assessment (CGA)

Comprehensive geriatric assessment (CGA) is a structured process that evaluates older adults from multiple perspectives and often incorporates the expertise of several disciplines (see Chapter 3, Clinical assessment). Typically these include medicine, nursing, social work, physical and occupational therapy, and dietary and mental health. However, CGA can be performed with only a portion of those disciplines represented, or even by the physician alone.

CGA often uncovers many important conditions and problematic social situations that would not otherwise be discovered. These findings will often determine which services are most appropriate for the older adult.

In addition to CGA extensive assessment is a regulatory requirement in certain care settings. This includes nursing home care (the Minimum Data Set, or MDS) and home care (the Outcome and Assessment Information Set, or OASIS). A "common assessment tool for post-acute care" is currently being developed by Medicare to overcome the problems of fragmented assessment for older adults who are transitioning out of acute illness.

# Settings of care

### Ambulatory care

Primary care in the ambulatory setting includes a team of health-care providers, led by the physician, who oversee a continuum of health-care services including preventive care, management of chronic health conditions, coordination of services among subspecialists, and urgent care of acute conditions.

Medical technicians administer health screens for vision, hearing, physical function, falls, abuse, and depression.

Nurses administer vaccines and injectable treatments and provide education on safe medication administration and adverse drug experiences. Advanced practice nurses and physician assistants provide timely follow-up on chronic conditions, fine tuning the care plan established by the physician.

Referrals are made to social workers, home health services, governmental agencies such as the local Office on Aging and Adult Protective Services, and community resources such as Meals on Wheels and transportation services when medical conditions result in physical disability that cannot be safely managed in the home environment.

Healthy older adults benefit from an annual assessment for preventable diseases and the early recognition of treatable conditions (see Chapter 3, Clinical assessment, and Chapter 32, Preventive medicine).

Primary health care for the older adult includes sensory assessment for vision, hearing, and dental health. It also involves screening for falls and trauma and for impairments in basic activities of daily living—bathing, dressing, toileting, mobility, feeding. The functions required for living independently in the community, such as medication administration, maintenance of the home environment, meal preparation, transportation, and management of finances, must also be assessed.

Specialists recommendations should be reviewed and approved by the primary care provider, who is best positioned to prioritize the health needs and avoid duplicative tests and drug–drug interactions. Medication reconciliation is a time-consuming but vital safety practice that educates the older adult, caregiver, or both to maintain an accurate list of medications, doses, and special instructions on time of dosing and potential food–drug interactions.

Computerized health records accessible across the continuum of health-care settings and to the older adult, but periodically reviewed and revised by the primary care provider as a "medical home" is a goal not yet achieved in U.S. health care, but a recognized goal by the Institute of Medicine.

### Subspecialty care

Just as too many cooks spoil the broth, health care delivered by multiple subspecialists without a coordinating primary care provider may result in costly duplicative tests and avoidable drug–drug interactions. Effective consults to medical, surgical, and diagnostic specialists by the primary care provider ask specific questions for the consultant to answer.

For example, the note "patient with dilated cardiomyopathy with decreasing exercise tolerance; patient has mild memory impairment and relies on caregiver to monitor medication use; please advise on how to adjust current medications" is a defined starting point for the cardiologist when accompanied by a the recent echocardiogram (ECG) findings and an accurate medication list. The primary care provider is best able to put in context the recommendations of the subspecialist, given the other medical conditions and treatments. In this example, the primary care physician must review the patient's and caregiver's ability to adhere to new medication and life style recommendations and balance efficacy with practical considerations.

## Acute care service

Because older people present with complex medical conditions are at high risk for complications, acute care services should be designed to meet their needs while minimizing risks. Whether it occurs in the physicians' office, emergency department, or home, proper assessment of the older patient will allow for the best management strategy.

### Emergency department

Older people often present to the emergency department (ED). In addition to a broad range of acute surgical and medical problems, other common problems among older adults referred to the ED include falls, fractures, and mental-status changes. When unstable medical conditions are identified it is often the most appropriate place for the older adult.

However, the ED is potentially inhospitable and hazardous for older people. The environment may be uncomfortable, disorientating, and lacking dignity and privacy. Often a direct admission to an inpatient unit is possible and allows the older adult to bypass the frequently chaotic environment of the ED. When ED use is unavoidable, a strategy to optimize care for older adults includes the following:

- Close liaison with the family to ensure that accurate information is obtained
- Attention to appropriate lighting and sensory input needs
- Quick through-put to inpatient floors for those patients admitted
- Attention to immobility risks (bed sores)

Routine screening of older adults in the ED followed by a nursing assessment for specific follow-up has demonstrated better rates of referral to the primary care physician and is associated with a lower rate of functional decline at 4 months.

### Hospital care

Hospital care is more common among older adults because of the high prevalence of chronic and complex illness. However, hospitalization of older adults is associated with several adverse outcomes, including functional decline, delirium, and falls. Exposure to opportunistic and drug-resistant organisms, as well as medication errors and pressure sores can also occur.

*Hazards of hospitalization*
- Delirium
- Pressure sores
- Poor nutritional intake (unfamiliar food and preparation)
- Poor hydration (encumbered access to water)
- Medication errors
- Exposure to resistant microorganisms

Targeted strategies have been designed to improve important outcomes in older adults. For example, the risk of delirium is reduced by ensuring adequate hydration, measures to maintain patient orientation, and non-pharmacological interventions to enhance sleep (e.g., massage, quiet environment, warm drink at bedtime). Frequent, structured prevention-oriented nursing rounds in the hospital reduce the frequency of call light use, increasing patient satisfaction with care and reducing the incidence of falls.

*ACE units*
Due to the high rate of hospitalization among older adults and the important risks associated with traditional inpatient care, an innovative approach to "specializing" care on inpatient units for older patients, the acute care for elders (ACE) unit, focuses on early rehabilitation, discharge planning, and delivering functionally oriented, patient-centered care. These units are located within hospitals. There is evidence to suggest that older patients who receive care in an ACE unit are less likely to be discharged to a nursing home.

*Hospital at home*
This model of care acknowledges the risks of standard hospitalization as well as patient preferences to stay at home. The "hospital at home" provides standard hospital services in the home, coordinated by a medical team that provides daily provision of care and monitoring. It has been shown to have shorter lengths of stay and lower cost than acute hospital care. Although "hospital-at-home" is a promising model for providing cost-effective acute care to older adults, it is not widely disseminated in the United States at this time.

### Assisted living facilities
Assisted living facilities (AL) are supportive housing that has also been called group homes, board and care homes, and residential care facilities. They provide care to older adults who require (or prefer) 24-hour care and supervision. However, these facilities typically do not have continuous, skilled nursing care. This is an important difference between AL and nursing homes (NH) (see Table 2.1).

Although regulations vary by state, there is typically an "affiliated" or "delegating" nurse who oversees the nursing and medication administration within the facility. Standard services provided by AL are listed in Box 2.1. Residents who reside in AL have a range of health-care needs. These include functional impairment, the full range of chronic medical conditions, and dementia (diagnosed in 40%–65% of AL residents).

AL is financed almost exclusively by private pay, with only a small portion covered by Medicaid. Nationally, the average annual cost of AL is $36,000; that cost rises to $51,000 for dementia-specific AL. When state funds are available to pay for AL through Medicaid waiver programs, they fund only the very poor ("Medicaid-eligible"). Therefore, a gap of affordability exists for many older adults who qualify for Medicaid but are not able to pay privately for AL.

---

### Box 2.1 Typical services in assisted living facilities

- Housekeeping
- Medication reminders or assistance
- Help with activities of daily living (ADLs)
- Transportation
- Security
- Health monitoring
- Care management
- Activities and recreation

---

**Table 2.1** Comparison of assisted living facilities and nursing homes[5]

|  | Assisted living (AL) | Nursing home (NH) |
|---|---|---|
| Number of beds in the U.S. | 1 million | 1.9 million |
| Average size | 9–65 beds depending on subtype* | 120 beds |
| Physician visits | Typically occur in office; visits required once a year | Typically occur in facility; visits required every 60 days |
| Predominant model of care | Social | Medical |
| Involvement of licensed nursing | Variable, often as supervisors rather than direct care providers | 24 hours/day |
| Nursing procedures, physical therapy, IV treatment | Provided by home health personnel or not at all | Provided by facility staff |
| Help with dressing, bathing, other ADLs | Provided by facility staff | Provided by facility staff |
| Payment sources | Private pay (including Social Security Disability) 85%; other public funds 2%; Medicaid and other public funds 15% | Private pay 44%; Medicaid 40%; Medicare 13% |
| Percent of facilities with ≥50% of beds in private rooms | 55%–75% depending on subtype* | 11% |

* "Small" AL (<16 beds), "Traditional" AL (board and care type; 16 or more beds), "New Model" AL (variable pay rates and care need requirements, RN/LPN on duty at all times)?

*Home care*

Most people needing personal care remain at home rather than moving into a nursing home. Their needs are provided by a caregiver who may be a spouse or other family member or other "informal" caregivers, or by professional "formal" caregivers (self-employed or employed by a private care agency or public body). In 2004, over 20% of U.S. households provided informal care to an adult. This informal (unpaid) care-giving is valued at 6 times that of formal (paid) care-giving. The "typical" unpaid caregiver is a 46-year-old woman with at least some college experience who provides more than 20 hours of care each week to her mother.[1]

Many older adults independently arrange their own home care (formal and informal).

Formal home care may also be arranged through a "home health agency" at the recommendation of a medical provider. This often occurs after a hospitalization or a notable decline in function. While home care agencies have been providing services to Americans for more than a century, the growth of the home health care industry has accelerated since Medicare began covering these services in 1965.

Home health agencies' services include skilled nursing, rehabilitation therapy, social work, and assistance by home health aides. Some older adults also receive home medical care (or "house calls"). These can be provided by primary care physicians (family or internal medicine) or geriatricians working within traditional, office-based practices. There are a small, but growing, number of physician practices that are exclusively house call based.

## Home health care

Home healthcare agencies are funded by Medicare to provide home care when a patient is **homebound** and has a **skilled need**.

| Descriptor | Definition | Exclusion |
|---|---|---|
| Homebound | Leaving the home requires considerable and taxing effort; andAbsences from the home are infrequent or of brief duration | Leaving the home for medical visits, adult day care, hemodialysis, religious services, or occasional errands or special events is allowable |
| Skilled need | A need that can only be safely and effectively met by a person with special training and certification (nurse, physical therapist, occupational therapist, speech therapist) | Visits solely for the purpose of venipuncture |

Once a skilled need has been identified, the agency can also receive payment for providing other services, such as personal care assistance and medical social work. These services are not covered in the absence of a skilled need.

## Medical House Calls

Few US physicians make house calls, but some evidence suggests that longitudinal home-based primary care for homebound older adults or a timely house call for an acutely ill, otherwise ambulatory patient may prevent hospitalization, functional decline, and long-term care placement. For Medicare reimbursement, clinicians must document the medical necessity of the home visit, although the patient does not have to meet the "homebound" criteria for home healthcare agency services.

Although most clinicians are not specifically trained in medical house calls during their training, the essential skills are identical to those needed for patient care in any setting: the ability to perform a thorough and accurate history and physical exam including vital signs, the medical knowledge to diagnose and treat acute and chronic illnesses, attention to details of the patient's environment, and a clear understanding of the patient's goals and preferences. House call physicians must be competent in basic ancillary procedures such as phlebotomy and electrocardiography, and should be well-versed in the primary care of many subspecialty problems, since homebound patients often have great difficulty accessing office-based subspecialty care and the number of subspecialist house calls is vanishingly small.

### What can you observe on a house call?
- Medications
- Functional status
- Nutrition
- Hygiene
- Home safety
- Neighborhood safety
- Caregivers and support

### What can you do on a house call?
- History and physical examination, including pulse oximetry
- Labwork (phlebotomy, urine collection)
- Electrocardiography
- Plain portable X-ray films (usually through a mobile radiology company)
- Joint injection
- Skin biopsy
- Hand-held Doppler ultrasound

### What can't you do on a house call?
- CT, MRI
- Procedures requiring other than local anesthesia

**What do you take on a house call?**
- Stethoscope, sphygmomanometer, pulse oximeter, EKG machine
- Oto-ophthalmoscope, reflex hammer
- Lab supplies (phlebotomy tubes, needles, gauze, bandages, specimen cups)
- Nail clippers, safety glasses
- Basic wound care supplies
- Sharps container

## Funding

Medicare home healthcare agency care and medical house calls are covered by Medicare Part B. In addition, physicians can bill Medicare for coordinating and supervising home health care. **Home care certification** fees reimburse for the time spent reviewing the plan of care and signing home care orders, while **care plan oversight** fees reimburse for the time spent communicating with other health care professionals when the physician is not in the presence of the patient, as long as such time adds up to at least 30 minutes per calendar month. Payments vary by geographic region.

## References

Levine SA, Boal J, Boling PA (2003). Home care. *JAMA* **290**(9):1203–1207.
Meyer GS, Gibbons RV (1997). House calls to the elderly–a vanishing practice among physicians. *N Engl J Med* **337**(25):1815–1820.

### Post–acute care inpatient services

Trends in U.S. health care are shortened hospital stays for medical conditions, during which diagnostic studies are completed and treatments are targeted to correct unstable vital signs. Intravenous (IV) fluids, antibiotics, and cardiac drugs are short-term treatments often begun during an acute hospital admission. When the patient is stable, discharge to a skilled nursing facility is arranged, where further medication adjustments and physical recovery to baseline physical function are goals of care.

Noninvasive surgical techniques have shortened postoperative recovery, but older adults with baseline physical debilities cannot routinely return to a home environment that may require ambulation on stairs or independence in personal care and meal preparation. Skilled nursing facilities, some hospital-based, some free-standing facilities, provide assistance with personal care, physical therapy targeted to improve mobility, occupational therapy targeted to improve personal care, meal preparation, and the tasks required to live independently. Speech therapy may also be required to address language, speech, and swallowing disorders.

Patients with certain acute medical conditions, stroke, brain injury, spinal cord injury, hip fracture, or exacerbations of chronic conditions such as Parkinson's disease, multiple sclerosis, and rheumatoid arthritis require a complex rehabilitation program under the direction of a physician certified in physical medicine and rehabilitation. The physical, occupational, and speech therapy may require 3 hours or more per day and the patient may qualify for inpatient rehabilitation hospital care.

Discharge from either a skilled nursing facility or an inpatient rehabilitation hospital is required when the individual achieves a functional level that is safe for discharge to the home environment, returns to baseline function, or reaches a plateau in physical recovery.

### Nursing homes

Multiple active medical conditions, physical debility, and dependence in two or more basic ADLs pose a threat to independent living for the older adult who lives alone or whose medical and nursing needs are greater than what can be managed in an AL environment. Examples include labile congestive heart failure and emphysema that require skilled nursing, multiple, stage IV pressure ulcers that require time-consuming dressings by licensed nurses, and dementia with aggressive behaviors that requires close observation and redirection to prevent harm to self and other residents.

Nursing facilities used to be homes for the aged, poorly staffed, and unsafe. The Omnibus Reconciliation Act of 1987 imposed significant federal oversight of licensed nursing facilities that receive federal payments from Medicare and Medicaid. To qualify for payment, a multidisciplinary assessment tool, called the 3871, is completed and signed by the licensed physician, documenting medical conditions and their treatments that require nursing facility care.

**1**. National Association for Home Care and Hospice (2008) *Basic Statistics about Home Care.* www.nahc.org. Accessed August 26, 2009.

# Regulation of geriatric services

The Center for Medicare Services provides federal oversight of health services funded by Medicare and Medicaid and sets reimbursements for health-care services. State and local health departments apply regulations relevant to more regional issues such as infection-control reporting and building codes.

Many states conduct unannounced surveys of health-care facilities such as nursing homes and hospitals as part of the renewal of the facility license. The Joint Commission Accreditation Health Care Facilities sets health-care standards to which many U.S. hospitals and some nursing facilities voluntarily subscribe. In addition, some health-care organizations participate in voluntary inspections by organizations that set health-care standards for specialty units, such as the Commission on Accreditation of Rehabilitation Facilities.

# Financing geriatric services

Medicare was enacted by legislative act in 1965 to provide payment for acute hospital services for adults age 65 years and older and for younger adults with chronic disability. It provides for 100 days of inpatient stay at a skilled nursing facility following a 3-day hospital stay and for short-term skilled nursing and rehabilitation services in the home to manage significant changes in health and physical function. All adults 65 years and older who contributed to Medicare through a mandatory payroll deduction are eligible for enrollment without monthly premiums, but with annual deductible and co-pays for all services.

Medicare Part B was added to provide payment for physician services in both the inpatient and ambulatory settings and for diagnostic studies, including radiographs and laboratory studies. Medicare Part B monthly premiums are deducted from Social Security income.

In 2006, Medicare Part D added a prescription drug plan for those who signed on to the additional reduction in monthly Social Security income to cover the Medicare Part D premium.

Medicare reimbursement for skilled nursing care ends when the need for skilled nursing or rehabilitation services is met, to a maximum of 100 days of care, but is renewable after 60 days without services. Medicare Part A acute hospital payment has a lifetime maximum of 180 days of coverage, regardless of the medical necessity of inpatient care.

Many older adults subscribe to additional health insurance, called Medigap policies, that cover the annual deductible and 20% co-payments associated for acute care, physician services, and diagnostic studies.

Nursing home care is not a Medicare benefit. Individuals and their families pay out of pocket for nursing home stays. When an individual's assets are depleted, he or she is eligible for Medicaid funding for nursing home stay (see Chapter 28, Financing health care).

## Further reading

Grumbach K, Bodenheimer T (2004). Can health care teams improve primary care practice? *JAMA* **291**:1246–1251.

Institute of Medicine. (2001) *Improving the Quality of Long-Term Care*. Washington, DC: National Academy Press.

Levine SA, Boal J, Boling PA (2003). Home care. *JAMA* **290**:1203–1207.

National Association for Home Care and Hospice (2008) *Basic Statistics about Home Care*. www.nahc.org. Accessed August 26, 2009.

Zimmerman S, Sloane PD, Eckert JK (2001). *Assisted Living: Needs, Practices, and Policies in Residential Care for the Elderly*. Baltimore, MD: Johns Hopkins University Press.

# Clinical assessment of older adults

**Lisa Boult**

# Introduction to assessment

Older adults vary greatly in their health and function, ranging from healthy and fully independent to chronically ill, frail, and disabled. Similarly, there is a spectrum of types of assessment that are appropriate for older adults.

While evaluations similar to those for younger adults may suffice for healthy, independent older people, more extensive evaluation, both of medical conditions and of other functional domains (including physical, psychological, and cognitive function) may be appropriate for those burdened by chronic disease and disability.

## Goals of assessment

- Be clear about the goals for both assessment and treatment; they may be different than those for younger people. This requires understanding the patient's priorities, values, and preferences about medical care.
- Consultative assessments should address the questions the referring practitioner wants answered.
- Older patients seeking help for a problem don't necessarily expect a cure; they may simply want to understand symptoms and be content to live with them.
- Some older adults, particularly the chronically ill, may prefer to forego onerous testing or aggressive treatment, even for potentially lethal conditions (for example, surgery for critical aortic stenosis or chemotherapy for cancer), opting instead for control of symptoms.
- Patients who are capable of making reasoned decisions about their care have the right to make those decisions, such as opting for comfort over longer life, even if their preferences are not what their family members (or physicians) would wish.

# Chronic disease and comorbidity

### Chronic disease

Many chronic diseases are associated with aging and some, like osteoarthritis, are present in most older adults. About 40% of adults over 65 have three or more chronic diseases and about 25% have four or more. The average number of diseases per person also increases with age.

Many chronic conditions are stable. Most patients adapt gradually and well to the limitations these conditions impose (e.g., not walking as far or as fast as before because of arthritic knees, or reading large-print books to compensate for poor vision).

Assessment and intervention can be helpful. Some problems, such as osteoarthritis and impaired hearing, are often accepted as a part of normal aging but can be easily treated, thus improving quality of life.

### Comorbidity

Even stable comorbid disease can decrease physiological reserve, impairing the body's ability to resist a physiological challenge. A seemingly minor insult or change, such as a new medication, a change in dosage of an old medication, an upper respiratory infection, or constipation, may suffice to cause new and seemingly unrelated symptoms or illness.

Acute medical problems may present with nonspecific signs and symptoms that reflect the complexity of the underlying pathology and cause acute decline without obvious cause. Acute events may have several interacting causes (multifactorial etiology) that need to be disentangled from one another.

Fragile patients are subject to the so-called cascade effect, in which one problem, or its treatment, leads to another problem, and so on, in a seemingly inexorable downward spiral. For example, a bed-bound patient with pneumonia is at high risk for thromboembolic disease; treatment of the embolic disease can predispose to bleeding, etc. To avert the cascade effect, think proactively about what is most likely to go wrong next and try to prevent it.

### Medications and polypharmacy

As older patients acquire chronic conditions, medications are prescribed for those conditions, making patients susceptible to polypharmacy and adverse effects of medications. Management of chronic conditions relies increasingly on recommendations found in evidence-based guidelines. These include the prescribing of medications not only for established or symptomatic disease but also for secondary and tertiary prevention, thereby increasing the number of medications patients take.

When several practitioners prescribe medication for the patient, the medication list may include redundant medications, medications with problematic interactions, medications that counteract each other's effects, or medications that exacerbate conditions other than the one they were prescribed for.

Limiting medications to those that are truly essential for preventing and treating disease or managing symptoms will help prevent adverse drug reactions and save money.

When a new problem arises in an older patient, always consider that it might result from a medication, even one that is usually safe. Scrutinize the medication list, including over-the-counter (OTC) medications. Not only new medications but also changes in dosage of old medications may be the culprits. When they do occur, statistically rare side effects often affect this fragile population.

# Setting the stage

### Medical appointments

- Getting to medical appointments may be physically and emotionally challenging for older patients, and they may be particularly reluctant to make the trip when they feel ill.
- Transportation services often convey older patients to appointments. Morning appointments usually require them to be ready early, which may be difficult. Late-morning or afternoon appointments are preferable for patients who cannot travel independently.
- Instructions about appointments should be clear. Ideally, appointments for cognitively impaired patients should be arranged so that caregivers can attend with them; patients with impaired vision may need a large-print reminder or a phone call.
- Patients should bring both medications and prescription lists to their appointments. Comparison of the medications that patients are actually taking with what their prescription lists say they are taking helps prevent medication-related morbidity.
- A patient's confusion about medications may indicate cognitive impairment and inability to self-administer medications safely.
- Requests for cognitive assessment are often made by concerned family members. Patients may be reluctant to attend, as they do not perceive or wish to face the problem.
- For debilitated or disabled patients, home visits or house calls may be preferable to office visits. They are less disruptive for the patient and may also provide otherwise elusive information (e.g., about family dynamics and the physical environment of the home).

### Rapport

- Establishing good rapport with the patient makes the assessment easier and more productive. Informal conversation can break the ice.
- Always introduce yourself, and address the patient formally (Mr/Mrs/Miss) unless invited to do otherwise. Be respectful and not patronizing or over-familiar.
- Older patients may have greater faith in a familiar physician than in a consultant met for the first time. Emphasize that you work as part of a team, and explain recommendations, noting that you will inform the patient's primary physician of recommended changes.

### Environment

- Patients may feel helpless and vulnerable if they are only partially clothed and seated on a high examining table during an interview. If possible, interview patients while they are dressed and sitting in a chair.
- Poor vision and hearing can make an interview more difficult and frightening for the patient. If possible, use a well-lit, quiet room.
- Ensure that hearing aids are in position and turned on. Use written questions if hearing is too impaired to allow conversation. (See also sections on hearing in Chapter 21, and on vision, Chapter 22.)

# Obtaining a history

## The patient interview

The medical history of an older person with many medical problems may be hard to unravel. Part of the interviewer's task is to discern which problems are new, which are serious or urgent, which are old and stable, and which are old but have recently changed.

- Patients with chronic back pain might answer "yes" to the closed question, "Do you have pain?", but the pain may be unchanged and unrelated to the reason for the current visit. Determine whether symptoms are different from usual.
- Allow time for the patient to volunteer symptoms and avoid interrupting. Sometimes it is necessary to politely redirect patients who digress.
- If an important symptom is mentioned in passing, return to it later.
- Patients may underplay issues that are emotionally upsetting (such as incontinence, failing memory, or abuse by a caregiver) or that they fear will increase the likelihood of their losing independence. Fostering an atmosphere of trust and collaborative problem-solving may encourage them to open up.

## Cognitive impairment

Patients with dementia or delirium may not be able to answer questions clearly or succinctly. Important elements of history may need to be elicited and separated from less relevant information.

- General questions such as "Do you feel sick?" and "Are you having any pain?" are a good place to start.
- Alternating open-ended questions with closed, clarifying questions that can be answered with a clear "yes" or "no" may help delimit the symptoms.
- A patient who feels embarrassed may become silent.
- Patients who are afraid that full evaluation may reveal their cognitive impairment may attempt to close down questioning and hasten the end of an evaluation. In such situations, it is especially important to pursue too-brief responses, persevere through the patient's gestures of impatience, and assess cognition.

# Other sources of information

Patients who are acutely ill or cognitively impaired may be unable to give a full and accurate history. Information must then be obtained from other sources.

### The family

Family members are a helpful source of information, especially at an initial assessment. Patients may underplay their symptoms, fearful that they will be perceived as unable to cope or as complainers. Family members' histories can complement those of the patient.

- The family may have different concerns from those of the patient, and both should be evaluated fully.
- Family members may wish to speak separately from the patient. This can be useful, but information about the patient should not be given to or sought from family members without the patient's permission.
- People with intact decision-making capacity have the right to assume risks, provided they understand the possible consequences of their choices (e.g., deciding to live at home rather than in a more supervised environment if they have a high risk of falling) (see Chapter 5, Falls and gait imbalance).

### Neighbors and friends

Older people with no family living nearby may be familiar to their neighbors or best known to their friends, who may be able to provide helpful information.

- Friends or neighbors may be informal caregivers, sometimes providing more care than family or formal caregivers.
- Common-law partners are often deeply involved in patients' lives, yet may be less visible (and feel less welcome) in the hospital or clinic than other family members.
- Rifts that exist between established family and new partners must be taken into account when care is planned.
- Neighbors may be aware of, or even have observed, a patient's unusual behavior (such as becoming lost or wandering at night). They may not be available to volunteer such information, so it should be sought if it is needed.

### Physicians, nurses, and other professional caregivers

Doctors and nurses may know patients very well and have insight about family dynamics, family members' concerns, and current arrangements for care. They can help clarify the current medication list and past medical history.

- If a patient arrives confused to a clinical appointment, the primary care physician should be informed and asked about recent cognitive function.
- Homebound patients and those with medical issues requiring home care (such as skin ulcers or urinary catheters) are usually well known to home care providers.

- Professional caregivers will be familiar with the usual functional and cognitive state of the patient; they may have alerted medical services about changes in function. If they are not present at medical visits, they should be called for further information.

## Ambulance crew

An ambulance crew may be present during the initial hospital assessment of a sick older patient. Ask crew members what they observed, or examine their written documentation, which will include clinical observations including vital signs. This source of information is underused.

## Nursing homes

When patients are admitted from institutional care a good history should be available. Information about usual functional state, past medical history, medications, and acute illness should arrive with the patient, but if it does not, it can be sought by telephone immediately.

## Old medical records

Obtain and review old medical records as early as possible. If the patient is not local, arrange for information (letters, discharge summaries, etc.) to be faxed, or speak to health professionals who know the patient.

# The physical examination

### Challenges: pain and functional impairment

Several factors can make the examining older patients more challenging than younger patients; these include physical constraints, pain and easy fatiguing, and cognitive problems.

- Less agile patients may undress slowly and have difficulty adopting optimal positions for examination (e.g., lying flat).
- Watching a patient undress, walk, and climb onto an examining table can provide important information about balance, strength, mobility, and dexterity.
- A patient's pain or fatiguing during the examination provides clues about stamina and constraints to activity at home.
- Difficulty following verbal instructions (e.g., during neurologic or visual field examination) may indicate cognitive impairment.

### Investigating new problems

When older patients present with new problems, the scope of the examination is wider than in younger people. **Symptoms may be poorly localized,** and more systems are possible loci of the problem.

- The physical examination often reveals the diagnosis underlying a vague or nonspecific presentation (for example, a previously unrecognized abdominal mass or a new arrhythmia).
- Abnormal physical signs are more prevalent in older adults. The chance of detecting incidental and previously unrecognized pathology (e.g., asymptomatic heart murmurs or skin lesions) is much higher in older than in younger patients.
- Previously unrecognized abnormal findings may have no impact on the problems being investigated. Some asymptomatic abnormalities can safely be watched rather than immediately investigated; many will never cause symptoms.
- Suboptimal examination is dangerous when inaccurate or incomplete findings are documented and then assumed to be accurate by others. If your examination was not complete, note that in the record and complete it later.
- Note general characteristics; include body shape and height, nutritional status, hydration, alertness, mood, cooperation, affect, insight, anxiety, hygiene, state of clothing, intellect and presentation, and speech.
- If the patient looks ill, state this and try to describe in what way.
- Check the blood pressure yourself, in both arms. In patients with hypertension, check postural blood pressures.
- In older adults, temperatures may be low, even with severe infections.
- Crackles heard at the lung bases that clear with deep inspiration or coughing often do not indicate pathology.

## Examining patients with impaired mobility

- Less complete examinations can occasionally be appropriate: it might be reasonable to listen to a chest through a thin shirt or nightgown, for example, but it is ineffective to examine an abdomen with the patient seated in a wheelchair.
- If necessary, seek the help of nurses, relatives, or other caregivers to assist with a complete examination. Electric beds and lifts can make examination more efficient and comfortable for the patient.
- Try to examine all aspects of one portion of the body at the same time. If the examination is well organized, patients should not have to sit up, roll over, or stand up more than once per examination.
- When a full skin examination is indicated, look under clothing (especially at the sacrum), in skin folds, between toes, and under wound dressings, wigs, and prostheses.

# Diagnostic testing

In general, cognitively intact older people accept and tolerate diagnostic procedures as well as younger patients. Exceptions include the following:
- Colonoscopy (increased risk of colonic perforation)
- Bowel preparation for colonoscopy or barium enema (higher risk of dehydration)
- Exercise tolerance tests (Arthritis or neurological problems may prevent a patient from walking briskly. Chemical stress testing is an alternative.)
- Use of intravenous contrast agents for radiological procedures (risk to kidneys)

It may be useful to discuss a proposed procedure with the person who will perform the test (often a radiologist), who might suggest how to modify the test or substitute a different procedure to ensure safety.
- Cognitively impaired or delirious patients may need to be accompanied to procedures and tests by a relative or member of the health-care team.
- For agitated patients, the cautious use of sedatives or anxiolytics is sometimes helpful (weigh risks against benefits).

## Simple investigations

Potentially useful tests in older people who present with new symptoms include the following:
- Complete blood count (CBC)
- Electrolytes, blood urea nitrogen (BUN), creatinine
- Glucose
- Complete chemistry panel
- Calcium and phosphate
- Erythrocyte sedimentation rate (ESR)
- Thyroid function
- Chest X-ray (CXR)
- ECG
- Urinalysis

These tests are inexpensive, well tolerated, rapidly available, and high yield. Coupled with a complete history and physical examination, they will often give sufficient information to guide initial management and further investigations.
- In non-urgent situations, consider awaiting results of initial tests and observing the results of initial treatment before ordering more tests. Further tests may be unnecessary.
- Do not request a test if it will not affect management.
- Note for the next provider which results are still pending.
- Don't order repeat tests automatically—some normal tests may not need to be repeated.

# Common blood test abnormalities

A series of screening blood tests in an older person often yields several results that fall outside normal laboratory ranges; these may occur in the absence of illness. Unless they are very abnormal or something in the presentation makes them particularly relevant, they can sometimes be disregarded. They fall into four broad categories.

## Different reference range in older patients

- *ESR:* In older adults, the upper limit of normal may be as high as age/2 in men and (age + 10)/2 in women (see Chapter 16, Hematology).
- *Hemoglobin:* This has been debated, but the reference range should probably be unchanged (see p. 468).

## Common result rarely implying important new disease

- *Thyroid-stimulating hormone (TSH):* During acute illness, TSH can be low, with normal free T4 and T3 (sick euthyroid syndrome) (p. 455). Repeat 2–4 weeks after acute illness has resolved.
- *Low-serum sodium:* Very low levels should be investigated (p. 418), but some patients have an asymptomatic, persistent, mild hyponatremia as result of medications or for unknown reasons.
- *Alkaline phosphatase (ALP):* If liver function tests are normal, an isolated elevated ALP can indicate Paget's disease (p. 506), which is often asymptomatic. ALP remains high for weeks after fractures, including osteoporotic compression fractures.
- *Hemoglobin* can temporarily be normal in acutely ill patients who are volume depleted and thus hemoconcentrated; it later falls to an abnormal level when they are rehydrated.
- *Asymptomatic bacteriuria* (p. 656): This is common in older patients and does not always indicate significant urinary infection. Check for symptoms and the presence of white cells on urine microscopy.

## False-negative results

- *Serum creatinine* in patients with low muscle mass can be misleadingly low and mask poor renal function (p. 394). Use a conversion formula to estimate glomerular filtration rate, e.g., when choosing drug dosages (see Chapter 13, Nephrology).
- *BUN* levels in the middle or upper range of normal can be seen in frail older patients with dehydration.

## False-positive results

- *D-dimer:* Bruising, infection, or inflammation can increase d-dimer.
- *Troponin:* Although troponin is specific to cardiac muscle, low-level release can occur with arrhythmias, pulmonary embolus, and heart failure.

# Comprehensive geriatric assessment (CGA)

In comprehensive geriatric assessment (CGA), members of an interdisciplinary geriatric team evaluate an older person's needs, performing formal assessments in their own disciplines, and then meet to create a plan for meeting those needs. Most CGA programs are consultative programs, in which the team makes recommendations to the patient's primary care physician, who then implements them. In geriatric evaluation and management (GEM) programs, the team implements its own recommendations before transferring care to the primary physician.

The goals of CGA are to improve the quality of care, optimize physical and psychological function, and improve quality of life. They also aim to prevent unnecessary hospital admissions, nursing home placement, caregiver burden, and costs of care.

## The team

The CGA team usually includes a nurse, a physician (often a geriatrician), a social worker, and sometimes a psychologist, pharmacist, dietician, occupational therapist, physical therapist, or speech therapist.

## Assessments

The goals of each program determine the domains it assesses. Most programs assess health status and several domains of function—cognitive, physical (including balance, gait, and mobility), and psychological (especially depression). Other frequently assessed domains are nutritional status, values and preferences about care, social support, quality of life, home environment, caregiver burden, and home safety.

## Interventions

CGA usually generates several recommendations for further management. These can include changes in medications (e.g., discontinuing unnecessary or problematic medications), suggestions about further testing (e.g., cognitive evaluation), referrals to specialist physicians or rehabilitation therapies, and referrals to community or home care agencies. Some programs incorporate systems for improving adherence to recommendations (see Adherence to recommendations, p. 44).

The principles of CGA have been adapted to programs designed with different goals and for different patient populations. Some address specific medical problems (e.g., heart failure or hip fracture), others are adapted for patients using a specific site of care (e.g., the emergency department), and still others are designed for use in collaboration with a particular specialty (e.g., oncology, to help determine which older patients are likely to tolerate aggressive treatment).

**Evidence**

Although the variety of CGA and GEM programs makes it difficult to generalize about their effectiveness, the evidence from many randomized trials and one large meta-analysis suggests that CGA can improve physical function, psychological function, satisfaction with care, and quality of life. Successful programs tend to

- Target interventions to populations most likely to benefit, usually frail or multi-morbid older patients
- Implement their own recommendations and plans of care
- Treat patients over an extended period of time rather than at a single visit

**Screening for functional problems**

CGA programs are less common in the United States than in other countries. Because CGA as such is not currently paid for by Medicare, most health-care organizations in the United States do not offer these programs. A single practitioner can, however, easily perform a screening assessment for functional problems (an abbreviated form of CGA) during regular office visits (see Table 3.1).

# Screening for functional problems

Primary care providers can fairly easily integrate functional assessment into routine office visits. This involves initially assessing each functional domain through a very brief screen (for example, screening for depression with the single question, "Do you often feel sad and depressed?") (see Table 3.1). A positive brief screen indicates the need for a more detailed assessment of that domain, one that can be performed by the same practitioner, perhaps at a later date, or that might prompt a referral to a specialist or therapist.

For example, a positive screen for hearing impairment (using the "whisper test" described below) might indicate a referral to an audiologist for hearing evaluation and perhaps a hearing aid. Different approaches to this kind of abbreviated functional assessment are described in three sources cited at the end of this chapter (Boult, 2000; Lachs et al., 1990; Moore and Siu, 1996).

**Table 3.1** Domains and procedures for functional screening

| Domain | Assessment procedure | Abnormal result [recommendation] |
|---|---|---|
| Vision | Test each eye with a Jaeger card* while patient wears corrective lenses (if needed). | Inability to read greater than 20/40 [Refer to optometrist or ophthalmologist] |
| Hearing | Conduct "whisper test:" Whisper a short, easily answered question into each ear from behind while out of the patient's direct view. | Inability to answer question[Check canals for cerumen; clean if necessary. Repeat test; if still abnormal, refer to audiologist] |
| Arm | Proximal: "Touch the back of your head with both hands." | Inability to perform task [Examine arm fully (muscles, joints, nerves), checking for weakness, pain, limited range of motion. Consider referral to physical therapy] |
| Gait, balance, mobility | Ask about falls in the previous 6 months.Observe patient after asking, "Rise from your chair, walk 10 feet, return, and sit down." | Falling. Inability to perform any part of task; over 30 sec to complete [Perform full musculoskeletal and neurological examination, paying attention to strength, pain, range of motion, balance, and gait. Consider referral for physical therapy] |
| Urinary incontinence | Ask, "Do you ever lose control of your urine?" | Yes [Ascertain frequency and quantity. Search for remediable causes, including local irritations, polyuria, and medication. Consider bladder-training exercises, medication, referral to urologist] |

| Domain | Assessment procedure | Abnormal result [recommendation] |
| --- | --- | --- |
| Nutrition | Weigh the patient. Inquire about recent weight loss. | Weight below acceptable range for height, or unintentional weight loss over 10 lb. in previous 6 months [Determine whether patient has difficulty obtaining food or cooking meals or in eating complete meals; if nutrition is adequate, consider medical evaluation] |
| Mental status | Ability to remember three objects after 1 minute. Ability to draw a clock showing the numbers on the clock and the hands saying "10 minutes after 11." | Inability [Assess alertness, attention, and mood; review medications. Perform further cognitive assessment, e.g., with MMSE*; further cognitive and laboratory testing as needed] |
| Depression | Ask, "Do you often feel sad and depressed?" | Yes [Ask about feelings of hopelessness, worthlessness, and sadness; review medications. Consider administering the Geriatric Depression Scale*; consider treatment (with or without medication) or referral] |
| Daily function (ADL)* and instrumental activities of daily living (IADL)* | ADL: Ask about independent ability to go from bed to chair, dress, eat, bathe, use the toilet, control bowel and bladder. IADL: Ask about independent ability to prepare meals, do housework, manage finances, manage medications, use the telephone, shop. | "No" to any question [Corroborate accuracy with family; determine reason for inability (e.g., motivation vs. physical limitations). Implement medical, social, environmental interventions] |
| Home environment | Ask about difficulty with stairs inside or outside the house, and about potential hazard inside the house (bathtubs, throw rugs, lighting). | Unsafe features [Arrange home safety evaluation and implementation of recommended changes] |
| Social support | Ask who would be available to help in an emergency. | Isolation or existing need for caregivers [List names in the medical record; refer for social services, if needed, for information about services in the community] |
| Preferences, values, advance directives | Ask whether the patient has a living will or durable power of attorney for health care (DPOAHC). | None [Ask about preferences and whom the patient would want to make medical decisions if he or she were to become incapacitated] |

Adapted from Lachs et al. (1990), Moore and Siu (1996), and Boult (2000), with additions by author.

*Katz S, Ford AB, Moskowitz RW, et al. Studies of illness in the aged. *JAMA* 1963; **185**:914–919. Lawton MP, Brody Em. Assessment of older people: self-maintaining and instrumental activities of daily living. *Gerontologist* 1969; **9**:179–186

# Planning care

## Problem lists

Complete problem lists are essential for formulating plans of care for medically complex older patients in any setting. They help prioritize problems and function as reminders about comorbidities. Plans of care include a list of the patient's problems (both functional and medical) and the plans for further investigating and treating those problems.

They can be generated at any stage in an illness (the earlier the better) and amended as old problems change or resolve and new problems appear.

- The first assessment of a medically complex older patient should prioritize medical and functional problems, so that acute and dangerous problems are addressed first. Less urgent problems can be addressed at later visits.
- Problem lists should include acute and chronic problems; inactive problems should be included and listed as inactive. **Chronic conditions should be described in terms of their stability and current management**.
- Problems can be symptoms (e.g., falls) rather than diagnoses.
- For each active problem possible causes, a plan for further investigation (if needed), and a plan for treatment should be included.
- Medically complex patients can have long problem lists. Stable and less serious conditions can be addressed periodically and not at each visit.
- Problems should be prioritized at each visit to ensure that new and medically serious problems are not missed because of disproportionate attention to more minor issues.

## Transitions of care and discharge summaries

Communicating medical and functional information is particularly crucial during a medically complex patient's transition from one site of care to another. Many patients make four or more such transitions each year, and for chronically ill older adults, these transitions can be dangerous.

- Severely ill patients may not be able to give clear histories at these times of transition, and people familiar with their history may be temporarily unavailable.
- A medical discharge summary may temporarily be the only source of information about the patient. It should include a complete problem list, a complete medication list, information about functional status and goals of care, and a list of test results that are still pending.

## Adherence to recommendations

Patients' adherence to recommendations will be better if rapport has been good during the assessment. When a new recommendation differs from what has been recommended to a patient in the past, or when testing or medication is recommended for asymptomatic conditions (e.g., carotid bruits), taking time to explain the rationale for each recommendation increases the likelihood of its being accepted.

- Making too many new recommendations (generally more than five) in a single visit can overwhelm patients and result in nonadherence. Prioritizing is essential.
- Writing out a list for the patient of planned diagnostic tests, medication changes, and other recommendations, along with their justification, increases the likelihood that recommendations will be followed.
- Offering to discuss recommendations with family members in person or by telephone is helpful. They may not be able to accompany a patient to an outpatient visit but may be vital to the patient's care.
- Patients with several chronic diseases may find that following a large number of recommendations is burdensome, expensive, and confusing. Recommendations should be prioritized in a way that is consistent with the patient's values and stated goals of care.

# Case example

### Example of a patient who might be referred for CGA

The hypothetical history, assessments, and recommendations that follow are not meant to be complete but are meant to illustrate an approach. The focus is more on function than on specific diseases.

The patient is an 81-year-old woman brought in by her daughter because of recent forgetfulness. Her history includes the following:

- Difficulty finding words, missed appointments, repeating questions
- Unintentional 13 lb. weight loss over the past year
- Treatment for hypertension with diuretic
- Treatment for hypothyroidism
- History of coronary artery disease (myocardial infarction and coronary bypass surgery in the past, with no recent symptoms)
- Wrist fracture in a fall 3 years earlier
- Living alone; driving short distances to shop
- Two recent traffic tickets for moving violations
- Two falls without injury in last 4 months
- Reluctance to leave the house because of urinary urgency and incontinence
- Care by a primary and two specialist physicians
- Seven prescription medications

*Findings from physical examination*

- Vagueness about medical history, difficulty giving clear answers
- Gaunt, with clothes a bit too big; fragile appearance
- Slightly elevated systolic blood pressure (BP)
- Difficulty hearing whisper
- Difficulty getting onto exam table
- Unsteadiness walking; poor balance
- Kyphosis

*Findings from functional assessment*

- Independent with ADLs; difficulty with all IADLs except light housekeeping and using the telephone
- MMSE (Mini-Mental State Examination): 22/30 (abnormal), losing points for short-term memory, visuospatial ability, orientation, attention, and calculation
- Clock-drawing: numbers all present but unequally spaced on clock; hands incorrectly drawn (abnormal)
- Inability to understand words spoken in whisper test
- Required 29 seconds to get up, walk 10 feet, and return to seat
- Unsteadiness turning around while walking
- Daily episodes of urinary urgency or incontinence
- Concern by family about ability to prepare meals—eating cereal for most meals
- Good social support but has not asked relatives for help
- Has not specified advance directives

*Partial problem list*

- Impaired cognition: problems noted with memory, orientation, visuospatial and possibly executive function
- Weight loss: evidence of difficulty preparing whole meals
- Probable osteoporosis: kyphosis (physical exam) and history of fracture
- Impaired balance and mobility
- Nonadherence to medication regimen (mixing up medications, forgetting what she has taken)
- Urge incontinence
- Social isolation
- Possible unsafe driving
- No advance directives specified or surrogate decision maker named

*Possible recommendations by the interdisciplinary team for the patient*

### 1. Cognitive impairment

- Further evaluation (diagnosis and monitoring) of the problem
- Treatment as indicated (e.g., improving antihypertensive treatment, stroke prevention, dementia-specific intervention)
- Monitoring of cognition and behavior by family
- Discontinuing inessential medications; simplifying regimen
- Assistance with medications by family, using compartmentalized pill box

### 2. Weight loss

- Assistance from family or home health aide as needed with shopping, food preparation
- Trial of adequate diet (and possible stabilization of weight) before medical workup for problem

### 3. Hearing impairment

- Audiology evaluation for possible hearing aids

### 4. Osteoporosis, risk of falls and fractures

- Referral to physical therapy—see point 8 below
- Calcium and vitamin D; further evaluation as needed

### 5. Urinary urgency and incontinence

- Consider change to nondiuretic antihypertensive medication
- Bladder training if memory allows; scheduled toileting

### 6. Absence of advance directives

- Clarify goals of care
- Assist with written advance directives, including appointment of durable power of attorney for heath care

### 7. Driving and transportation

- Possibly unsafe because of impaired cognitive function, mobility
- Arrange for professional evaluation of driving safety
- Help family arrange for alternate forms of transportation if needed

### 8. Impaired mobility, balance, falls
- Refer to physical therapy for gait and balance training, training with gait aid (e.g., cane), if needed
- Home evaluation for safety to check for hazards

### 9. Social isolation
- Discuss with family
- Discuss participation at senior centers, adult day programs, other social settings

## Further reading

Boult C (2000). Comprehensive geriatric assessment, In Beers MH, Berkow R, eds. *The Merck Manual of Geriatrics*. Whitehouse Station, NJ: Merck Research Laboratories, pp. 40–46.

Kane RL, Kane RA, eds. (2000). *Assessing Older Persons: Measures, Meaning, and Practical Applications*. New York: Oxford University Press.

Lachs MS, Feinstein AR, Cooney LM Jr, et al. (1990). A simple procedure for general screening for functional disability in older patients. *Ann Intern Med* **112**:699–706.

Moore AA, Siu AL (1996). Screening for common problems in ambulatory elderly: clinical confirmation of a screening instrument. *Am J Med* **100**:438–443.

Stuck AE. Siu AL, Wieland GD, et al. (1993). Comprehensive geriatric assessment; a meta-analysis of controlled trials. *Lancet* **342**:1032–1036.

# Chapter 4

# Rehabilitation

**Richard Zorowitz**

# Rehabilitation

Rehabilitation is a process of care aimed at restoring or maximizing physical, mental, and social functioning. It is appropriate for the following conditions:
- Acute reversible insults, e.g., hip fracture
- Acute nonreversible or partially reversible insults, e.g., stroke, acquired brain injury, spinal cord injury
- Chronic or progressive conditions, e.g., amputation, Parkinson's disease, amyotrophic lateral sclerosis, multiple sclerosis

**Rehabilitation involves both *facilitation* of functional recovery and *compensation* of reduced function. Rehabilitation is an active process done by the patient, not to him or her. It is hard work for the patient (akin to training for a marathon), not "convalescence" (akin to a vacation).**

Rehabilitation is the "secret weapon" of the geriatrician, though poorly understood by most physicians. An invaluable tool box used in rehabilitation contains a selection of non-evidence-based, common-sense interventions comprising the following:
- *Positive attitude:* Good rehabilitation physicians are optimists because they have seen very frail and disabled older people do well.
- *Positive team culture:* An enabling culture encourages independence. Patients usually are dressed in their own clothes. Intravenous and urinary catheters are removed where appropriate. Patients are encouraged to eat meals communally and not in their hospital rooms.
- *Interdisciplinary coordinated team:* The patient, caregivers, and team agrees on functional goals so that approaches to therapy are consistent.
- *Functionally based treatment:* Treatment focuses on maximizing independent mobility, activities of daily living (ADLs), language and communication, and swallowing. Medical issues are addressed to optimize cardiovascular conditioning or prevent complications that interfere with rehabilitation.
- *Individualized holistic outcome goals:* Functional goals incorporate psychosocial and environmental components that are often neglected. Goals in activity and participation build on neurological or musculoskeletal impairments.

## Settings

Inpatient rehabilitation facilities are only one place in which rehabilitation takes place. Successful rehabilitation can also occur in the following places:
- Specialty wards (e.g., stroke units, orthopedic floors)
- Day hospitals
- Nursing and residential homes
- The patient's home
- Outpatient therapy facilities

# The process of rehabilitation

### 1. Selection of patients (p. 56, 57)

### 2. Initial assessment

Know your patient on different levels (e.g., their medical conditions, premorbid function, motivation and expectations, complex psychosocial factors). Assess their activity and participation limitations, not just impairments.

### 3. Goal setting (p. 52)

### 4. Therapy

- Mobility: mainly through physical therapy (p. 62) or nurse-led therapy (p. 71) Mobility consists of transfers, balance, and ambulation. Endurance often is a key issue in allowing a patient to return to the community.
- Activities of daily living (ADLs): Self-care is coordinated by occupational therapy (p. 100) and by nurses.
- Language: mainly speech–language pathology. Language issues include aphasia, apraxia, dysarthria, and cognitive-communication impairment.
- Nutrition and swallowing: mainly through speech-language pathology. May include nursing, occupational therapy, and dietician.
- Adjustment to disability: mainly through (neuro)psychology. Adjustment issues include depression and anxiety.
- Bowel, bladder and skin dysfunction: mainly through nursing, but may be assisted by physical and occupational therapy.
- Environmental modification is addressed through aids and adaptations.
- Caregiver training: Caregivers should be identified prior to the patient's entering the inpatient rehabilitation facility. Training must start soon after admission.

### 5. Reassessment

This usually occurs at weekly interdisciplinary team conferences (p. 59). Goals are adjusted and new goals are set as appropriate. Points 3, 4, and 5 are repeated in a cycle until the patient has reached his or her targeted functional goals or has reached a functional plateau. Discharge occurs thereafter.

### 6. Discharge planning (p. 61)

This should be started prior to the patient's admission to the inpatient rehabilitation facility by identifying psychosocial and environmental issues. Efforts usually escalate toward the end of the inpatient admission. A home visit and family meeting are often held to clarify issues.

### 7. Follow-up and maintenance

This consists of post-discharge home, outpatient, or day-hospital visits. Ideally, continuity by the same team is preferred, but in reality other teams often take over care in the community. Good communication throughout the continuum is vital.

# Aims and objectives of rehabilitation

It is essential that the patient, caregivers, and rehabilitation team clearly list functional goals that can be realistically achieved. They are met through the agreement and statement of targets at two hierarchical levels: aims and objectives.

## Aims

Aims are best set by the team, in discussion with the patient and caregiver. One or two patient-centered targets encompass the broad thrust of the team's work—a team "mission statement" for that individual. For example:
- To achieve discharge home, with the support of spouse, in 3 weeks
- To transfer easily with the assistance of one person, thus allowing return to residential home in 2 weeks.

## Objectives

Objectives are best set by individual team members in discussion with patient and caregiver. Several more focused targets usually reflect specific disabilities and help focus the team's specific interventions. For example:
- To walk 150 feet independently with a single-point cane at 3 weeks
- To achieve night-time urinary continence at 2 weeks

Both the aims and objectives should have five characteristics, summarized by the acronym *SMART*:
- **S**pecific, i.e., focused, unambiguous
- **M**anageable, i.e., amenable to the team's influence
- **A**chievable
- **R**ealistic, acknowledging time and/or resource limitations. It is futile and demoralizing to set targets that cannot be achieved. Conversely, the team (and patient) should be stretched—i.e., the target should not be inevitably achievable.
- **T**ime-limited. Specify when the target should be achieved. Many patients are motivated and cheered by the setting of a specific date (especially for discharge).

Setting dates for specific functional achievements prompts further actions, e.g., ordering of equipment for the home.

## Estimated date of discharge (EDD)

Specifying an EDD from the point of admission is useful for patients, caregivers, and interdisciplinary team members.
- It emphasizes to the patient that the inpatient rehabilitation stay is not indefinite and that the aim is to return the patient to the home environment.
- It can be intrinsically motivating for the patient and team.
- It prompts caregivers and interdisciplinary team members to think ahead to pre- and post-discharge phases of care.

# Measurement tools in rehabilitation

## Principles

The most widely used standardized measurement instruments are structured questionnaires that deliver a quantitative (numerical) output. They vary in precision, simplicity, and applicability (to patient groups or clinical settings). For each domain of assessment several tools of differing size are usually available, reflecting tensions between brief assessments (speed, easy to use, well tolerated) and a more prolonged evaluation (precision improved, give added layers of information).

Measurement tools are helpful at single points (especially entry and exit to a therapy program) and in assessing progress.

## Advantages

- Quantifies a "snapshot" of functional ability
- Transfers standardized information across facilities
- Facilitates communication between professionals and settings of care
- Permits a less biased, more objective view of the patient
- Facilitates a structured approach to assessment and clinical audit

## Disadvantages

- May be time consuming
- May conceal considerable complexity—e.g., patients scoring the same may be very different due to "floor" or "ceiling" effects
- May have intra-individual, intra-rater, and inter-rater variability that conceals measures of meaningful clinical change—e.g., 3 or 4 points change in the 20-point Barthel Index of daily activities is needed before a team can be absolutely confident that the patient has changed
- May be confusing since many scales are available, some of which are not in general use

# Measurement instruments

### Activities of daily living (ADL)

Use a scale appropriate to the patient's level of function:
- Personal ADLs. Include key personal tasks, typically transfers, mobility, continence, feeding, washing, dressing (see Barthel Index in Appendix)

### Cognition

Several screening and assessment tools are in common use:
- Mini-Cog (see Appendix)
- The 30-point Mini-Mental State Examination (MMSE) provides sufficient precision to be used for serial assessment, e.g., tracking recovery from delirium, or therapeutic response to cholinesterase inhibitors in dementia, and takes <10 minutes to administer.

### Depression

An example is the Geriatric Depression Scale (GDS). Several versions are available, but the 15-item version is most common (see Appendix). It takes 10–15 minutes to administer. Some questions are superficially distressing, but well tolerated by most patients. Sensitivity is 80%, although specificity is only 60%.

### Pressure sore risk

Prompt, systematic evaluation of patients at risk is required. The most widely used instrument is the Braden Scale for Predicting Pressure Sore Risk, which allows nurses and other health-care providers to reliably score a patient's level of risk for developing pressure sores.

### Disease-specific scales

All of the common diseases have dedicated scales, usually developed for research use, and then introduced variably into clinical practice. They are often more complex than those used in general clinical practice, with corresponding disadvantages: they are time consuming and less easily transferable to the next site of care.

# Selecting patients for inpatient rehabilitation

Selecting patients for admission to an inpatient rehabilitation facility is an important yet complex and time-consuming task (see Box 4.1). Most hospital units operate at full capacity, so selection of patients who will optimally benefit is important.

## Who should select patients?

Review of referrals is often completed by experienced rehabilitation professionals, e.g., a physiatrist (physical medicine and rehabilitation [PM&R] physician), but may be performed by internists, neurologists, or nurses. In some cases, a team assessment is done in a conference setting.

## Who to choose?

Two factors must be considered:
• Which patients will benefit most?
• What does the interdisciplinary team need to keep it positive and functioning well?

In many ways the "best" rehabilitation patient is one who has had an acute event from which he or she is recovering (e.g., stroke, fracture) and is motivated andable to participate in therapy with enthusiasm, and has a clear goal in mind (usually to return home). Rapid results and fast turnover keep variety and interest going for the team; however, this patient may, in fact, get better in almost a supported setting with adequate time to convalesce (e.g., skilled nursing facility with therapy to improve stamina and confidence and social support on discharge).

Contrast this with a frail older woman with multiple medical problems, moderate cognitive impairment, and difficulty managing at home alone before undergoing a prolonged hospital inpatient stay with repeated complications. She has declined physically and mentally. When asked, she wishes to go home, though this may not be realistic. Her daughter thinks she should go to a nursing home for "her own safety." It is easy to write this patient off, deny them rehabilitation, and arrange nursing home placement. This is the kind of complex patient that most needs the expertise of the rehabilitation team. In any other specialty, the most complex cases are dealt with by the specialist; the same should be true of rehabilitation. These types of patients often do remarkably well and should at least be offered a trial of rehabilitation.

Even patients with no recovery potential can benefit from aspects of the team's expertise, whether this entails compensatory strategies, teaching skills to caregivers, or arranging complex discharge packages. In general, the harder a problem seems to be, the less likely it is that it will be sorted out in a nonspecialist setting and the more likely that the patient will benefit from an interdisciplinary rehabilitation team.

In practice, patients often are somewhere between the two extremes.

**Box 4.1 Information required for patient selection**

This should be gleaned from all available sources (including primary nurse, hospital notes—medical, nursing and therapy, family, caregivers, primary care provider, specialists, etc.) and may involve telephone calls and/or several visits. Regardless of who does the assessment, the following information should be acquired.

*Premorbid features*

- *Physical problems*—list of medical conditions, activity level; list of medications
- *Functional limitations*—assess by conversation: Did you use an assistive device or orthosis? Do you require assistance in ADLs or iADLs? Can you ascend and descend stairs? Formalize by estimating function using the Functional Independence Measure (FIM). Ask about physical ability and personal care.
- *Psychosocial status*—Assess by conversation: Whom do you live with (and how fit and willing to help are they)? Where do you live (rural or in town)? What is the physical setup of your home (e.g., one or more stories, stairs to enter the home, stairs inside the home, location of bedroom and bathroom on first or other floors)? Does anyone help out (e.g., caregivers, neighbors, family, friends)? What do you on a regular basis (e.g., walk to a store or restaurant for lunch, attend day care center, etc.)?
- *Cognitive state* may range from mild memory problems (may predispose to delirium) to significant dementia. Ask about any difficulties the problem causes in everyday life.

*Acute features*

- Nature of acute insult—is it reversible (e.g., amputation vs. stroke)?
- Interacting comorbidities
- What is the expected recovery curve? This varies with the disease: a patient with a large MCA stroke may show very slow progress at the outset and then show steady but slow progress after several weeks. A patient with a femoral neck fracture, by contrast, is likely to improve rapidly after surgery and continue to make quick progress. A patient with sepsis is likely to improve steadily after treatment is completed. If the assessor has limited knowledge of the disease, information should be obtained from the specialist caring for the patient.

*Patient wishes*

- Do they understand the problems they face?
- Do they know what they wish to do when they leave the hospital (e.g., go home as soon as possible, return to their residential home, not go home unless they are able to function as before)?

# Patients unlikely to benefit from rehabilitation

- Patients with plateaued function who are awaiting placement
- Patients for whom the process of waiting for a rehabilitation bed will delay discharge (e.g., when expected recovery to discharge fitness is under a week)
- Patients with a single requirement for therapy or function (e.g., transfers, ambulation on stairs)
- Patients who are medically unstable, requiring active medical diagnosis or treatment
- Patients without therapy need (e.g., comatose patients)
- Terminal-care patients (palliative care or hospice teams likely able to support discharge planning when needed)

## Dementia and rehabilitation

Dementia can be frustrating and difficult (but also very rewarding). Therapists often prefer patients who can carry over what they have learned from one therapy session to another. Nurses may find patients with behavioral problems disruptive to the unit. Patients may become disinherited and unaware of dangerous situations. Anxiety of caregivers may be high. However, there is still much that can be done.

In general, dementia alone is not a reason for refusing rehabilitation. Repeated exercise can build stamina and increase the potential for learning. Rehabilitation settings may allow some time for spontaneous recovery to occur. The more complex the patient, the greater the need for an interdisciplinary team. The team may be the best way to advocate for the rights and wishes of the demented patient.

## How to conduct an interdisciplinary team meeting

Interdisciplinary team meetings serve primary functions of communication, goal setting, reviewing progress, and discharge planning. They also contribute to wider aims:

- Team building—Discussions of patient care are vital for team bonding.
- Education—Team members share knowledge and insight into each other's jobs.

Team meetings usually take place weekly in inpatient settings but can be less frequent in community or outpatient settings. Most commonly the team meets in a room away from patients and caregivers. Sometimes, the patient and/or caregivers are brought into the room.

Theoretically, any member of the team can lead the meeting, but in practice a nurse, therapist, or physician takes this role. The leader is responsible for the following:

- *Timing*—Enough time should be allocated to discuss each patient. Essential information should be shared to resolve problems. Anecdotes should not be included in the discussion unless the details absolutely influence decisions. The order of patients should be varied each week to allow equal time for discussion.
- *Involving all team members*—Each member should have an unimpeded opportunity to comment on each patient. The team should establish an order in which each member take turns to present (see next page). Don't allow assumptions that everyone knows certain information or that it is unimportant. Ask members to clarify jargon or code that may not be universally understood.
- *Ensuring decisions are made* and goals are set. Good leadership limits discussion to essential details so that a positive action plan can be established. Prompt discussion with questions like "So what are we going to do about this?" or "Who is going to take that on?" or "When will that actually happen?" The leader prevents discussions from going in circles or resulting in disputes. Where there is agreement on goals, make sure they are SMART (p. 52).
- *Maintaining morale*—Remember, case conferences can be stressful. Keep discussions professional. Positive feedback on performance and acknowledgment that individuals and the team have done well are very important.
- *Encourage feedback*—It is interesting and educational to hear follow-up on discharged patients. Ensure that thank you letters, etc. are shared as well as news on deaths and readmissions.

### How to conduct an interdisciplinary team meeting (cont'd.)

The conventional order of presentation is as follows:
1. Doctor—diagnosis, current management, and changes planned; prognosis, particularly if symptoms are limiting therapy
2. Social worker—background, discharge discussions, external liaison (e.g., with home health agency, funding panels etc.)
3. Nursing—nursing requirements, mood and behavior, continence, sleeping, relatives' and visitors' comments.
4. Speech–language pathologist—swallowing difficulties, obstacles in language and cognition that prevent the patient from making functional progress
5. Occupational therapist—functional assessments (e.g., dressing, kitchen), cognition, and home visits
6. Physical therapist—mobility, equipment, progress and potential
7. Psychologist—cognition and adjustment issues
8. Recreational therapist—leisure activities

This order allows discussions to flow naturally from medical background to discharge plans (social worker) and psychosocial issues that bear on functional goals (therapists). The order may be different depending on the team. However, watch for one person dominating the discussion and avoid discussing discharge goals before going through the logical steps or else important elements will be missed.

Notes of the meeting should be written and shared with all team members for review. At a minimum record the date, current status, notes about the content of discussion (even if solutions are not found), goals, and plans. You have failed if you summarize a 20-minute important discussion as "continue" or "aim home next week"!

## How to plan a complex discharge

There is no such thing as a "safe discharge," only a safer one. There is widespread misconception that hospitals and nursing homes are "safe" whereas home is dangerous. In reality, the rate of falls in institutions is higher (there is just someone there to pick the person up), and the increased exposure to infection (e.g., MRSA, flu) can be life threatening.

The *timing of discharge* is sometimes obvious (e.g., when the patient is safe enough to return home with caregivers or by him- or herself), but can be controversial. Some patients want to go before the interdisciplinary team feels they are ready. Others (or their caregivers) wish to stay longer (usually because of unrealistic expectations or dislike of the chosen discharge destination). Communication is the key to avoiding this situation. Patients and caregivers should understand that discharge is not the end of recovery following an illness, but a part of the continuum of recovery.

Start to *plan discharge* prior to admission to the inpatient rehabilitation facility, e.g., by obtaining background social history and patient aspirations. Estimated discharge dates and destination should be established as soon as possible to focus goal-planning. It is better to revise a projected discharge date or destination than to have none at all.

Involve *care givers early in the prcoess*—family meetings will ensure effective two-way communication. This also reduces the chance that a care giver who has unresolved questions will arrive just before the planned discharge and block or alter the plans.

Common pitfalls that cause a discharge to fail are as follows:

- Care availability (especially night times)—Check well in advance with the social worker that the caregivers you plan for are available.
- Modifications and equipment—Ideally, any environmental modifications should be in place before your patient is discharged to prevent lengthy delays. Simple measures, such as moving a bed downstairs, may take significant time. For more complex alterations (e.g., stairway elevator, walk-in showers) obtain a realistic estimate of time to complete the task. Patients may need time before they move to their definitive living environment.

# Physical therapy

## Training

See the American Physical Therapy Association Web site at www.apta.org

## The role of the physical therapist

- Aimed at improving physical functioning by exercise, reducing pain, and providing appropriate assistive devices
- May teach facilitative or compensatory strategies
- The patient may need sufficient motivation, muscle strength, and energy to participate—it is an active, *not* a passive, process.
- The duration of therapy may be short initially, but increases as the patient tolerates more.
- Cognitive impairment may limit learning and carryover of skills from session to session, but stamina may be improved with repeated sessions.
- Rehearsal of skills improves function and teaches patients to perform exercises independently (often with written instructions). Physical therapy assistants, nursing staff, and relatives all can assist in this rehearsal process.
- Involved in training caregivers in assisting transfers and ambulation.

## Range of interventions

*Increasing range of movement*
- Perform and teach active, active assisted, or passive range-of-motion exercises
- Increase joint mobility
- Prevent pain and contractures

*Increasing strength of muscles*
- Strengthen muscles to improve stamina
- Target specific areas of weakness using resistive exercises
- Teach falls prevention

*Improve coordination*
- Rehearse skills and improve coordination using repetition
- Improve sitting balance

*Transfers*
This is the ability to get from one place (bed) to another (chair).
- Depends on the patient's ability.
- Dependent patients may require devices (e.g., Hoyer lift).
- Patients with good sitting balance may transfer with the assistance of one or two people and a sliding board, or perform a lateral transfer.
- Patients with good standing ability may perform stand-pivot transfers.

*Ambulation*
- Exercises are aimed at improving strength, standing balance, and endurance.
- Realistic goals should be set—i.e., safe household distances may be adequate if supervision or assistance is available.
- Balance training usually takes place in the parallel bars, then with assistive devices.

### Heat treatment
- Use packs, hydrotherapy pools, ultrasound, etc., to treat pain and improve joint mobility.

### Other treatments
- Cold treatments, electrical stimulation for pain relief (e.g., TENS)

### Provision of aids
- Usually assistive devices (e.g., cane, walker)
- May include orthotic devices (e.g., ankle foot orthosis)

# Assistive devices

Assistive devices increase stability and facilitate improved confidence and function that may decrease the number of falls. In general, identifying the need for an assistive device should prompt consideration of the cause of functional decline (is it reversible?), an assessment for prescription (correct device, correct size), education (use of the device, how to get up after falls), and treatment (strength and balance training).

All assistive devices without wheels should be fitted with rubber tips to optimize grip and should be checked for wear regularly.

## Cane

A cane may be single-pointed ("straight"), three-pointed ("tripod"), or four-pointed (quad cane, hemi-walker). The three- or four-pointed canes offer additional stability compared to that of the single-point cane. Held in the hand on the less affected side, the cane unloads the more affected limb. The level of hand placement should be at the greater trochanter; this positions the elbow most efficiently at 20–30 degrees of flexion.

The choice of handle is important; e.g., a *T-top* improves grip and reduces pressure. Weight is centered over the base of the stick, providing a little more stability. A *round top* is hooked over the arm when not in use, but is less stable.

## Walker

A walker is a device made of lightweight alloy metal that is self-stabilizing (usually based around four points in contact with the floor). Walkers provide unloading of the lower limbs and greater stability than a cane. Various sizes are available. Some are difficult to transport, others fold up for easy storage. Walkers may be used indoors or outdoors.

The handgrips should be at wrist level, with the elbows slightly flexed (15 degrees). Shorter frames may be used in patients who fall backward. To use a non-rolling walker, lift and move it 4–12 inches (10–30 cm) in front of the body. Lean forward, taking some weight through the arms. Take one equal step with each leg into the center of the walker.

A weighted walker has weights low on the frame to provide additional counterbalance against falls.

A *wheeled (rolling)* walker has wheels at the front that permits faster walking and an improved gait pattern, but provides a slightly less stable base.

A *platform* walker has forearm rests that enable weight bearing through the forearms instead of the hands, and provides additional support when weight bearing through the hands or wrists is impaired.

## Crutches

A full assessment by a therapist is needed before selecting crutches. Crutches may be of the axilla or elbow type. Both are available with various features that should be individually prescribed. For example, closed elbow cuffs provide added security and enable the user to let go of the handgrip to open a door without the crutch falling to the floor.

## Rolling walkers

A rolling walker has three or four wheels and hand-operated brakes (for added stability). Three-wheeled versions usually fold, permitting storage in a car. Rolling walkers with additional features, such as bigger wheels (for uneven ground) or a seat or attached basket for shopping or other house and garden tasks, are larger than most standard walkers and usually used outdoors.

# Occupational therapy

### Training

The occupational therapist (OT) completes a 5- or 6-year post-baccalaureate occupational therapy degree. A certified occupational therapy assistant (COTA) completes a 2-year OTA associate degree at one of approximately 280 accredited programs at colleges and universities throughout the United States. See the American Occupational Therapy Association (AOTA) Web site at www.aota.org.

### Role of the occupational therapist

The AOTA defines *occupational therapy* as a "skilled treatment that helps individuals achieve independence in all facets of their lives." Occupational therapy focuses on enabling people to perform activities of daily living (ADLs). The very word *occupation* denotes an activity that "occupies" our time.

Occupational therapy assists people in developing the "skills for the job of living necessary for independent and satisfying lives."

### Skills vs. habits

- A *skill* is the ability to start, carry out, and complete a task effectively (e.g., making a cup of coffee).
- A *habit* is a task that is actually carried out (e.g., a person may be able to make a meal, but does not do so when alone as they do not feel hungry).

### Components of personal ability

- Assessed by direct observation during tasks, formal testing, and information taken from caregivers, family members, and other professionals.
- Cognition—one has the ability to understand the task and why it is performed. It may be limited by dementia, poor concentration span, poor problem-solving skills, etc. Assessed with cognitive tests
- Psychology, or the motivation to do and complete the task. This is limited by depression, apathy, impaired coping skills, etc.
- Sensorimotor ability, especially in the upper limb function

# Occupational therapy assessments and interventions

## Assessments

- Washing and dressing should be performed in the morning, when the patient normally carries out these tasks.
- Kitchen—Evaluate the patient's competence and safety for required tasks (e.g., the patient may need to make a meal on a gas stove, or pour a hot drink from a prepared thermos).
- Home visits are done with or without the patient, to study the layout and potential problems of a patient's own home.

### Home assessment visits

A visit should be conducted with the patient, to see them in their own environment.

- It can be accomplished with an OT alone, but usually with another member of the interdisciplinary team (e.g., physical therapist, care manager).
- It may be useful to include intended caregivers (volunteer or professional), as concerns can be addressed during the visit.
- It can be done in the community while the patient is still at home, from an inpatient rehabilitation facility prior to discharge, or after discharge as follow-up to identify and address all possible problems and dangers.
- It may be surprising. Patients may perform either considerably better than expected (because they are in a familiar environment) or considerably worse (especially when a new physical limitation has occurred, such as stroke, as being at home emphasizes how different life will now be).
- It should incorporate a standard format for assessing all aspects of the property.

A report of the visit should contain observations on patient performance and a list of recommendations regarding reorganization of furniture (e.g., bring bed downstairs) and equipment and care required. The report should be typed and circulated to all interdisciplinary team members.

## Interventions

Interventions should include teaching new skills (e.g., putting on clothing with an arthritic shoulder) and relearning habits (e.g., heating up a microwave meal at lunchtime). The interdisciplinary team member should observe how much can be done by the patient themselves, and how much help is needed from caregivers. The interdisciplinary team member should assess the need and suitability of equipment, as well as training of caregivers in its use. Commonly used equipment includes devices for the following needs and activities:

- Access—ramps, rails, banisters, stair glide, perching stool (high stool to enable seated access to a kitchen work surface)
- Transfers—transfer board, Hoyer lift, leg lifter
- Mobility—wheelchair, scooter, etc.
- Bathing and dressing—bath chair and bench, accessible bath and shower, long shoe horn, reacher, button hook, dressing stick

- Toileting and continence—raised toilet seat, commode, urinal, bedpan
- Eating and drinking—cutlery and cups with large or weighted handles, aids to improve safety with hot water (kettle holders, full-cup alarms), tap turners
- Splints for wrists and hands (prevent pain) and for ankles and feet (foot drop)
- Sensory aids—enhanced signals (e.g., large dials on a clock), altered signals (e.g., flashing light for the deaf)

# Physicians on the rehabilitation team

Physicians (e.g., physiatrist or neurologist) are commonly part of the inpatient rehabilitation team, but may be missing from community rehabilitation teams when a primary care physician (e.g., general internist or geriatrician) may be consulted about specific issues.

Rehabilitation unit rounds may be less frequent than those on acute wards but usually take place daily in inpatient rehabilitation facilities. Since the patient is usually medically stable, communication with the patient and family may predominate over medical management.

In a rehabilitation setting the doctor's main duties to the patient are as follows:
• Selection of patients
• Optimize and stabilize medical treatments (e.g., monitor blood pressure and blood glucose, ensure adequate pain management)
• Rationalize drug therapy (e.g., facilitate sleep or stop daytime sedation)
• Anticipate and treat complications (e.g., pressure sores, *Clostridium difficile* colitis)
• Diagnose and treat depression
• Identify and manage comorbid conditions (e.g., bowel and bladder incontinence)
• Initiate secondary prevention (e.g., aspirin for stroke, bisphosphonates for osteoporosis)
• Make secondary referrals to other specialists (e.g., dermatology, orthopedics)

Additional duties of the team include the following:
• Education
• Team building
• Context setting—Physicians often cross health-sector boundaries, whereas therapists and nurses can be fixed in teams or on wards. They should share information about the patients on the waiting list and about those who are not admitted to the inpatient rehabilitation facility and why. This overview can help the team understand admission rationales, rationing of beds, etc.

# Nurses on the rehabilitation team

A registered nurse with at least 2 years of practice in rehabilitation nursing can earn distinction as a Certified Rehabilitation Registered Nurse (CRRN) by successfully completing an examination that validates expertise. See the Association of Rehabilitation Nurses Web site at www.rehabnurse.org.

The role of rehabilitation nurses in the recovery of a patient is often underestimated. Of all the members of the professional team, they spend the most time and often have the most intimate relationship with patients and their caregivers. Their wide role encompasses the following:

- Rehabilitation aide. They rehearse with the patient new tasks learned with therapists (e.g., transfers, dressing). It usually takes longer and more skill to encourage a patient to wash and dress themselves independently than it does to do it for them. This is the fundamental difference between rehabilitation and medical nursing.
- Overall performance assessors vs. snapshot. They can detect performance differences between what a patient can do with the therapist and what the patient does when on their own, when tired, or when caregivers are visiting.
- Communication and liaison. Nurses are the first call for members of the interdisciplinary team, patient, and caregivers. They may learn of emotive information that is sometimes more readily revealed in nonthreatening discussions.
- Nocturnal assessment. Nurses and aides are best able to monitor sleep, nocturnal confusion or wandering, and nocturnal continence and toileting.
- Continence management
- Pressure and wound care management
- Medication administration and monitoring of self-medication
- Inpatient rehabilitation facility management

Some nurse specialists have roles that overlap with those of the doctor, e.g., in selecting patients for rehabilitation, chairing interdisciplinary and family meetings, and prescribing. This is especially true in some community inpatient rehabilitation facilities that can be run exclusively by nurse practitioners.

# Social work and case management

Professional social workers assist individuals to restore or enhance their capacity for social functioning while creating societal conditions favorable to their goals. In the rehabilitation environment, their role encompasses the following:

- Help people overcome the effects of poverty, discrimination, abuse, addiction, physical illness, divorce, loss, unemployment, educational problems, disability, and mental illness
- Help to prevent crises and counsel individuals, families, and communities to cope more effectively with the stresses of everyday life
- Identify resources that allow patients with disabilities to remain in the community
- If patients cannot live in the community, the social worker helps them apply for medical and financial assistance, as well as identify short-term and extended-care facilities.

See the National Association of Social Workers Web site at www. naswdc.org.

The rehabilitation case manager usually is a registered nurse who is certified as a case manager. Their role encompasses the following:

- Advocating for the appropriate medical treatment at the appropriate time
- Coordinating referrals to specialty physicians, second opinions, physical and occupational therapy, functional capacity evaluations, and work hardening programs
- Synthesizing and implementing a rehabilitation plan to maximize functional recovery and attempt return to the community and work force, as appropriate

See the American Case Management Association Web site at www. acmaweb.org.

# Speech–language therapy and dieticians

## Speech-language pathologist (SLP)

Speech–language pathologists must have masters or doctoral degrees. See the American Speech–Language–Hearing Association Web site at www. asha.org.

### Assessment and treatment of speech disorders

This forms a large part of SLPs' work, commonly following stroke, or head and neck surgery. Therapists are experts in communication disorders, and their assessments are useful in treating aphasia, apraxia, dysarthria, and cognitive-communication impairment. They provide facilatory and compensatory therapy; advice to the patient, caregivers, and staff; augmentative communication; and communication with tracheostomy and ventilator care.

### Assessment and treatment of swallowing disorders

This forms the remainder of inpatient work. The patient receives a careful bedside evaluation. On the basis of this evaluation, the SLP may recommend videofluorography or fiber-optic endoscopy, if necessary.

Useful interventions include patient positioning, changes in the texture or consistency of food and fluid, and caregiver supervision or prompting with food boluses. A period of nothing by mouth (NPO) may be necessary if the patient cannot swallow safely. Enteral feeding should be considered if safe oral feeding cannot be achieved.

## Dieticians

Dieticians are trained at the baccalaureate degree level, followed by internship and certification. See the American Dietetic Association's Web site at www.eatright.org.

Malnutrition in older people is common, underdiagnosed, and undertreated. Prevalence and severity are especially high with acute or chronic comorbidities and in inpatients. Community-dwelling older people may have an insufficient diet, depleted in fruit and vegetables ("meat-and-potatoes" diet). While dieticians are experts in the assessment and treatment of nutritional problems, other members of the interdisciplinary team must also be alert to the possibility of malnutrition and initiate interventions and dietician referral. Screening tools are useful.

Effective interventions include offering attractive food tailored to the individual, asking the family to bring in food, offering food frequently, and providing a staff member or caregiver at the bedside to assist with feeding. Modern packaging (prepackaged margarine, snack boxes, and drinks) can be obstructive if patients cannot open them.

When "normal" feeding is impossible, e.g., after acute stroke, the dietician can provide assessment, monitoring, and advice to the patient and caregiver regarding alternative means of feeding.

# Pharmacy

Pharmacists must have at least 2 years of specific undergraduate college study, followed by 4 academic years of professional pharmacy study, leading to the Doctor of Pharmacy (Pharm.D.) degree. See the American Pharmacists Association Web site at www.pharmacist.com.

Pharmacists are involved in the preparation, prescribing, packaging, and dispensing of medicines and are a key part of the system delivering quality drug use to out- and inpatients. They are the gatekeepers of many hospital formularies (limited drug lists optimizing costs and effectiveness). They advise on all aspects of prescribing, especially interactions and dosing.

Issues that pharmacists may help to resolve or reduce include the following:

- High frequency of adverse drug reactions (up to 17% of hospital admissions)
- Under- and overuse of medications, e.g., preventatives in asthma
- Poor concordance or adherence
- Poor administration technique, e.g., inhalers
- Frequent and complex changes in medication
- Poor communication with primary care physicians after discharge
- Absence of full medication history on admission
- Reconciliation of medication available in the inpatient facility or on a patient's insurance formulary.

# Neuropsychologist

Psychology is the study of the mind and behavior and embraces all aspects of the human experience. A *neuropsychologist* specializes in studying brain–behavior relationships, i.e., they attempt to infer damage to specific parts of the brain from observations of the behavioral deficits that follow brain injury or disease.

Neuropsychologists have extensive training in the anatomy, physiology, and pathology of the nervous system. They study brain–behavior relationships under controlled and standardized conditions, using valid and reliable tests that have acceptable levels of sensitivity and specificity in order to identify and treat cognitive and neurobehavioral dysfunction.

Tests also allow clinicians to monitor the course of recovery and the patient's potential for return to the community.

See the American Psychological Association Web site at www.apa.org.

# Recreational therapy

*Therapeutic recreation* is defined by the U.S. Department of Labor as a "profession of specialists who utilize activities as a form of treatment for persons who are physically, mentally or emotionally disabled." Differing from diversional or recreation services, recreational therapy uses various activities as a form of active treatment to promote the independent physical, cognitive, emotional, and social functioning of persons disabled as a result of trauma or disease, by enhancing current skills and facilitating the establishment of new skills for daily living and community functioning.

In addition, recreational therapists assist the patient in developing or redeveloping social skills, discretionary time skills, decision-making skills, coping abilities, self-advocacy, discharge planning for reintegration, and skills to enhance general quality of life. Recreational-therapy services offer a diversity of rehabilitation benefits addressing the needs of individuals with a range of disabling conditions.

Recreational therapists are standard treatment team members in psychiatric rehabilitation, substance abuse treatment, and physical rehabilitation services. However, because most of these therapies have not been validated in controlled clinical trials, in some countries they are considered "alternative medicine" and are not reimbursable by health insurance.

See the American Therapeutic Recreation Assocation's Web site at http://atra-online.com/cms.

# Certified rehabilitation counselor

Rehabilitation counseling is a systematic process that assists patients with physical, mental, developmental, cognitive, and emotional disabilities in the community to maximize their vocational and avocational living goals in the most integrated setting possible. This involves assessment and appraisal; diagnosis and treatment planning; vocational counseling; facilitating adjustments to the medical and psychosocial impact of disability; case management, referral, and service coordination; program evaluation and research; interventions to remove environmental, employment, and attitudinal barriers; consultation services among multiple parties and regulatory systems; job analysis, job development, and placement services, including assistance with employment and job accommodations; and consultation about and access to rehabilitation technology.

See the Web site at http://www.crccertification.com. Similar functions are performed by Certified Disability Management Specialists (www.cdms.org).

# Vocational therapist/counselor

Vocational rehabilitation enables a disabled person to secure, retain, and advance in suitable employment. Advocates in this field formulate, implement, and periodically review national policy on vocational rehabilitation and employment of disabled people, and promote employment opportunities for disabled people in the open labor market.

Vocational counselors also promote cooperation and coordination between the public and private bodies engaged in vocational rehabilitation, and they evaluate vocational guidance, training, placement, employment, and other related services to enable disabled persons to secure, retain, and advance in employment.

The Rehabilitation Services Administration (RSA) of the Office of Special Education and Rehabilitation Services (OSERS) in the U.S. Department of Education oversees grant programs that help individuals with physical or mental disabilities to obtain employment and live more independently through the provision of such supports as counseling, medical and psychological services, job training and other individualized services.

RSA's major Title I formula grant program provides funds to state vocational rehabilitation (VR) agencies to provide employment-related services for individuals with disabilities, giving priority to individuals who are significantly disabled.

See the website at:

http://www.ed.gov/about/offices/list/osers/rsa/index.html

# Orthotist and prosthetist

An *orthotist* makes and fits braces and splints (orthoses) for patients who need added support for body parts that have been weakened by injury, disease, or disorders of the nerves, muscles, or bones. They work under a physician's orders to adapt purchased braces or to create custom-designed braces.

Orthotics are often named for the body part(s) they cross, such as AFO (ankle–foot orthosis) or KAFO (knee–ankle–foot orthosis). Orthotics such as Halo braces (a brace that surrounds the head and is held in place with small screws in the skull) or TLSO (thoracolumbar spinal orthosis) may be used to stabilize portions of the spine and prevent further damage to the spinal cord after injury.

A *prosthetist* makes and fits artificial limbs (prostheses) for patients with disabilities. This includes artificial legs and arms for patients who have had amputations due to conditions such as cancer, diabetes, or injury. While prosthetics are not usually used in patients with neurological conditions, amputation may be a comorbid condition in patients with neurological impairment.

See the American Board for Certification in Orthotics, Prosthetics, and Pedorthics Web site at www.abcop.org.

# Falls and gait imbalance

**Danelle Cayea**

# Falls

A *fall* is an event that results in a person unintentionally coming to rest at a lower level (usually the floor). Falls are common and important, affecting one-third of people living in their own home each year. Falls result in fear, injury, dependency, institutionalization, and death. Many can be prevented and their consequences can be minimized.

## Factors influencing fall frequency

### Intrinsic factors

Maintaining balance—and avoiding a fall—is a complex, demanding, multi-system skill. It requires muscle strength (power–weight ratio), stable but flexible joints, multiple sensory modalities (e.g., proprioception, vision) and a functional peripheral and central nervous system. Higher-level cognitive function permits risk assessment, giving insight into the danger that a planned activity may pose.

Older adults with any of the following conditions have a higher than average risk of falling: arthritis, depressive symptoms, orthostasis, impairment in cognition, vision, balance, gait, or muscle strength, or the use of four or more prescription medicines.

### Extrinsic factors

Contributing environmental factors may include lighting, obstacles, the presence of grab rails and the height of steps and furniture, appropriate footwear, and the softness and grip of the floor.

### Magnitude of stressor

All people have the susceptibility to fall. The likelihood of a fall depends on how close to a "fall threshold" a person sits. Older people, especially those with disease, are closer to the threshold and are more easily and more often pushed over it by stressors. These can be internal (e.g., transient dizziness due to orthostatic hypotension) or external (e.g., a gust of wind, or a nudge in a crowded shop). They may be minor or major (no-one can avoid falling in hurricane-force winds or during complete syncope).

If a person has a higher risk of falling and their insight is preserved, they can reduce risk to some extent by limiting hazardous behaviors and minimizing stressors (e.g., avoiding stairs or uneven surfaces, using an assistive device, or asking for help from another person).

## Factors influencing fall severity

In older people, the adverse consequences of falling are greater, due to the following:

- **Multisystem impairments** that lead to **less effective self-protective mechanisms.** Falls are more severe and injury rates per fall are higher.
- **Osteoporosis** and increased fracture rates
- **Secondary injury** due to post-fall immobility, including pressure sores, burns, dehydration, and pneumonia
- **Psychological adverse effects** including loss of confidence and fear of falling

A fall is often a symptom of an underlying serious acute problem. Falls are almost always multifactorial. Think:

- **Why today?** Often the fall is a manifestation of acute or subacute illness, e.g., sepsis, dehydration, or adverse drug effect.
- **Why this person?** Usually a combination of intrinsic and extrinsic factors increases vulnerability to stressors and leads to falls.
- For every fall, identify the intrinsic factors, extrinsic factors, and acute stressors that have led to it.
- Within each of these categories, think of how their influence on the likelihood of future falls can be reduced.

## Assessment following a fall

Think of fall(s) if a patient presents with the following:

- Having tripped
- A fracture or non-fracture injury
- Having been found on the floor

Patients who have fallen are often mislabeled as having syncope, which is an infrequent cause and may limit the search for multiple causal factors.

Practice opportunistic screening—ask all people age 70 and older on initial exam and annually whether they have fallen recently.

## History

Obtain a corroborative history, if possible. In many cases, a careful history differentiates between falls due to the following:

- Frailty and unsteadiness
- Syncope or near syncope
- Acute neurological problems (e.g., vertigo, seizures, vertebrobasilar insufficiency)

Gather information about the following factors:

- Fall circumstances (e.g., timing, physical environment)
- Symptoms before and after the fall
- Use of drugs, including alcohol
- Previous falls, fractures, and syncope, even as a young adult
- Previous near-misses
- Comorbidity (cardiac, neurological [stroke, Parkinson's disease, seizures], cognitive impairment, diabetes)
- Functional performance (difficulties bathing, dressing, or toileting)

## Drugs associated with falls

Falls may be caused by any drug that is either directly psychoactive or may lead to systemic hypotension and cerebral hypoperfusion. Polypharmacy (>4 drugs, any type) is an independent risk factor.

Drugs having the strongest link to an increased risk of falling include the following:

- Benzodiazepines and other hypnotics
- Tricyclic antidepressants
- Selective serotonin-reuptake inhibitors (SSRIs)
- Antipsychotics
- Anticonvulsants
- Class IA antiarrhythmics

- Diuretics
- Digoxin
- Skeletal muscle relaxants

## Examination

This can sometimes be focused if the history is highly suggestive of a particular pathology. But perform at least a brief screening examination of each system.

- *Functional:* The "get up and go" test provides information about balance and gait and is performed by asking the patient to stand from a chair, walk 10 feet, turn around, walk back, and sit back down. This test can also be used for comparison at different time points and for screening (completion time >16 seconds correlates with increased fall risk). Assess gait, use of walking aids, and hazard appreciation.
- *Cardiovascular:* Always check lying and standing BP. Check pulse rate and rhythm. Listen for murmurs (especially of aortic stenosis).
- *Musculoskeletal:* Assess footwear (stability and grip). Remove footwear and examine the feet. Examine the major joints for deformity, instability, or stiffness.
- *Neurological:* Assess to identify stroke, peripheral neuropathy, Parkinson's disease, vestibular disease, myelopathy, cerebellar degeneration, visual impairment, and cognitive impairment.

## Tests

Many tests are of limited value, but the following are considered routine:
- CBC
- Vitamin $B_{12}$
- Urinalysis (UA) and urine culture
- Glucose
- Electrolytes
- BUN and creatinine
- Thyroid function tests
- Vitamin D

Vitamin D deficiency is common in older adults. Recent evidence suggests that replacement reduces fall. Therefore, checking the vitamin D level is worthwhile for most patients.

If a specific cause is suspected, then test for it—for example:
- 24-hour ambulatory cardiac monitoring only if there are frequent episodes suggestive of arrhythmia and there is a known history of cardiac disease

## Interventions to prevent falls

The complexity of treatment reflects the complexity of etiology.
- Older people who fall more often have remediable medical causes.
- Do not expect to make only one diagnosis or intervention—making minor changes to multiple factors is more powerful.
- Tailor the intervention to the patient. Assess for relevant risk factors and work to modify each one.

### Reducing fall frequency

Priorities are likely to include the following.

*Drug review*
- For each drug, weigh the benefits of continuing the drug against the benefits of reducing or stopping it. Stop use if risk outweighs benefit.

Reduce the dosage if benefit is likely from the drug class but the dosage is excessive for that patient.
- Taper psychotropic medications.
- Try and reduce the overall number of drugs.

*Treatment of orthostatic hypotension*
- Diagnose and treat the underlying cause.
- If possible, reduce the number of blood pressure–lowering drugs, relax salt restriction, ensure adequate hydration, and apply pressure support stockings.

*Muscle strengthening and balance and gait training*
- Get an evaluation by a physical therapist. Exercise classes or disciplines such as Tai Chi can be helpful.

*Assistive device*
- Provide an appropriate aid (i.e., cane) and teach patient how to use it.

*Standardized home assessment and modification*
- This should be done by an occupational therapist.

*Adequate vision*
- Ensure that the patient has adequate vision through an ophthalmology referral, provision of adequate lighting, and avoidance of multifocal lenses while walking to enhance depth perception.

*Adequate footwear*
- Supportive thin-soled shoes help those with proprioceptive deficits.

*Reducing stressors*
This involves decision making by the patient or caregivers. The cognitively able patient can judge risk/benefit and usually modifies risk appropriately— e.g., by limiting walking to indoors, using a walking aid properly and reliably, and asking for help if a task (e.g., getting dressed) is particularly demanding. However:
- Risk can never be abolished.
- Enforced relative immobility has a cost to health.
- Patient choice is paramount. Most patients will have clear views about risk and how much their lifestyle should change.
- Institutionalization does not usually reduce risk (see below).

## Preventing adverse consequences of falls
Despite risk reduction, falls may remain likely. In this case, consider the following:
- **Osteoporosis detection and treatment**
- **Teaching patients how to get up**, usually by a physical therapist
- **Alarms**—i.e., a pendant alarm (worn around the neck). Often these alert a distant call center that summons help to the home (ambulance).
- **Supervision**. Regular visits to the home (by caregivers, neighbors, or family) can reduce the duration of lying on the ground after a fall.
- **Change of accommodation**. This sometimes reduces risk, but it is not a panacea. A move from home to a supervised setting rarely reduces risk, as these environments are unfamiliar to the person and often have hard flooring surfaces. The staff cannot provide continuous supervision.

## Preventing falls in the hospital

Falls in the hospital are common, as acutely ill older people with chronic comorbidity are admitted into an unfamiliar environment. Multifactorial interventions have the best chance of reducing falls (but cf. Box 3.1):

• Treat infection and dehydration and implement a protocol to reduce the risk of delirium.
• If delirium is present, consider assigning a sitter or allowing a caregiver to stay with the patient.
• Stop high-risk drugs and avoid starting them.
• Provide good-quality footwear and an accessible walking aid.
• Provide good lighting and a bedside commode for those with urinary or fecal urgency or frequency.
• Keep a call bell close to hand.
• Place highest-risk patients in rooms in sight of the nurses' station.

### Box 3.1  Interventions that are rarely effective and may be harmful

• *Bedrails.* Injury risk is substantial: patients may try to climb over the rails, falling even greater distances onto the floor below.
• *Restraints.* These increase the risk of physical injury, including fractures, pressure sores, and death. They also increase agitation.
• *Hip protectors.* These are impact-absorptive pads stitched into undergarments. Increasing evidence suggests that they are not effective, largely because of practical issues and resulting poor compliance—they are difficult to put on and can be uncomfortable, and multiple pairs are needed if incontinence is a problem.

### Further reading

Leipzig RM, Cumming RG, Tinetti ME (1999). Drugs and falls in older people: a systematic review and meta-analysis: I. Psychotropic drugs. *J Am Geriatr Soc* **47**:30–39.
Leipzig RM, Cumming RG, Tinetti ME (1999). Drugs and falls in older people: a systematic review and meta-analysis: II. Cardiac and analgesic drugs. *J Am Geriatr Soc* **47**:40–50.
Tinnetti M (2003). Preventing falls in elderly persons. *N Engl J Med* **348**:42–49.

# Syncope and presyncope

*Syncope* is a sudden, transient loss of consciousness and postural tone due to reduced cerebral perfusion. The patient typically slumps or falls. Unconsciousness, usually lasting less than a minute, may be associated with one or more tonic–clonic jerks, which do not indicate an underlying seizure disorder. Once the patient is horizontal, gravity restores cerebral perfusion and consciousness is fully recovered.

*Presyncope* is a feeling of light-headedness that would lead to syncope if corrective measures were not taken (usually sitting or lying down).

These conditions

- Are a major cause of morbidity in the older population (occurring in a quarter of institutionalized older people) and are recurrent in a third. Risk of syncope increases with advancing age and in the presence of cardiovascular disease.
- Account for 5% of hospital admissions and many serious injuries.
- Cause considerable anxiety and can cause social isolation as sufferers limit activities, in fear of further episodes.

## Causes

These are many. Older people with decreased physiological reserve are more susceptible to most causes. It is important to distinguish between true syncope and nonsyncopal attacks such as seizure, where the loss of consciousness is due to altered electrical activity in the brain.

Stroke and transient ischemic attack (TIA) very rarely cause syncope, as they cause a focal, not a global, deficit. Brain stem ischemia is the rare exception.

Causes of true syncope can be subdivided as follows.

### Peripheral factors

- **Orthostatic hypotension** may be caused by the upright posture, eating, straining, prolonged standing, especially in hot places, and may be exacerbated by low circulating volume (dehydration), hypotensive drugs, or intercurrent sepsis. Orthostatic hypotension is the most common cause of syncope.

### Neurally mediated syncope

- **Classical vasovagal syncope** is common in young and old people. Vagal stimulation (pain, fright, distress, prolonged standing) leads to hypotension and syncope. The patient may have an autonomic prodrome (pale, clammy, light-headed) followed by nausea or abdominal pain, then syncope. This condition is benign, with no implications for driving. Diagnose with caution in older people with vascular disease, where other causes are more common.
- **Situational syncope** occurs immediately after urination, defecation, cough, or swallowing.
- **Carotid sinus syndrome**

*Cardiovascular factors*
- **Pump problem**—myocardial infarction (MI) or ischemia, arrhythmia (tachycardia (ventricular tachycardia [VT], supraventricular tachycardia [SVT], fast atrial fibrillation [AF]), bradycardia, Mobitz II type 2 or type 3 heart block)
- **Outflow obstruction**—e.g., aortic stenosis
- **Pulmonary embolism**—one-quarter of older adults may present with collapse.

## History

The history often yields the diagnosis, but accuracy can be difficult to achieve—the patient often remembers little. Witness accounts are valuable and should be sought.

Ensure that the following points are covered:
- **Situation:** Was the patient standing (orthostatic hypotension), exercising (aortic stenosis, ischemia, or arrhythmia), sitting or lying down (likely seizure), eating (postprandial hypotension), on the toilet (defecation or micturition syncope), coughing (cough syncope), in pain or frightened (vasovagal syncope)? Have they recently used alcohol?
- **Prodrome:** Was there any warning? Palpitations suggest arrhythmia; sweating with palpitations suggests vasovagal syndrome; chest pain suggests ischemia; light-headedness suggests any cause of hypotension. Gustatory or olfactory aura suggests seizures. However, associations are not absolute; e.g., arrhythmias often do not cause palpitations.
- **Was there loss of consciousness?** There is much terminology (fall, blackout, "fell-out," collapse), and different patients mean different things by each term. Syncope has occurred if there is loss of consciousness with loss of awareness due to cerebral hypoperfusion; however, many (~30%) patients will have amnesia for the loss of consciousness and simply describe a fall.
- **Description of attack**—ideally from an eyewitness. Was the patient pale and clammy (likely systemic and cerebral hypoperfusion)? Were there ictal features (tongue biting, incontinence, twitching)? Prolonged loss of consciousness makes syncope unlikely. A brain deprived of oxygen from any cause is susceptible to seizure; jerking or twitching after the loss of consciousness does not necessarily indicate that a seizure disorder is the primary problem. Assess carefully before initiating anticonvulsant therapy.
- **Recovery period**—ideally reported by an eyewitness. Rapid recovery often indicates a cardiac cause. Prolonged drowsiness and confusion often follow a seizure.

## Examination

Full general examination is required. Ensure that the pulse is examined, murmurs sought, and a postural blood pressure is obtained.

## Investigation

- **Blood tests**—check for anemia, sepsis, renal disease, and myocardial ischemia.
- **ECG**—for all older patients with loss of consciousness or presyncope. Look specifically at PR interval, QT interval, trifascicular block

(prolonged PR, right bundle branch block [RBBB], and left axis deviation [LAD]), ischemic changes, and LVH (occurs in aortic stenosis).

- **Other tests** depend on clinical suspicion. An echocardiogram may be useful as ejection fraction is a highly predictive marker of sudden cardiac death. Head imaging, in the absence of head trauma, is generally not useful. An electroencephalogram (EEG) may be done if seizures are suspected, a Holter monitor if arrhythmias are suspected. Tilt testing is a very labor-intensive test and should not be requested unless symptoms sound orthostatic but diagnosis is proving difficult.

## Treatment

- Treat the cause
- Often not found (~40% in elderly) or multifactorial, so treat all reversible factors
- Review medication (e.g., diuretics, vasodilators, cholinesterase inhibitors, tricyclic antidepressants)
- Education about prevention and measures to abort an attack if there is a prodrome. Advise against swimming or bathing alone, and inform patient about driving restrictions (see Chapter 30, The older driver, p. 727).

## Further reading

Brignole M, Alboni P, Benditt D, et al. (2004). Guidelines on management (diagnosis and treatment) of syncope: update 2004. Executive summary. *Eur Heart J* **22**:2054–2072.

Hood R (2007). Syncope in the elderly. *Clin Geriatr Med* **23**:351–361.

# Balance and dysequilibrium

Balancing is a complex activity, involving many systems.

## Input

There must be awareness of the position of the body in space, which comes from the following:

- **Peripheral input**—information about body position comes from peripheral nerves (proprioception) and mechanoreceptors in the joints. This information is relayed via the posterior column of the spinal cord to the central nervous system.
- **Eyes** provide visual cues as to position.
- **Ears** provide input at several levels. The otolithic organs (utricle and saccule) provide information about static head position. The semicircular canals inform about head movement. Auditory cues localize a person with reference to the environment.

## Assimilation

Information is gathered and assessed in the brain stem and cerebellum.

## Output

Messages are then relayed to the eyes to allow a steady gaze during head movements (the vestibulo-ocular reflex) and to the cortex and the cord to control postural (antigravity) muscles.

When all this functions well, balance is effortless. A defect(s) in any one contributing system can cause balance problems or dysequilibrium:

- **Peripheral nerves**—neuropathy is more common. Specifically, it is believed that there is a significant age-related loss of proprioceptive function.
- **Eyes**—age-related changes decrease visual acuity. Disease (cataracts, glaucoma) is more common (see Chapter 22, Eyes p. 587).
- **Ears**—age-related changes decrease hearing and lead to reduced vestibular function. The older vestibular system is more vulnerable to damage from drugs, trauma, infection, and ischemia (see Chapter 21, Ears p. 567).
- **Joint receptors**—degenerative joint disease (arthritis) is more common in older people.
- **Central nervous system**—age-related changes can slow processing. Disease processes (ischemia, hypertensive damage, dementia) are more common with age.
- **Postural muscles** are more likely to be weak because of inactivity, disease, medication (e.g., steroids), or reduced muscle mass of aging.

In the older person, one or more of these defects will occur commonly. In addition, skeletal changes may alter the center of gravity, and cardiovascular changes may lead to arrhythmias or postural change in blood pressure, exacerbated further by medications.

## An approach to dysequilibrium

- Etiology is usually multifactorial.
- Consider each system separately and optimize its function.

- Look at provoking factors (medication, cardiovascular conditions, environmental hazards, etc.) and minimize them.
- Work on prevention:
  - Alter the environment (e.g., improve lighting).
  - With the physical therapist, develop safer ways to mobilize and increase strength, stamina, and balance.
- Small adjustments to multiple problems can make a big difference—i.e., when appropriate, combine cataract extraction, a walking aid, vascular secondary prevention, a second stair rail, brighter lighting, and a course of physical therapy.

If falls persist despite simple (but multiple) interventions, refer to a specialist.

# Dizziness

A brain that has insufficient information to be confident of where it is in space generates a sensation of dizziness. This can be due to reduced sensory inputs or impairment of their integration. Dizziness is common, occurring in up to 30% of older people.

However, the term *dizziness* can be used by patients and doctors to mean many different things:
- Movement (spinning) of the patient or the room—vertigo
- Dysequilibrium or unsteadiness
- Light-headedness—presyncope
- Mixed—a combination of these sensations
- Other—e.g., malaise, general weakness, headache

Distinguishing these is the first step in management, as it will indicate possible causal conditions. This relies largely on the history. Discriminatory questions include the following:
- Please try to describe exactly what you feel when you are dizzy?
- Does the room spin? (vertigo)
- Do you feel light-headed, as if you are about to faint? (presyncope.)
- Does it occur when you are lying down? (if so, presyncope is unlikely)
- Does it come on when you move your head? (vertigo more likely)
- Does it come and go? (Chronic, constant symptoms are more likely to be mixed or psychiatric in origin.)

## Causes

The individual conditions most commonly diagnosed when a patient complains of dizziness are as follows:
- Benign paroxysmal positional vertigo
- Labyrinthitis
- Posterior circulation stroke
- Orthostatic hypotension
- Carotid sinus hypersensitivity
- Vertebrobasilar insufficiency
- Cervical spondylosis
- Anxiety and depression.

In reality, much dizziness is multifactorial, with dysfunction in several systems. This means that precise diagnosis is more difficult (and often not done) and treatment is more complex.

Making small improvements to each contributing problem can add up to a big overall improvement (perhaps making the difference between independent living or institutional care).

### How to manage multifactorial dizziness: clinical example

Mrs A is 85 and has fallen several times. She complains of dizziness; specifically she feels "fuzzy headed," usually when standing. When this occurs, if she sits down promptly it will pass, but often she doesn't make it and her legs "just give way." She also feels "fuzzy" in bed sometimes when turning over. Past medical history includes hypertension (she takes hydrochlorothiazide 25 mg and metoprolol 100 mg) and osteoarthritis. She lives alone in an apartment.

*Examination*

She is thin and has a kyphotic spine. Pulse is 50/min; supine blood pressure is 130/80, falling to 100/70 on standing. There is limited movement at the hips and cervical spine. Neck movement causes unsteadiness.

*Investigations*

Blood tests are normal with exception of low vitamin D level. ECG shows sinus bradycardia; X-rays show severe degenerative change of the hip joints and cervical spine, with some vertebral wedge fractures.

*Diagnosis and treatment plan*

This is a multifactorial problem. Some of the relevant factors include

- Postural instability, caused by arthritis, kyphosis, and low muscle mass
- Presyncope, caused by bradycardia and mild postural drop
- Possibly vertebrobasilar insufficiency due to cervical spine degeneration
- Extrinsic factors (e.g., poor lighting) are almost certainly contributing.
- Vitamin D deficiency

Approach this problem by listing each contributing factor and identifying what can be done to improve it. For example:

| Contributing factor | Management |
| --- | --- |
| Osteoarthritis | Optimize analgesia |
| | Consider referral for hip joint replacement |
| | Physical and occupational therapy (provision of walking aids; strength and balance training) |
| Kyphosis | Consider bisphosphonate, and supplemental calcium and vitamin D to prevent progression |
| | Walking aids will improve balance |
| Low muscle mass | Take a dietary history |
| | Consider nutritional supplements combined with resistance exercise training |
| | Gait and balance training; encourage exercise |
| Bradycardia and postural drop | Consider stopping (or reducing) antihypertensives |
| | Monitor blood pressure |
| Environment | Occupational therapy review to |
| | Provide grab rails and shower chair |
| | Improve lighting and flooring |
| | De-clutter the home |

# Vertebrobasilar insufficiency

Vertebrobasilar insufficiency (VBI) is a collection of symptoms attributed to transient compromise of the vertebrobasilar circulation. There is often associated compromise of the anterior cerebral circulation.

## Symptoms

These arise from functional impairment of the midbrain, cerebellum, or occipital cortex and can include the following:
- Abrupt onset, recurrent dizziness, or vertigo
- Nausea and/or vomiting
- Ataxia
- Visual disruption (diplopia, nystagmus)
- Dysarthria
- Limb paresthesia

## Causes

Impairment of the posterior cerebral circulation leads to VBI:
- Atherosclerosis of the vertebral or basilar arteries
- Vertebral artery compression by cervical spine osteophytes (due to degenerative joint disease), at times triggered by neck movement
- Obstructing tumor

## Diagnosis

This is based mainly on the history, supported if necessary by investigations. Invasive tests such as angiography are very rarely indicated.
- Check for vascular risk factors.
- Cervical spine X-ray may show osteophytes, although these are common and very nonspecific.
- CT brain may demonstrate tumor or ischemic change. MRI is more sensitive for posterior circulation ischemic change.
- MR angiography may reveal occlusive vertebral artery disease.
- Doppler ultrasound may be used (rarely) to examine vertebral artery flow.

## Treatment

- Vascular secondary prevention measures
- Limiting neck movements, if these are a precipitant for symptoms, can be useful. Soft collars can be worn and act mainly as a reminder to the patient to avoid rapid head turns.
- There is no evidence that anticoagulants are effective.

**Box 5.1 "Drop attack"**

This term refers to unexplained falls with no prodrome, no (or very brief) loss of consciousness, and rapid recovery. The proportion of falls due to "drop attack" increases with age.

There are several causes:
- Cardiac arrhythmia
- Carotid sinus syndrome
- Orthostatic hypotension
- Vasovagal syndrome
- Vertebrobasilar insufficiency from atherosclerosis or compression by cervical spondylosis

The first four causes listed usually lead to syncope or presyncope, with identifiable prior symptoms (e.g., dizziness, pallor); those episodes would not be termed "drop attacks." However, such prior symptoms are not universal and may not be recollected, leading to a "drop attack" presentation.

In most cases, following appropriate assessment, cause(s) can be identified and effective treatment(s) begun.

Making a diagnosis of "drop attack" alone is not satisfactory. Assess more completely and, where possible, determine the likely underlying cause(s).

# Orthostatic (postural) hypotension

Orthostatic hypotension (OH) is common. About 20% of community-dwelling and 50% of institutionalized older people are affected.

- OH is an important, treatable cause of dizziness, syncope, near-syncope, immobility, falls, and fracture. Less frequently it leads to visual disruption, lethargy, neck- or backache, or dyspnea on exertion.
- OH is often most marked after meals, exercise, at night, and in a warm environment, and abruptly precipitated by increased intrathoracic pressure (cough, defecation, or micturition).
- It is often episodic (coincidence of precipitants) and covert (ask direct questions; walk or stand the patient and look for it). OH may occur several minutes after standing.
- Some older people with orthostasis are asymptomatic, but this may still increase their risk of falls.

## Diagnosis

Thresholds for diagnosis are arbitrary. A fall in BP of ≥20 mmHg systolic or 10 mmHg diastolic on standing from supine is said to be significant.

## Causes

- **Drugs:** vasodilators, diuretics, negative inotropes or chronotropes (e.g., beta-blockers, calcium channel blockers), antidepressants, antipsychotics, opiates, levodopa, alcohol
- **Chronic hypertension** (reduced baroreflex sensitivity and left ventricular [LV] compliance)
- **Volume depletion** (dehydration, acute hemorrhage)
- **Sepsis** (vasodilation)
- **Autonomic failure** (pure, diabetic, Parkinson's disease, etc.)
- **Prolonged bed rest**
- **Adrenal insufficiency**
- **Raised intrathoracic pressure** (bowel or bladder evacuation, cough)

## Treatment

- Treat the cause. Stop, reduce, or substitute drugs incrementally.
- Reduce consequences of falls (e.g., pendant alarms).
- Have patient modify behavior by standing slowly and step-wise, and lying down at prodrome.
- If patient is salt or water depleted (e.g., diuretics, diarrhea) supplement with
  - Na (liberal use of salt with meals)
  - Water (oral or IV fluid as isotonic dextrose or saline)
- Consider starting drugs if non-drug measures fail:
  - Alpha-1 agonists, e.g., midodrine (2.5 mg tid, titrated to maximum 40 mg/day); only FDA-approved drug for orthostatic hypotension
  - Fludrocortisone (0.1–0.2 mg/day)
  - Desmopressin 5–20 mcg at bedtime
- In all cases, monitor electrolytes and for heart failure and supine hypertension. Use caution if supine BP rises >180 mmHg systolic. Dependent edema alone is not a reason to stop treatment.

The following may help:
- Full-length compression stockings
- Head-up tilt to bed (decreases nocturnal natriuresis)
- Perform physical countermaneuvers such as crossing legs, stooping, squatting, and tensing muscles
- Avoid prolonged recumbency
- Minimize postprandial hypotension

### Postprandial hypotension
This is significant when associated with symptoms and fall in BP ≥20 mmHg within 75 minutes of meals. A modest fall is normal (usually asymptomatic) in older people. It is often more severe and symptomatic in hypertensive people with orthostatic hypotension or autonomic failure.

### Diagnosis
Measure BP before meals and at 30 and 60 minutes after a meal. Symptoms and causes overlap with OH.

### Treatment
- Avoid hypotensive drugs and alcohol with meals.
- Lie down or sit after meals.
- Reduce osmotic load of meals (small frequent meals, low simple carbohydrates, high fiber/water content).
- Caffeine before a meal is sometimes used.

### How to measure postural blood pressure

1. Lay the patient flat for ≥5 minutes.
2. Measure lying blood pressure with a manual sphygmomanometer.
3. Stand the patient upright rapidly, if necessary with assistance.
4. Check BP promptly (within 30 seconds of standing).
5. While the patient is standing, repeat BP measurement continually—at least every 30 seconds for >2 minutes.
6. Record
   - Supine BP
   - Nadir of systolic and diastolic BP
   - Symptoms

- **Lying-to-standing measurements** are more sensitive than sitting-to-standing or lying-to-sitting ones. The latter are sometimes all that is possible for less mobile patients, even with assistance.
- **Consider repeat assessment** at different times of day; orthostatic hypotension is more common after a meal and when the person is relatively fluid depleted (early morning).
- **Consider referral to a specialist** for prolonged upright head-up tilt table testing if symptoms suggest syncope or near-syncope after more prolonged standing.

### Further reading
Freeman R (2008). Neurogenic orthostatic hypotension. *N Engl J Med* **358**:615–624.

# Carotid sinus syndrome

Carotid sinus syndrome (CSS) is episodic, symptomatic bradycardia and/ or hypotension due to a hypersensitive carotid baroreceptor reflex, resulting in syncope or near-syncope. It is an important and potentially treatable cause of falls.

CSS is common in older patients and rarely occurs under age 50 years. Series report a prevalence of 2% in healthy older people and up to 35% of those over 80 who fall. It is a condition that has been identified recently, and not all physicians are convinced that we fully understand the normal responses of older people to carotid sinus massage or the significance of the spectrum of abnormal results.

Normally, in response to increased arterial blood pressure, baroreceptors in the carotid sinus act via the sympathetic nervous system to slow and weaken the pulse, lowering blood pressure. This reflex typically blunts with age, but in CSS it is exaggerated, probably centrally. This hypersensitivity is associated with increasing age, atheroma, and the use of drugs that affect the sinoatrial node (e.g., beta-blockers, digoxin, and calcium channel blockers).

Typical triggers include the following:
• Neck turning (looking up or around)
• Tight collars
• Straining (including cough, micturition, and defecation)
• Meals, i.e., postprandial
• Prolonged standing

Often, however, no trigger is identified.

There are three subtypes:
• **Cardioinhibitory** (sinus pause of >3 seconds)
• **Vasodepressor** (BP fall >50 mmHg)
• **Mixed** (both sinus pause and BP fall)

The diagnosis is made when all three of the following factors are present:
• Unexplained attributable symptoms
• A sinus pause of >3 seconds and/or systolic BP fall of >50 mmHg in response to 5 seconds of carotid sinus massage (see How to Perform Carotid Sinus Massage, next page)
• Symptoms are reproduced by carotid sinus massage.

CSS is often associated with other disorders (vasovagal syndrome and orthostatic hypotension), probably because of shared pathogenesis (autonomic dysfunction). This makes management more challenging.

## Treatment
• Stop aggravating drugs when possible.
• Pure cardioinhibitory carotid sinus hypersensitivity responds well to AV sequential pacing, resolving symptoms in up to 80%.
• Vasodepressor-related symptoms are harder to treat (pathogenesis is less well understood) but may respond to increasing circulating volume with fludrocortisone or midodrine, as for orthostatic hypotension.

## How to perform carotid sinus massage

1. Because this is a potentially hazardous procedure:
   • Perform it in conditions that optimize test sensitivity—e.g., on a tilt table, at a 70- to 80-degree tilt, massaging on the right-hand side.
   • Ensure that resuscitation facilities are available (full cardiac arrest trolley, another health professional close by, telephone).
2. Check for contraindications—do not perform after a recent MI (increased sensitivity), in cerebrovascular disease, or if there is a bruit present unless carotid Doppler is normal.
3. Advise the patient about possible side effects—arrhythmias (most common if taking digoxin) and neurological symptoms (usually transient, occurring in about 0.14% of tests).
4. The patient should be relaxed, with the head turned to the left, lying on a couch with the body resting at 45 degrees (or on a tilt table at 70–80 degrees).
5. Attach the patient to a cardiac monitor with printing facility (to provide documentary evidence of asystole). The fall in BP is usually too brief to be detected by conventional (sphygmomanometric) methods, but continuous ("beat-to-beat") BP monitoring (using, e.g., Portapres or Finapres devices) enables the detection of pure vasodepressor CSS.
6. Identify the carotid sinus—the point of maximal carotid pulsation in the neck.
7. Massage with steady pressure in a circular motion for 5–10 seconds.
8. Look for asystole and/or hypotension during massage or shortly (seconds) afterwards.
9. If clinical suspicion is high, and the result of right-sided massage is negative, repeat on the left side (do not do this routinely).

# Pharmacology and medication use

**Lynsey Brandt**

# Drugs and older patients

The most common intervention performed by physicians is to write a prescription. Older patients have more conditions requiring medication, and polypharmacy is common.

In the developed world:
- Patients over age 65 typically make up around 13% of the U.S. population yet purchase 33% of all prescription drugs.
- 66% of patients over 65 and 87% of patients over 75 are on regular medication.
- 34% of patients over 75 are on three or more drugs.
- Nursing home patients are on an average of eight medications.

*Polypharmacy* is a term indicating the use of multiple medications. The exact number of medications that constitutes polypharmacy is variable, ranging from 3 to 5 in some studies, to 9 or greater medications as determined by the Centers for Medicare & Medicaid Services.
- Risk factors for polypharmacy include increased age, white race, use of multiple physicians and pharmacies, and declining health status.
- Consequences of polypharmacy include increased risk of medication nonadherence, adverse drug reactions, drug interactions, geriatric syndromes (falls, urinary incontinence, cognitive impairment), and increased health-care costs.

Good prescribing habits are essential for any medical practitioner. This is especially true when prescribing for older adults.

# Rules of prescribing

## 1. Is it indicated?

*Treatment of new symptom*

Some symptoms seem to trigger a reflex prescription (e.g., constipation—laxatives; dizziness—meclizine). However, before starting a medication, consider the following:

• What is the diagnosis? (e.g., dizziness due to postural BP drop?)
• Can something be stopped? (e.g., opioid analgesia causing constipation)
• Are there any non-drug measures? (e.g., increase fiber for constipation)

*Optimizing disease management*

For example, a diagnosis of cardiac failure triggers consideration of loop diuretics, spironolactone, angiotensin-converting enzyme (ACE) inhibitors, and beta-blockers.

• Ensure the diagnosis is correct before committing the patient to multiple drugs (this may be difficult where there is no clear diagnostic gold standard, e.g., with TIAs).
• Do not deny older patients disease-modifying treatments simply to avoid polypharmacy.
• Do not deny treatment because of potential side effects. While these may affect functional ability or cause significant morbidity (e.g., low blood pressure with beta-blockade in cardiac failure) and need to be discontinued, this should usually occur after a trial of treatment with careful monitoring if the potential benefit of the medication outweighs the risk.
• Conversely, do not start treatment to improve mortality from a disease if the patient has limited life span for other reasons (e.g., cholesterol medication in a patient with advanced dementia).

*Preventative medication*

For example, glycemic control and cholesterol lowering.

• There is a limited evidence base in older patients—be guided by comorbidities and estimated life expectancy.
• Ensure the patient understands the rationale for treatment.

## 2. Are there any contraindications?

• Review past medical history (drug–disease interactions are common).
• Contraindications are often relative so a trial of treatment may be indicated, but warn the patient, document risk, and review the impact e.g., of ACE inhibitors, when there is renal impairment.

## 3. Are there any likely interactions?

• Review the medication list.
• Ask about over-the-counter (OTC) and herbal medication use.
• Computer prescribing assists with drug–drug interactions, automatically flagging potential problems.

### 4. What is the best drug?

Choose the broad category of drug (e.g., which antihypertensive) by considering which one will work best in this patient (e.g., ACE inhibitors work less well in African Americans), which is least likely to cause side effects (e.g., calcium channel blockers may worsen lower extremity edema), and if there is any potential for dual action? (E.g., a patient with angina could have a beta-blocker for both angina and blood pressure control.)

Within each category of medication there are many choices:

- Develop a personal portfolio of drugs with which you are very familiar.
- Hospital formularies will often dictate choices for inpatients.
- Cost should be a consideration; use generic drugs when possible.
- Pharmaceutical companies may advertise the benefits of a new brand-name medication. Unless this is a novel class of drug, it is likely that existing medications have a greater proven safety record with similar benefit. Older patients have greater potential to suffer harm from new drugs and are unlikely to have been included in clinical trials. Time will tell if there are real advantages; in general, it is best to avoid new agents until clear therapeutic advantage and safety are established.
- Avoid being the first, or last, of your peers to use a new drug.

### 5. What dose should be started?

- "Start low and go slow."
- Drugs are usually better tolerated at lower doses and can be increased if there are no adverse reactions.
- In most cases, benefit is seen with drug initiation, and further increments of benefit occur with dose optimization (e.g., ACE inhibitors for cardiac failure, where 1.25 mg ramipril is better than 10 mg with a postural drop in blood pressure).
- However, do not under-treat—use enough to achieve the therapeutic goal (e.g., beta-blockers for angina).

### 6. How will the impact be assessed?

Schedule follow-up, looking for the following:

- Efficacy of the drug (e.g., has the bradykinesia improved with a dopamine agonist?) Medication for less objective conditions (e.g., pain, cognition) requires the setting of clear therapeutic goals and careful questioning of the patient and family or caregivers. In some cases, monitor blood tests to assess efficacy (e.g., lipid panel on statin).
- Any adverse events, reported by the patient spontaneously, elicited by direct questioning (e.g., headache with dipyridamole), or checked by blood tests where necessary (e.g., thyroid function on amiodarone)
- Side effects can be subtle and easily missed. For example, decreased appetite or alertness in a patient with dementia may have many potential causes. Even seemingly innocuous medications such as aspirin or iron may affect appetite, and a previously effective antidepressant may dampen alertness. A trial off the medication and careful reassessment are often worthwhile.
- Any capacity to increase the dose to improve the effect (e.g., ACE inhibitors in cardiac failure).

## 7. What is the time frame?

Many older patients remain on medication for a long time; 88% of all prescriptions in patients over age 65 are chronic. Sixty percent of prescriptions are active for over 2 years, 30% over 5 years, and 6% over 10 years. This may be appropriate (e.g., with antihypertensives) and, if so, the patient should be aware of this and continue to refill the prescription.

Some drugs should not be prescribed long term, e.g., meclizine, which causes sedation.

Medication should be regularly reviewed and discontinued if ineffective or no longer indicated, e.g., some psychotropic medications (e.g., lithium, antidepressants, antipsychotics) were intended for long-term use at initiation, but the patient may have had no psychiatric symptoms for years (or even decades). They can contribute to falls, and cautious withdrawal may be indicated.

Some medications prescribed for older adults should be considered for eventual discontinuation rather than long-term use. Special attention should be given to the following agents:

- Acetylcholinesterase inhibitors (e.g., donepezil) may have limited clinical effect with long-term use.
- Antipsychotic medications (e.g., quetiapine) are often initiated for an acute behavioral disturbance that subsides. You should attempt to gradually decrease the dose.
- Proton pump inhibitors: long-term use is associated with pneumonia, *Clostridium difficile* infections, and hip fractures.
- Urinary antispasmodics (i.e., oxybutynin) have limited efficacy and many anticholinergic side effects.

# Pharmacology in older patients

### Administration challenges

- Packaging may make tablets hard to access—childproof bottles and tablets in blister packets can be difficult to open with arthritic hands or poor vision.
- Labels may be too small to read with visual impairment.
- Tablets may be large and difficult to swallow or have an unpleasant taste (e.g., potassium supplements).
- Liquid formulations can be useful, but accurate dosage becomes harder to maintain (especially where manual dexterity is compromised).
- Any tablet needs around 60 mL of water to wash it down and prevent adherence to the esophageal mucosa, which is a large volume for some patients. Other tablets (e.g., bisphosphonates) require even larger volumes.
- Regimens of multiple tablets with different instructions (e.g., before or after food) are confusing and may be taken in a suboptimal way.
- Some routes (e.g., topical to back) may be impossible without assistance.
- Pharmacists with experience compounding medications can sometimes reformulate prescriptions in forms that are easier to take (e.g., it may be possible to create a suspension that is more easily swallowed than a large tablet).

### Absorption

Many factors are different in older patients (increased gastric pH, delayed gastric emptying, reduced intestinal motility and blood flow). Despite this, absorption of drugs is largely unchanged with age. Exceptions include iron and calcium, which are absorbed more slowly.

Enteral feedings alter absorption of some medications (e.g., phenytoin).

### Distribution

Some older people have a very low lean body mass, so if the therapeutic index for a drug is narrow (e.g., digoxin) the dose should be adjusted.

There is often an increased proportion of body fat compared with that of water. This reduces the volume of distribution for water-soluble drugs, giving a higher initial concentration (e.g., digoxin). It also leads to accumulation of fat-soluble drugs, prolonging elimination and effect (e.g., lidocaine, diazepam).

There is reduced plasma protein binding of drugs with age, which increases the free fraction of protein-bound drugs such as warfarin and furosemide.

### Hepatic metabolism

Specific hepatic metabolic pathways (e.g., conjugation) are unaffected by age. Reduced hepatic mass and blood flow (e.g., right-sided congestive heart failure) can affect overall function, which slows metabolism of drugs (e.g., theophylline, acetaminophen, diazepam, nifedipine).

Drugs that undergo extensive first-pass metabolism (e.g., propranolol, nitrates) are most affected by the reduced hepatic function.

Many factors interact with liver metabolism (e.g., nutritional state, acute illness, smoking, other medications).

Patients with congestive heart failure can develop hepatic congestion, which leads to impaired hepatic metabolism of some drugs.

## Renal excretion

Renal function declines with age (glomerular filtration rate [GFR], tubular excretion—see Chapter 13, Nephrology), which has a profound impact on the elimination of drugs that are predominantly handled renally. Renal mass declines by 20%–25% from age 30 to 80. GFR, measured by creatinine clearance, decreases by approximately 10% per decade of life after age 30.

When assessing renal function in elderly individuals, do not be misled by a normal serum creatinine. Because of low muscle mass with resultant decreased production of creatinine, an elderly patient with normal serum creatinine may have severe renal dysfunction.

Estimate creatinine clearance (see Chapter 13, How to estimate the glomerular filtration rate, p. 403). In general, when creatinine clearance is <60 mL/min, dose adjustment is necessary.

Drugs, or drugs with active metabolites, that are mainly excreted by the kidney include allopurinol, digoxin, furosemide, gabapentin, gentamicin, lithium, metformin, ranitidine, and tetracyclines.

Where there is a narrow therapeutic index (e.g., digoxin, aminoglycosides), then dose adjustment for renal impairment is required. Impaired renal function is exacerbated by dehydration and urosepsis, both common in older patients.

# Drug sensitivity

Many older patients will have altered sensitivity to some drugs (see Box 6.1), for example:
- Receptor responses may vary with age. Alterations in the function of the cellular sodium/potassium pumps may account for the increased sensitivity to digoxin seen in older people. Decreased beta adrenoceptor sensitivity means that older patients mount less of a tachycardia when given agonists (e.g., albuterol) and may become less bradycardic with beta-blockers.
- Altered coagulation factor synthesis with age leads to an increased sensitivity to the effects of warfarin.
- The aging central nervous system shows increased susceptibility to the effects of many centrally acting drugs (e.g., hypnotics, sedatives, antidepressants, opioid analgesia, antiparkinsonian drugs, and antipsychotics).

Certain adverse reactions are more likely in older people. Because of this altered sensitivity:
- Baroreceptor responses are less sensitive, making symptomatic hypotension more likely with antihypertensives.
- Thirst responses are blunted, making hypovolemia due to diuretics more common.
- Thermoregulation is blunted, making hypothermia more likely with prolonged sedation.
- Allergic responses to drugs are more common because of altered immune responses.

---

### Box 6.1 **Drugs requiring possible dose alteration**

Despite variations in drug handling, most drugs have a wide therapeutic index and there is no clinical impact. Only for drugs with a narrow therapeutic index or for older patients who show very marked increased sensitivity may dose alteration be required:
- ACE inhibitors (p. 122)
- Aminoglycosides (dose determined by weight, and reduced if impaired renal function)
- Benzodiazepines (start with low dose, e.g., 0.25 mg lorazepam)
- Digoxin (older patients with low body weight rarely require more than 62.5 mcg maintenance dose [see p. 288]).
- H2 antagonists
- Nonsteroidal anti-inflammatory drugs (see p. 126).
- Opiates (start with 1–2 mg morphine to assess impact on the central nervous system [CNS])
- Oral hypoglycemics (increased sensitivity to hypoglycemia with decreased awareness—avoid long-acting preparations such as glyburide, and start with lower doses of shorter-acting drugs (e.g., glipizide 2.5 mg)
- Warfarin (load more cautiously—see p. 132).

# Taking a drug history

An accurate drug history includes the name, dose, timing, duration, and reason for all medication (see Table 6.1). Studies have suggested that patients will report their drug history accurately around half of the time, and this figure falls with increasing age.

### Reasons for problems arising
- Inadequate information to the patient at the time of prescribing
- Multiple medications
- Multiple changes if side effects develop
- Use of both generic and brand name drugs
- Variable doses over time (e.g., dopamine agonists, ACE inhibitors)
- Cognitive and visual impairment
- Over-the-counter drugs

### Useful sources of information
- The patient's actual drugs—ask the patient to bring the medications in a bag to outpatient appointments or when admitted.
- Many seasoned patients will carry a list of their current medication, written either by them or a health-care professional.
- Computer-generated printouts of current medication from the primary care provider or pharmacy
- A telephone call to the primary care provider
- Family members or caregivers will often know about medication, especially if they help administer them.
- Medical notes will often contain a list of medications at the last hospital admission.

These can be extremely useful, but they have limitations. A prescription issued does not mean that it was necessarily dispensed or that the medication is being taken correctly and consistently. Previously prescribed medications may still be taken and patients may occasionally use someone else's medication (e.g., a spouse).

### Good habits
- Every time a patient is seen (in the clinic, day hospital, admission) take time to review the medications and make an up-to-date list.
- Include a list of current medications with each correspondence.
- If changes are made, or a new medication is tried and not tolerated, document the reason for this and communicate this to all people involved in care (especially the primary care physician).
- Always include allergies and intolerances in the drug history.

### Solutions
1. Take the drug history with meticulous care—ask directly about the following:
- Inhalers. Ask the patient to describe and/or demonstrate how he or she uses the medicine.
- Topical medication (creams, eye drops, patches, etc.).

- Medications used occasionally or "as needed"
- Intermittent-use medication (e.g., monthly $B_{12}$ injections, depot antipsychotics, weekly bisphosphonates. etc.)
- Over-the-counter medication (a growing number of drugs are available this way, including proton pump inhibitors and nonsedating antihistamines)
- Herbal and traditional remedies

2. Clarify how often occasional-use medication is taken—analgesia may be used very regularly, or not at all.

3. Be nonjudgmental. If you suspect poor adherence to medications (e.g., persistent hypertension despite multiple prescriptions), the following questions can be useful to elicit an accurate response:
- Most of us miss taking medication sometimes. Can you tell me when you might miss your medications?
- Which tablets do you find useful?
- Do any of the tablets disagree with you?—if yes, then, How often do you manage to take it?
- What triggers you to remember? (e.g., take with each meal, leave by toothbrush).

4. Scrutinize computer-generated lists carefully. Remember to look at when the prescription was last issued and estimate when they would be due to run out (e.g., 28 tablets to be taken once a day, last issued 3 months ago means that the drug has either run out or not been taken regularly). You may also obtain refill information by contacting the patient's pharmacist.

5. The gold standard is to ask the patient to bring in all of the medications that they have at home—both old and new. Go through each medication and ask them to explain which ones they take, and how often. This practice allows for the following:
- Comparison with a list of medications that they are supposed to be taking
- Old drugs can be discarded (if necessary retain them and discard).
- An estimate of adherence (by looking at the date of dispensing and number of tablets left)
- Clarification of doses, timings, and rationale for treatment. If time permits, it is useful to generate a list for the patient to carry with them (see p. 537 for example).
- Education of the patient and family, where needed (e.g., reason for taking a particular medication)

## How to improve adherence

### Simplify prescription regimens

- Convert to once-a-day dosing, where possible (e.g., change captopril three times daily to ramipril once daily).
- Try to prescribe medications to be taken at the same time of day—this may challenge firmly held views (e.g., warfarin must be taken at night).
- Try to use medications that have dual indications for the patient (e.g., beta blockade for both hypertension and angina).
- Optimize the dose of one medication before switching to or adding another agent.
- Consider a daily-dose reminder system (e.g., pill box) or a monitored dosage system.

### Educate the patient and family

- Do they understand the reason for taking the medication and how to take it correctly? Are there any problems the patient is attributing to the medication (perhaps incorrectly)?
- Medication summaries (see Table 6.1) can assist with this.
- Warn of predictable side effects that are likely to pass (e.g., nausea with citalopram, headache with dipyridamole).
- Promote personal responsibility for medication.
- Enlist support of the family and caregivers in monitoring adherence.

### Monitor

- Check pill boxes and see if meds are being taken.
- Look at how often a refill prescription has been requested.
- Monitor serum drug levels when indicated (e.g., digoxin, phenytoin, and lithium).

Some medications will produce changes detectable at physical examination (e.g., bradycardia with beta-blockade, black stool with iron therapy).

**Table 6.1** Example of a patient drug summary sheet

| Medication | Brand name | Reason | Dose | Morning | Lunch | Evening | Duration |
|---|---|---|---|---|---|---|---|
| Aspirin | | Thins blood, prevents heart attack | 81 mg | X | | | Lifelong |
| Simvastatin | Zocor | Lowers cholesterol, prevents heart attack | 40 mg | | | X | Lifelong |
| Ramipril | Altace | Lowers blood pressure, prevents heart attack | 5 mg | | | X | Lifelong |
| Atenolol | Tenormin | Lowers blood pressure, prevents angina attacks | 50 mg | X | | | Lifelong |
| Isosorbide mononitrate | Ismo | Prevents angina attacks | 20 mg | X | X | | Lifelong |
| NTG spray | | Treats angina | 1 puff | | | | As needed |
| Amoxicillin | Amoxil | Antibiotic for chest infection | 500 mg | X | X | X | 7 days |

# Adverse drug reactions

These are more common and complex with increasing age—up to 3 times more frequent in patients over 80. Drug reactions account for considerable morbidity, mortality, and hospital admissions (one study estimated a quarter of U.S. hospital admissions relate to medication complications).

Older people are not a homogeneous group, and many will tolerate medications as well as younger people, but a number of factors contribute to the increased frequency:

- **Altered drug handling and sensitivity** occur with age, made worse by poor appetite, nutrition, and fluid intake.
- Frailty and multiple diseases make **drug–disease interactions** more common, for example:
  - Anticholinergics may precipitate urinary retention in a patient with prostatic hypertrophy.
  - Benzodiazepines may precipitate delirium in patients with dementia.

Also, the likelihood of **drug–drug interactions** increases with the large numbers of drugs prescribed for multiple conditions in older adults (see Box 6.2). Mechanisms for drug interactions include the following:

- *Pharmacodynamic:* When there are additive or opposing effects of drugs. For example, an osteoporotic patient is prescribed a bisphosphonate, then sustains a vertebral crush fracture and is given a nonsteroidal drug that exacerbates gastric irritation and causes a gastrointestinal bleed (additive toxicity), or a nonsteroidal agent is given, leading to sodium retention, counteracting the effect of the diuretic in a patient with congestive heart failure (opposing effects).
- *Pharmacokinetic:* When one drug alters the absorption, distribution, metabolism, or excretion of another drug. This occurs most commonly with drugs that are substrates, inducers, or inhibitors of the cytochrome P450 enzyme system.
- *Plasma protein binding:* When two drugs are highly protein bound, they may displace each other from binding sites, leading to an increased free (active) fraction of drug (e.g., amiodarone, warfarin).

---

### Box 6.2 Medications with frequent drug interactions in older adults

- Amiodarone
- Antifungals (azole)
- Digoxin
- Fluoroquinolones
- Phenytoin
- Selective serotonin reuptake inhibitors (SSRIs)
- Warfarin

Grapefruit juice has also been shown to affect the metabolism of many drugs, due to inhibition of intestinal and hepatic enzymes. Drugs that interact with grapefruit juice include calcium channel blockers, HMG-CoA reductase inhibitors (statins), antiarrhythmics, benzodiazepines, and others.

**Errors in drug taking** make adverse reactions more likely. Mistakes increase with the following:

- Increasing age (controversial)
- Increasing numbers of prescribed drugs (20% of patients taking 3 drugs will make errors, rising to 95% when 10 or more drugs are taken)
- Cognitive impairment
- Living alone

## Strategies to minimize adverse drug reactions

- Prescribe sensibly—see pp. 526–528.
- Consider possible drug–drug and drug–disease interactions whenever a new drug is started. Consult the pharmacist or drug-interaction software when prescribing new agents, especially those known to have frequent interactions.
- For every new problem, consider if an existing medication could be the cause. Try to avoid the so-called prescribing cascade where side effects are treated with a new prescription, rather than discontinuing the offending drug. If multiple medications are possible culprits, then stop one at a time and watch for improvement.
- Optimize adherence (see pp. 536–537).
- Minimize the number of prescribers and encourage the patient to use one pharmacy.
- Use extreme caution at times of care transitions. Studies have shown that transitions of care frequently lead to medication errors. Communication between providers, provision of accurate medication lists, and review of all medications at time of "hand-off" should be performed to ensure an optimal transition.

# Inappropriate medications in older adults

In 1991, Beers and colleagues surveyed expert clinical geriatricians and published an article on medications that are inappropriate in older adults. This led to eventual development of the "Beers List" of inappropriate medications in older adults.

Use of medications on the Beers List may increase the risk of morbidity and mortality. It should be used as a guide when selecting agents for older patients. Note that some patients may be able to tolerate medications on this list. It is important to consider each individual patient when prescribing medications.

An excerpt from the Beers List is given below. For the complete list, refer to Fick et al.[1]

It is important to recognize that medication not on the Beers List present significant risk in older patients. In one study, warfarin, digoxin, and insulin were associated with 33% of emergency department visits related to adverse medication reactions, whereas drugs on the Beers List accounted for 3.6% of visits.

### Beers list of inappropriate medications in the elderly (excerpt)

| Medication class | Rationale for inappropriateness |
|---|---|
| Amphetamines | Hypertension, angina, dependence |
| Antihistamines | Anticholinergic side effects |
| Benzodiazepines | Sedation, risk of falls |
| Muscle relaxants | Anticholinergic, sedation, weakness |
| Tricyclic antidepressants | Sedation, anticholinergic effects |

1. Fick et al. (2003) Updating the Beers criteria for potentially inappropriate medication use in older adults. *Arch Intern Med* **163**:2716–2724.

## How to manage drug-induced skin rashes

Skin rash is a common side effect in older patients. It is thought to be due to altered immune function. It is rarely life threatening, but it can cause considerable distress.

### Make the diagnosis

- Variable in appearance, but most commonly toxic erythema—symmetrical, erythematous, itchy rash, trunk > extremities, lesions may be measles-like, urticarial, or resemble erythema multiforme
- Certain drugs may produce predictable eruptions:
  - Acneiform rash with lithium
  - Bullous lesions with furosemide
  - Target lesions with penicillins and phenytoin
  - Psoriasis-like rash with beta-blockers
  - Urticaria with penicillin, opiates, and aspirin
  - Fixed drug eruption (round, purple plaques recurring in the same spot) with acetaminophen, laxatives, sulfonamides, and tetracyclines
- Toxic epidermal necrolysis is a rare, serious reaction to drugs such as nonsteroidals, allopurinol, and phenytoin. The skin appears scalded. Large areas of epidermis may shear off, causing problems with fluid and electrolyte balance, thermoregulation, and infection.
- Take a careful drug history to elicit a temporal relationship to medication administration—e.g., within 3 days of starting a new drug (may be as long as 3 weeks), or if rash is becoming worse every morning after a regular drug is given.

### Stop the drug

- Stop multiple medications one at a time (stop drugs started closest to the onset of the rash first), and watch for clinical improvement.
- Symptoms may get slightly worse before improving.
- The rash usually clears within 2 weeks.
- Advise the patient to avoid the drug in the future.

### Soothe the skin

- Emollients, cooling agents like calamine and topical steroids help.
- Oral antihistamines are often given with variable success. Sedating antihistamines (e.g., hydroxyzine 25 mg) may help sleep. Use only with caution in older patients because of risk of delirium and falls.

### Treat the complications

These are more likely if extensive and prolonged. Risks include the following:
- Hypothermia
- Hypovolemia
- Secondary infection

>>Consider dermatology referral if patient is not improving after 2 weeks off the suspected drug.

From Budnitz DS, Shehab N, Kegler SR, Richards CL (2007). Medication use leading to emergency department visits for adverse drug events in older adults. *Ann Intern Med* **147**(11):755–765.

# ACE inhibitors

Common indications include blood pressure control, vascular risk reduction, heart failure, and diabetic nephropathy.

## Cautions

### Renal disease

- Use ACE inhibitors with extreme caution if there is a known history of renal artery stenosis, as renal failure can be precipitated. If clinical suspicion of this is high (renal bruit, uncontrolled hypertension that is unexplained), consider investigating for renal asymmetry with an ultrasound before starting treatment.
- Renal impairment per se is not a reason to withhold ACE inhibitors (indeed, they are effective treatment for some types), although the dose may need to be reduced.
- Monitor renal function before and after treatment (see How to Start ACE Inhibitors, next page). Sudden deterioration may indicate renal artery stenosis and the ACE should be stopped pending investigation.
- In the setting of acute illness (dehydration, sepsis, etc.), temporary withdrawal of the ACE inhibitor may be needed (see How to Start ACE Inhibitors, next page).

### Hypotension

- Early ACE inhibitors (e.g., Captopril) were associated with a risk of first-dose hypotension so many patients were given an in-hospital test dose.
- This is rare with newer ACE inhibitors, and cautious outpatient initiation is acceptable (see How to Start ACE Inhibitors, next page).
- Older patients are more prone to postural hypotension. Check blood pressure lying and standing, and ask about postural symptoms (e.g., light-headedness).
- The risk of hypotension is greater with volume-depleted patients— e.g., those on high-dose diuretics, on renal dialysis, dehydrated from intercurrent illness, or in severe cardiac failure. Correct dehydration before initiation where possible.
- ACE-induced hypotension is common in patients with severe aortic stenosis, so ACE inhibitors should probably be avoided (unless under cardiology supervision).
- Start low, and go slow. Monitor carefully. This approach may take multiple clinic visits, but avoids complications.

### Cough

- Many ACE inhibitors cause a persistent dry cough. Always warn the patient about this, as it can cause considerable distress. Forewarned is forearmed, and many patients will be prepared to accept this side effect if the ACE inhibitor is the best choice for them.
- Changing to an angiotensin receptor blocker (ARB) removes the cough in most cases, but there is greater evidence supporting ACE inhibitors for reduction of cardiovascular risk.

- There is a risk of hyperkalemia when ACE inhibitors are used with potassium-sparing diuretics, e.g., spironolactone (in heart failure), or with nonsteroidal agents.
- Be aware, and monitor electrolytes. Most patients tolerate a potassium level of up to 5.5 mmol/L.
- The tendency toward hyperkalemia can be useful in patients who are also on potassium-losing diuretics (e.g., furosemide) as the two may balance each other out.

## How to start ACE inhibitors

- Screen for contraindications (see p. 122).
- Check baseline renal function and electrolytes.
- Warn patient about possible cough and postural symptoms.

### An example of initiation and titration

*Week 1*
- Start ramipril 1.25 mg at night.

*Week 2*
- Check renal function and blood pressure (lying and standing) and check for postural symptoms.

*Week 4*
- Increase ramipril to 2.5 mg at night.

*Week 6*
- Check renal function and blood pressure (lying and standing) and check for postural symptoms.

*Week 8*
- Increase ramipril to 5 mg at night.

Continue titrating the dose upward as tolerated, but most older patients will develop postural symptoms at higher doses, increasing the risk of falls. The goal should be for safe optimization.

Once established on an ACE inhibitor, periodic renal monitoring is sensible (perhaps every 6 months).

## If a patient becomes acutely ill

- Dehydration increases susceptibility to ACE-induced renal failure and hypotension.
- Correct the dehydration first—treat cause, give fluid supplementation, and stop diuretics.
- Temporary cessation of ACE inhibitor may be needed if dehydration is prolonged (>24 hours).
- Monitor renal function daily.
- Remember to restart the ACE inhibitor after recovery.

# Amiodarone

Indications include rate control and prevention of supraventricular cardiac arrhythmias (commonly atrial fibrillation) and prevention of paroxysmal ventricular arrhythmias.

Intravenous amiodarone is included on the Advanced Cardiac Life Support protocols (ACLS) for cardiac arrest.[1]

## Cautions

- Interacts with many drugs, including warfarin, which is often co-prescribed for atrial fibrillation stroke prophylaxis. A steady state will be reached if both drugs are taken regularly, but careful INR monitoring is needed with initiation.
- Can cause abnormal thyroid function tests in either direction. Baseline thyroid function should be taken before initiation and then at 6-month intervals. Measure thyroid-stimulating hormone (TSH), free T4, and free T3.
- Photosensitivity can occur, so amiodarone is unlikely to be suitable for avid gardeners or outdoor workers.
- Corneal microdeposits often occur that can cause a glare with night driving. If this is likely to be a problem, avoid the medication. These are reversible.
- Liver function can become abnormal—check at baseline and every 6 months.
- Pulmonary problems may occur (fibrosis, alveolitis, and pneumonitis) and any new respiratory symptoms on treatment should trigger a chest X-ray.
- Peripheral neuropathy may occur—be alert for early signs of this and stop the drug promptly to avoid progression.
- For dosing recommendations, refer to product literature or other suitable drug reference.

1. 2005 American Heart Association Guidelines for Cardiopulmonary Resuscitation and Emergency Cardiovascular Care. *Circulation* 2005; **112**(24, Suppl).

# Analgesia in older patients

Older patients are more likely to suffer chronic pain than are younger ones, owing to the increased frequency of conditions such as osteoarthritis, osteoporosis, etc.

Pain management is more challenging, and a standard "pain ladder" approach is not always useful because of the altered sensitivity of the older patient to certain classes of analgesic medication. Furthermore, inadequate analgesia has been shown to be a risk factor for development of delirium in older adults.

## Nonsteroidal anti-inflammatory drugs (NSAIDs)

These include aspirin (especially at analgesic doses).

*Potential problems*

- Fluid retention causing worsening hypertension, cardiac failure, and ankle swelling.
- Renal toxicity—there is a risk of acute tubular necrosis, exacerbated by intercurrent infection or dehydration.
- Peptic ulceration and gastrointestinal bleeding—there is a greater risk with increased age, and the bleeds tend to be more significant.
- Age itself is probably not an independent risk factor for most complications of NSAID treatment, but factors such as comorbidities, co-medications, hydration, nutritional status, and frailty are linked to an increased risk, all of which are more common with advancing age.

*Guidance for use in older patients*

- NSAIDs should be used with extreme caution in older patients and avoided altogether in the very frail.
- They should be given for a short period only.
- Use low-dose, moderate-potency NSAIDs (e.g., ibuprofen 1.2 g daily).
- Never use two NSAIDs together.
- Consider short-term prescription of a gastric-protective agent (e.g., omeprazole) for the duration of the therapy.
- Avoid using ACE inhibitors and NSAIDs together. They have opposing effects on fluid handling and are likely to cause renal toxicity in combination.

## Opioid analgesia

These constitute a wide range of drugs sharing many common features, but with qualitative and quantitative differences.

*Potential problems* include constipation, nausea and vomiting, confusion, drowsiness, respiratory depression, and falls.

*Guidance for use in older patients*

- Most of these are dose dependant, and careful up-titration will obtain the right balance of analgesic effect and adverse effects.
- Constipation is common (worse in older people) but can be managed with good bowel regimen (see Chapter 12, Constipation, p. 380).
- Most adverse effects are reversible once the medication is reduced or discontinued.

## How to manage pain in older patients

*Diagnose the cause*
Chronic abdominal pain may be due to constipation that will respond to bowel care rather than analgesia.

*Consider non-drug measures*
- Weight loss and physical activity help with many pains (e.g., arthritis).
- Temperature treatments (e.g., hot/cold packs applied to painful joint)
- TENS units
- Alternative therapies (e.g. acupuncture, aromatherapy) can help.
- Complementary medicine is sought by many patients. A tolerant and supportive perspective by the physician can enhance pain treatment.
- Avoidance of (nonessential) activity that provokes pain if possible
- Consider consultation with a physical medicine specialist to optimize physical function while avoiding painful activity.
- For additional formation, see the American Geriatrics Society pain guideline: AGS Panel on Persistent Pain in Older Persons (2002). The management of persistent pain in older persons. *J Am Geriatr Soc* **50**:S205–S224.

*Consider targeted therapy*
For example, consider topical capsaicin for post-herpetic neuralgia, local nerve blocks for regional pain, massage for musculoskeletal pain, joint replacement for arthritic pain, or radiotherapy for pain from bony metastases.

*Regular acetaminophen*
- Well tolerated and with few side effects
- Before moving from this, ensure that the maximum dose is being taken regularly (i.e., 1 g taken four times a day) for optimal analgesic effect. Many patients will find taking an occasional acetaminophen ineffective. Explain that regular dosing increases analgesic effect.

*Opioid analgesia*
- Second-line therapy in older patients
- Options to deal with mild to moderate (e.g., codeine) and severe pain (e.g. morphine, oxycodone, fentanyl).
- Compound preparations are useful when adding an opioid to regular acetaminophen as it limits the number of tablets taken. For example, Tylenol with codeine (codeine and acetaminophen) has variable doses of codeine (15 mg, 30 mg, or 60 mg per tablet), allowing up-titration of the opioid component. Patients using these products must be counseled not to exceed the maximal daily dose of acetaminophen.
- All opioids affect the same receptors, so use as a continuum. If regular maximum-dose codeine is not working, step up to the next level of opioid strength (e.g., oxycodone 2.5 mg or morphine 5 mg).

**How to manage pain in older patients (cont'd.)**

- Remember to consider equianalgesic dosing when converting from one opioid to another. Consult a reference, such as http://www.globalrph.com/narcoticonv.htm, to calculate appropriate doses.
- Various formulations for the delivery of strong opiates. Liquids are useful if swallowing is a problem (e.g., morphine sulfate oral solution). Slow-release tablets (e.g., morphine sulfate extended release) and transdermal patches (e.g., fentanyl) provide constant analgesic effect for continuous pain. Parenteral opiates are used in terminal care (subcutaneous injections of morphine for intermittent pain; 24-hour infusion pumps for constant pain).
- Monitor for side effects—prescribe bowel regimen with initiation.

*Other drug options*

- Some older patients without contraindications can be given short courses of NSAIDs.
- COX-II inhibitors have a limited role given emerging data on thrombotic complications.

*Psychological factors*

- Depression is often coexistent (consequent or causal). Treatment can help with overall pain management.
- Positive mental attitude and learning to live with a degree of discomfort may be preferable to side effects of analgesic medication.

# Steroids

Oral steroids (usually prednisone) are given for many conditions in older patients, commonly chronic obstructive pulmonary disease (COPD) exacerbations, polymyalgia rheumatica, rheumatoid arthritis, and colitis. Treatment may be long term, and although the benefits of treatment usually outweigh the risks, awareness of these can often minimize harm.

## Cautions

- Osteoporosis is most marked in the early stages of treatment. Older people have diminishing bone reserves, and there is a strong argument for putting all steroid-treated older patients on bone protection at the outset, unless the course is certain to be very short (<2 weeks). This should consist of daily calcium and vitamin D, and possibly a bisphosphonate (weekly preparations, e.g., alendronate 35–70 mg, improve adherence).
- Steroids can precipitate **impaired glucose tolerance** or **frank diabetes**. Monitor sugar levels periodically (perhaps weekly finger-stick blood glucose) in all steroid users. They will also worsen the sugar control in known diabetics, necessitating more frequent monitoring.
- **Hypertension** may develop because of the mineralocorticoid effect of prednisone; this should be monitored regularly.
- **Skin changes** occur and are particularly noticeable in older patients with less resilient skin. Purpura, bruising, thinning, and increased fragility are common.
- **Muscle weakness** occurs with prolonged use, particularly in proximal distribution. This leads to problems rising from chairs, climbing stairs, etc. and may result in functional decline for a frail older person with limited physical reserve.
- There is an **increased susceptibility to infections** on steroids, and the presentation may be less acute, making diagnosis harder. Candidiasis (oral and genital) is particularly common and should be treated promptly (see p. 640).
- High doses (as used in treatment of giant cell arteritis) can cause **acute confusional states**, and older people are particularly at risk. As treatment is often initiated as an outpatient, be sure to warn the patient and caregivers about this.
- **Cataracts** may develop with long-term steroid use. If vision declines, refer to an ophthalmologist.
- **Peritonitis may be masked** by steroid use—the signs are less evident clinically. Remember to have a higher index of suspicion of occult perforation in a steroid-treated older patient with abdominal pain. There is also a weak association between steroid use and peptic ulceration.
- Adrenocortical suppression means that the **stress response will be diminished** in chronic steroid users. If such a patient becomes acutely ill (e.g., septic), the exogenous steroid dose will need to be temporarily increased (e.g., stress dose steroids). In addition, patients on chronic steroids should be considered for perioperative stress dose steroids.

## Stopping treatment

Many patients are on fairly low doses of steroids for a long period. It can be difficult to completely reduce the dosage, as steroid withdrawal effects (fevers, myalgia, etc.) can often be mistaken for disease recurrence. Withdrawal often needs to be done very slowly (perhaps reducing by as little as 1 mg a month). There is no such thing as a "safe" dose of steroid, so for every patient you see on steroids, ask the following:

- Can the dose be reduced?
- Could a steroid-sparing agent (e.g., azathioprine) be used instead?
- Is the patient taking adequate bone protection?
- What is the blood pressure and blood glucose?

# Warfarin

Common indications (see Table 6.2) range from absolute (pulmonary embolus, deep vein thrombosis, artificial heart valve replacement) to relative (stroke prophylaxis in atrial fibrillation).

## Cautions

Risk is higher if the patient is unable to take medication accurately; it is not suitable without supervision for cognitively impaired patients or those who self-neglect. If there is an absolute indication, then consider supervised therapy (by a spouse, family, or caregiver via a dispensing system) or (rarely) a course of low-molecular-weight heparin instead.

Risk is also higher if there is a high probability of trauma, e.g., recurrent falls, in which case warfarin may be inappropriate. The patient's primary physician should be consulted to determine risk.

Bleeding is the major adverse event, ranging from an increased tendency to bruise to major life-threatening bleeds. The most significant adverse events include intracerebral hemorrhage and gastrointestinal (GI) blood loss.

Warfarin does not cause gastric irritation, but may accelerate blood loss from pre-existing bleeding sources. Ask carefully about history of nonsteroidal use (including aspirin) and GI symptoms (indigestion, heartburn, weight loss, abdominal pain, altered bowel habits, rectal bleeding, etc.). If any are present then quantify risk with further testing—full blood count and iron studies might indicate occult blood loss.

If the warfarin is not essential, then a full GI workup may be appropriate before starting warfarin in robust patients. In patients for whom GI workup would pose unacceptable risk, consider warfarin with an empiric proton pump inhibitor.

Epistaxis is common in older patients and may become more significant on warfarin. It is often due to friable nasal vessels that are amenable to treatment by ear, nose, and throat (ENT) surgeons. Also consider use of topical estrogen therapy to reestablish nasal mucosal epithelium.

Comorbidity may increase sensitivity to warfarin (e.g., abnormal liver function) and should be screened for if there is suspicion.

## Management of elevated INR

- If there is no sign of bleeding and INR is <5, simply stop the warfarin and monitor the INR as it falls. Do not give vitamin K at this point, as anticoagulation will be difficult for weeks afterward.
- For INR 5–9 with no bleeding, you may either stop warfarin temporarily or stop warfarin and give a small dose (1–2.5 mg) of oral vitamin K.
- For INR >9 without bleeding, stop warfarin and give 5–10 mg oral vitamin K.
- If there is bleeding, then reverse warfarin with vitamin K (5–10 mg slow IV infusion) and/or fresh frozen plasma.
- Recall risk of anaphylaxis with vitamin K IV route.
- Always investigate the reason for an elevated INR and correct this factor if possible.

**Table 6.2** Usual INR goals

| Indication | Target | Duration |
|---|---|---|
| Atrial fibrillation | 2.5 | Lifelong |
| Venous thromboembolism | 2.5 | Varies. Usually 6 months. Lifelong if recurrent or with ongoing precipitant (e.g., malignancy) |
| Recurrent venous thromboembolism while on warfarin | 2.5 | Lifelong. May consider changing from warfarin to low-molecular-weight heparin in patients with malignancy |
| Mechanical prosthetic heart valves | Varies with type of valve | Lifelong |

For most recent guidelines, refer to the Seventh ACCP Conference on Antithrombotic and Thrombolytic Therapy. *Chest* (2004) **126**(3 Suppl):163S–696S.

## How to initiate warfarin

Discuss risks and benefits of treatment with the patient—the indication is rarely absolute. See p. 301 for an example. Consider referral to anti-coagulation clinic.

### Ensure that the patient is told the following:

- There will be frequent blood tests and monitoring.
- Many medications interact with warfarin, so before taking any new medication (including over the counter) always check compatibility with the doctor, dentist, or pharmacist.
- Use acetaminophen or opioid-based analgesia (never NSAIDs) to minimize risk of bleeding.
- Note that acetaminophen also has the potential to cause supratherapeutic INRs. This is a dose-dependent effect, and patients on warfarin should be advised to limit acetaminophen use to 2 g/day.
- Alcohol interacts with warfarin metabolism and should be taken in moderation and on a regular basis (avoid binge drinking).
- If trauma occurs, bleeding may last longer. Apply pressure to wounds and seek medical help if it does not stop.
- Counsel patient regarding diet and importance of maintaining consistent intake of foods containing vitamin K.
- Because of a potential drug–food interaction, patients should be told to limit grapefruit juice intake to three glasses daily.

### Induction

- Check baseline clotting.
- Prescribe warfarin to be taken at 6 PM.
- Medical notes should state indication, target INR, and duration of therapy.
- The normal adult induction dose (10 mg day 1, 10 mg day 2, then an INR) is rarely appropriate in older patients who are more sensitive to its effects.
- Reduce the dose if the patient is frail, has a low body weight, has multiple comorbidities, or has a deranged baseline clotting.
- For most older patients 5 mg/5 mg/INR is a safer approach.
- If there are multiple factors causing concern, 5 mg/INR is better.
- There is no rush. If the indication is absolute, the patient should also be on therapeutic heparin until the INR is in range. It is much easier to increase the dose of warfarin than to deal with bleeding from an overdose.
- The INR will then need checking daily, then alternate days until a pattern becomes clear.
- The INR testing can gradually be done less frequently, stretching to once per month in long-term users.

# Herbal remedies

Use of herbal supplements by older adults is common. Some studies estimate that between a third and a half of older patients use alternative therapies. As many as 60% of those who use complementary and alternative medicine (CAM) do not discuss this with their physician.

Each patient should be asked about use of herbal products. Patients should be advised that herbal products are not regulated by the U.S. Food and Drug Administration (FDA) and are therefore not subject to the same testing standards. Some products may not contain a reliable quantity of active ingredient and may contain impurities.

Patients who use herbal remedies should seek out reputable manufacturers who follow good manufacturing practices.

Herbal substances can have adverse effects and drug interactions. For additional information, refer to www.naturaldatabase.com, or http://nccam.nih.gov/camonpubmed.

Some of the most commonly used herbal remedies are listed in Box 6.3.

## Box 6.3 Common herbal remedies

*Echinacea*
- Use: immune stimulant
- Adverse effects: allergic reactions, hepatitis, asthma, vertigo
- Drug interactions: immunosuppressants

*Garlic*
- Use: hypertension, hypercholesterolemia, antiplatelet agent
- Adverse effects: bleeding, GI upset, hypoglycemia
- Drug interactions: NSAIDs, antiplatelet drugs, anticoagulants

*Gingko*
- Use: memory problems
- Adverse effects: bleeding, seizures, headaches, dizziness, GI upset
- Drug interactions: NSAIDs, antiplatelet drugs, anticoagulants, monoamine oxidase inhibitors (MAOIs), trazodone

*Ginseng*
- Use: performance enhancement (physical, mental)
- Adverse effects: hypertension, tachycardia
- Drug interactions: NSAIDs, antiplatelet drugs, anticoagulants

*Glucosamine/chondroitin*
- Use: osteoarthritis
- Adverse effects: nausea, diarrhea, heartburn
- Drug interactions: hypoglycemic agents (reduced efficacy)

**Box 6.3 Common herbal remedies (cont'd.)**

*Kava kava*
- Use: anxiety, sedative
- Adverse effects: sedation, hepatotoxicity
- Drug interactions: anticonvulsants, benzodiazepines, ethanol

*Saw palmetto*
- Use: reduce symptoms of prostate hypertrophy
- Adverse effects: constipation, diarrhea, decreased libido, headaches, hypertension, urinary retention, GI distress
- Drug interactions: finasteride

*St John's wort*
- Use: antidepressant, anxiolytic
- Adverse effects: nausea, allergic reactions, dizziness, headache, photosensitivity
- Drug interactions: cytochrome P-450 drugs, anticoagulants, antivirals, SSRIs, oral contraceptives, statins

*Valerian*
- Use: anxiety, insomnia
- Adverse effects: sedation
- Drug interactions: barbiturates, CNS depressants

# Breaking the rules

Much prescribing in geriatric practice relies on individually tailored assessment and practical decision-making. While much of what is described in the preceding pages is appropriate for many, there are always times when the rules must be broken in the best interests of the individual patient. This approach requires experience, and the patient should always be followed up to assess the impact of the decision.

Polypharmacy causes problems but is not universally regarded as bad—depriving patients of beneficial treatments because they are old or already on multiple other medications can also be detrimental. In a recent study of medication changes during a geriatric admission, the total number of drugs was the same at admission and discharge, but they had often been changed. In other words, there was active evaluation of medication going on, the goal being not just to limit the number of drugs but to optimize and individually tailor treatment.

Where side effects are very likely but the drug is definitely indicated, it may be appropriate to co-prescribe something to treat the expected adverse effect, for example:

• Steroids and bisphosphonates
• Opiates and laxatives
• Furosemide and a potassium-sparing diuretic (or an ACE inhibitor)
• Nonsteroidal agents and a gastric protection agent

While certain disease drug interactions are very likely and should be avoided, others may be an acceptable risk. For example:

• Beta-blockers are to be used with caution with asthma, yet they have such a good impact on cardiovascular risk reduction that these cautions should not be absolute. Often the "asthma" is in fact COPD with little beta-receptor reactivity, so cautious beta-blockade initiated in the hospital while monitoring lung function may be appropriate.
• Diabetics often have cardiovascular disease and the risk of beta-blockade is usually outweighed by the benefits.
• Fludrocortisone (for postural blood pressure drop) will worsen hypertension and cause ankle swelling, yet if the postural drop is so profound that the patient cannot mobilize, it may be appropriate to accept the hypertension and associated risk.
• Amlodipine may worsen ankle swelling in a patient with chronic venous insufficiency, but if this is the best way of controlling hypertension, it may be appropriate to accept a cosmetic problem.

# Chapter 7

# Neurology

### Richard O'Brien

# The aging brain and nervous system

As in other systems, distinguishing the effects of "normal" aging on cognition, strength, and gait from disease processes in which age is an important risk factor is often difficult (see Table 7.1). See Chapter 9, Psychiatry (p. 195) for discussion of cognitive aging.

Histological changes in the brain include the following:
- Each neuron has fewer connecting arms (dendrites).
- Around 20% of brain volume and weight are lost by the age of 85.
- There is deposition of pigment (lipofuscin) in the cells and oxidative damage in mitochondria.
- The presence of senile plaques and neurofibrillary tangles increases with age, but they are not diagnostic of dementia.

**Table 7.1** Consequences of age-related changes in the brain

| Age-related change | Consequences |
| --- | --- |
| Loss of neurons (cannot be regenerated)<br>Decrease in brain weight (by around 20% at age 85) | Cerebral atrophy common on brain scans (although this doesn't correlate well with cognitive function) |
| Some neurons become demyelinated and have slowed nerve conduction speed and increased latency (time taken to recover before transmitting next impulse) | Reflexes with long nerve tracts (e.g., ankle jerks) can be diminished or lost<br>Minor sensory loss, e.g., fine touch or vibration sense, may be lost distally |
| Neurotransmitter systems alter (e.g., cholinergic receptors decrease) | Increased susceptibility to some neuromodulating drugs |
| Increasing frequency of periventricular white-matter changes seen on cerebral imaging | Probably not a normal finding<br>Significance unclear—assumed to be representative of small-vessel vascular disease but poor postmortem correlation |

# Tremor

Tremor is more common with increasing age. It can be disabling and/or socially embarrassing. It is important to try to make a diagnosis, as treatment is available in some cases.

Examine the patient first at rest and distracted (relaxed with arms supported on lap, count to 10 backwards), then with outstretched hands, and finally during movement (finger to nose). Tremors fall roughly into three categories:

1. **Rest tremor** disappears on movement and is exaggerated by movement of the contralateral side of the body. The most common cause is Parkinson's disease. It is usually associated with rigidity and decreased facial movements.
2. **Postural tremor** is present in outstretched limbs, may continue during action but disappears at rest. The most common cause is benign essential tremor.
3. **Action tremor** is exaggerated with movement. When tremor is maximal at extreme point of movement it is called an intention tremor. The most common cause is cerebellar dysfunction.

## Benign essential tremor

- The classic postural tremor of old age, worse on action (e.g., static at rest but person spills tea from teacup) may have head nodding (titubation) or jaw or vocal tremor, legs rarely affected. May be asymmetrical.
- About half of cases have a family history (autosomal dominant).
- It presents in middle age, occasionally earlier, and worsens gradually.
- It is often more socially embarrassing than physically impairing.
- It is improved by alcohol, gabapentin, primidone, and beta-blockers, but these are often unacceptable treatments in the long term. It is worth considering beta-blockers as a first choice in treatment of patients with coexisting hypertension.

## Parkinson's disease (see p. 146)

## Cerebellar dysfunction

The typical intention tremor is associated with ataxia.

**Acute** onset is usually vascular in older adults.

**Subacute** presentations occur with tumors (including paraneoplastic syndrome), abscesses, hydrocephalus, drugs (e.g., anticonvulsants), hypothyroidism, or toxins.

**Chronic** progressive course is seen with the following:

- Alcoholism (due to thiamine deficiency—always give thiamine 100 mg/day orally or IV preparation if in doubt, it might be reversible)
- Anticonvulsant (e.g., phenytoin—may be irreversible if severe, more common with high plasma levels but can occur with long-term use at therapeutic levels)
- Paraneoplastic syndromes (e.g., ovary anti-Yo, bronchus anti-Hu) anti-cerebellar antibodies can be found
- Multiple sclerosis
- Idiopathic cerebellar atrophy
- Many cases defy specific diagnosis. Consider multisystem atrophy (see Parkinson's-plus syndromes, p. 150).

## Other causes of tremor (see Table 7.2)

**Table 7.2** Diagnosing other causes of tremor

| Diagnosis | Recognition and characteristics | Management |
|---|---|---|
| Thyrotoxicosis | Fine resting tremor<br><br>This is actually more common in younger patients. | See p. 458 |
| Rigors | Sudden-onset coarse tremor with associated malaise and fever | Diagnose and treat underlying cause |
| Asterixis (tremor and incoordination) with hepatic, renal, or respiratory failure | Coarse postural "give-way" tremor in a sick patient with physiological disturbance<br><br>A less dramatic, often fine tremor can occur with metabolic disturbance such as hypoglycemia, hypocalcemia | Diagnose and treat underlying condition |
| Withdrawal of drugs e.g., alcohol, benzodiazepines, SSRIs, barbiturates | Always consider when patient develops tremor ± confusion soon after admission | For alcohol consider sedation with, e.g., lorazepam 0.5–2 mg every 4–6 hr. Give thiamine 100 mg/day (PO, IM, or IV). For therapeutic drugs recommence and consider gradual, controlled withdrawal at later date |
| Drug side effects, e.g., lithium, cyclosporine anticonvulsants | | Check that serum levels are in therapeutic range. Consider different agent |
| Anxiety/stress—increased sympathomimetic activity | Fine tremor | Rarely necessary to consider beta-blockers |
| Orthostatic tremor—rare, benign postural tremor of legs | Fine tremor of legs on standing diminished by walking or sitting<br><br>Can palpate muscle tremor in legs. Patient feels unsteady but rarely falls | Provide perching stools, etc., to avoid standing for long period of time |

# Neuropathic pain

This describes pain originating from nerve damage or inflammation. It is often very severe and debilitating and seems to be more common in the elderly. The pain is usually sharp or stabbing and is often intermittent, being precipitated by things like movement and cold.

Traditional analgesics (acetaminophen, NSAIDs) are not very effective and there is a long list of "neuromodulating" drugs that may give superior pain control but often have important side effects (mainly sedation). Nonpharmacological treatments such as TENS (transcutaneous nerve stimulation) can be helpful.

## Postherpetic neuralgia

Severe burning and stabbing pain occur in a division of nerve previously affected by shingles (p. 644). Pain may be triggered by touch or temperature change. Shingles and subsequent persisting neuralgia are much more common in the elderly. It can go on for years, be difficult to treat, and have a major impact on quality of life.

### Prevention

Start antiviral therapy within 72 hours of rash (e.g., famcyclovir 250 mg three times a day). Evidence that additional oral prednisone is beneficial in the acute setting either for treatment of the rash or prevention of postherpetic neuralgia is not convincing.

### Treatment

The mainstays of treatment are antidepressants with noradrenergic modulating abilities, such as amitriptyline or duloxetine. These should be introduced early on if pain persists after the rash has healed. These drugs should always be started at low doses in the elderly, but eventual doses may be similar to those for younger patients.

Drugs to be used in combination with antidepressants include the anticonvulsants gabapentin and pregabalin. Again, start low but keep pushing the dosages. Topical lidocaine has also proven effective. Referral to a pain clinic is warranted if pain control is difficult, as they may try nerve blocks or spinal stimulators.

## Trigeminal neuralgia

This causes unilateral, severe, stabbing facial pain, usually at V2, V3 rather then V1. Triggers include movement and temperature change. It occurs over years, with relapse and remission. Depression and weight loss can result.

Differential diagnoses include temporal arteritis, cluster headache, toothache, parotitis, and temporomandibular joint arthritis. Consider neuroimaging, especially if there are physical signs, i.e., sensory loss or other cranial nerve abnormality suggestive of secondary trigeminal neuralgia. Bilateral trigeminal neuralgia suggests multiple sclerosis.

Treatment revolves around anticonvulsants, especially carbamazepine and oxcarbazepine. A role for baclofen also exists in this disorder.

Patients not responding to medications should be referred to a specialized center for surgical decompression of the fifth cranial nerve.

Neuralgia can also occur with the following:

- Malignancy
- Cord compression
- Neuropathy

# Parkinson's disease (PD)

PD is a common idiopathic disease (prevalence 150/100,000) associated with inadequate dopamine neurotransmitter in the brain stem. Loss of neurons and Lewy body formation occur in the substantia nigra. The clinical syndrome is distinct from Lewy body dementia (p. 150) but there is overlap in some pathological and clinical findings, leading to suggestions that they might turn out to be related conditions.

The clinical diagnosis of PD is based on the following:

- **Bradykinesia** (slow to initiate and carry out movements, expressionless face, fatigability of repetitive movement)
- **Rigidity** (cogwheeling = tremor superimposed on rigidity)
- **Tremor** ("pill rolling" of hands—worse at rest)
- **Postural instability**
- **Gait disorder** (small steps)

Other clinical features:

- Usually an asymmetrical disease
- Autonomic features (e.g., postural hypotension, dribbling, and constipation) are late but common in older adults.
- There are no pyramidal or cerebellar signs, but reflexes are sometimes brisk.
- Dementia and hallucinations can occur in late stages, but drug side effects can case similar problems.
- Dysphagia can lead to nutrition and swallowing problems.

## Investigations

Diagnosis is clinical, but a trial of dopamine supplementation with quantified parameters (e.g., 2 minutes walking distance, sit-to-stand time, foot or finger tapping or grooved pegboard test) before and after the treatment period can aid diagnosis and help titrate dopamine treatment.

Brain imaging (e.g., CT) can be used to exclude other conditions that may mimic PD (e.g., vascular disease, normal-pressure hydrocephalus).

## Treatment

### Drugs

While there is some controversy about the ideal drug treatment strategy, the following is a reasonable way to start treatment:

- **Sinemet** 25/100, 1 pill twice a day with meals, advance to 1 pill 3 to 4 times a day 1 hour before meals
- **Dopamine agonists** (ropinirole, pergolide, cabergoline) are added if Sinemet treatment is not adequate. Psychiatric side effects (confusion, hallucinations), postural hypotension, and nausea often limit therapy.
- **Monoamine oxidase inhibitors (MAOIs)** such as selegiline can be added as well. Patients should not be on antidepressants if they are put on MAOIs.

Second-line agents such as the following should be given by specialists in the field:

- **COMT inhibitor** (entacapone) will smooth fluctuations in plasma levodopa concentrations. Give with each levodopa dose—sometimes patient will need levodopa dose decrease. It stains urine orange.
- **Amantidine** is a weak dopamine agonist that can reduce dyskinetic problems.

Psychiatric features (e.g., hallucinations) can often be decreased by reducing dopaminergic therapy. When this fails or is intolerable, some patients may respond to antipsychotics such as quetiapine or olanzapine. In some cases clozapine, an antipsychotic with no extrapyramidal effects, must be used. This should only be prescribed by a specialist because of bone marrow effects. If features suggest Lewy body dementia, a trial of anticholinesterases (Aricept®) may be warranted.

### Surgery
Ablation (e.g., pallidotomy) and stimulation (electrode implants) are used in highly selected populations. Older patients are often excluded because of the high operative risk.

### Other therapeutic options
- A course of physiotherapy can be helpful to boost mobility.
- Occupational therapy plays a vital role in aids and adaptations for disability.
- Speech and language therapists, along with dieticians, can help when swallowing becomes a problem.
- Depression is common—be vigilant and treat actively but beware of using antidepressants, which can exacerbate movement disorder and postural hypotension.

## How to treat challenging symptoms in Parkinson's disease

| | |
|---|---|
| **Wearing off**—progression of disease: patients require higher doses or more frequent dosing to produce same effect | Possible that levodopa itself is toxic to neurons and enhances progression. In younger patients or for milder disease, start with selegiline or dopamine agonists. |
| **Dyskinesias** | Reduce levodopa dose, if possible (either alone or with addition of an agonist). Add amantadine. |
| **Motor fluctuations** with choreodystonic "on" phases and freezing "off" phases develop and worsen with duration of treatment. | Use reduced levodopa dose more frequently (dose fractionation) or controlled-release preparations or add entacapone or add dopamine agonist |
| Other drug **side effects** (confusion and hallucinations, constipation, urinary retention, nausea and vomiting) are a particular problem in the elderly and often limit treatment to sub-ideal levels. | Domperidone (30 mg three times per day po) is the best antiemetic. |
| In general, **patients prefer dyskinetic side effects** to "off spells"—relatives and caregivers may find the opposite easier to cope with, especially if patient is confused or falling when "on". | Ensure that you talk to the patient as well, even if it is easier to talk to the caregiver. Compromise may be necessary. |
| **Quantifying response** to treatment is very difficult. | Get patient or caregiver to fill in a 24-hour chart. A formal, quantified drug trial by therapists can be very helpful. |
| **End-stage disease** | Ultimately, drug responsiveness is so poor and side effects so marked that decreasing and withdrawing therapy may be appropriate. Palliative treatment and social support are important. |

# Diseases masquerading as Parkinson's disease

The majority of slow, stiff, or shaky older patients do not have true PD. As many as 1 in 4 diagnoses of PD made by primary care physicians are incorrect. It is important to get the diagnosis right, or you will subject patients needlessly to the harmful side effects of medications. Coexistence of more than one syndrome can further complicate diagnosis (see Table 7.3).

*Atherosclerotic pseudoparkinsonism/multi-infarct dementia*

This is due to neurovascular damage—consider it in those with stroke or TIA or with atherosclerotic risk factors, e.g., hypertension. There is a short-stepping, wide-based unstable gait with relative preservation of arm and facial movements (lower body Parkinsonism). A head scan may show lacunae or white matter change.

*Benign essential tremor*

This condition is often inherited (autosomal dominant), worse on action (spills tea from teacup), and improved by alcohol and beta-blockers. The patient may have head nodding or vocal tremor.

*Lewy body dementia*

Lewy bodies are widely present throughout the cortex, not predominantly in substantia nigra as with true PD. Psychiatric symptoms, e.g., visual hallucinations, tend to precede physical ones. Dementia and the motor features of Parkinsonism start simultaneously.

*Drug-induced Parkinsonism*

Neuroleptics are the most common cause, but remember that prochlorperazine for dizziness and metaclopramide for nausea are also causes. Some irritable bowel treatments contain neuroleptics.

*Other causes*

Alzheimer's disease, normal-pressure hydrocephalus, and even severe polyarthritis can sometimes cause diagnostic confusion. Patients with hydrocephalus on CT or MRI that is not explained by global atrophy should be referred for a diagnostic spinal tap (which measures response of gait to a 30 cc spinal fluid drainage).

## Parkinson's-plus syndromes

This is a confusing array of rare disorders that includes the following:
- **Multisystem atrophy** (aka Shy-Drager syndrome, olivopontocerebellar atrophy) includes autonomic failure (orthostatic hypotension) along with parkinsonism, ataxia, and pyramidal signs.
- **Progressive supranuclear palsy** (aka Steele–Richardson–Olszewski disease) includes up- and down-gaze palsy, axial rigidity and falls, dysarthria and dysphagia, and frontal lobe dementia.

**Table 7.3** Clues to distinguish Parkinson's disease

|  | True PD | Pseudo-PD (esp. atherosclerotic) |
|---|---|---|
| Response to L-dopa | Good | Poor or transient |
|  | Develop dopa dyskinesias | Dopa dyskinesias unusual |
| Age of onset | 40–70 years | 70+ years |
| Tremor | Unilateral or asymmetrical | Absent or mild |
|  | Resting tremor prominent |  |
| Progression | Slow progression, long history | Rapid progression |
| Dementia | Only at late stage | Prominent or early |
| Instability or falls | Late | Early and prominent |
| Dysphonia, dysarthria, or dysphagia | Late | Early and prominent |
| Other neurology (pyramidal signs, downgaze palsy, cerebellar signs) | Rare | Common |

## Further reading

Tuite PJ, Krawczewski K (2007). Parkinsonism: a review-of-systems approach to diagnosis. *Semin Neurol* **27**(2):113–122.

# Epilepsy

Primary epilepsy most commonly presents around the time of puberty, but the incidence of new seizures is actually higher in those over 70 (>100 per 100,000) because of the increasing amount of secondary epilepsy (caused by, e.g., cerebrovascular ischemia, subdural hematomas, dementia, brain tumors; see Box 7.1).

In addition, fits can be precipitated by the following:
- Metabolic disturbance (e.g., hyponatremia)
- Drugs (e.g., ciprofloxacin)
- Infection (at any site but particularly with meningitis or encephalitis)
- Withdrawal from alcohol or drugs such as benzodiazepines
- Wernicke's encephalopay (due to thiamine deficiency in malnourished patients, e.g., alcoholics)

Many of these conditions are more common in older patients who also have a lower fit threshold for any given level of stimulus.

## Diagnosis
- See also Falls (Chapter 5, p. 82).
- An eyewitness account is the most useful diagnostic tool.
- Look particularly for post-event confusion or drowsiness, tongue biting, or incontinence.
- Patient with syncope may have several tonic–clonic jerks, but rarely experience post-event confusion or drowsiness, tongue biting, or incontinence.
- Remember that cerebral hypoperfusion from any cause (e.g., bradycardia) can cause myoclonic jerks, so epilepsy can coexist with other causes of syncope. In these cases, treatment of the primary syncope or hypoperfusion is more effective than antiepileptics.

## Investigations
- Routine blood screening, chest X-ray, and ECG are useful to look for precipitants and differential diagnoses.
- An MRI scan is vital to exclude a structural lesion.
- EEGs can be helpful when positive but very commonly have nonspecific changes and low sensitivity, i.e., a normal EEG does not rule out epilepsy.

## General management
- Ensure the patient is not taking medication that lowers the seizure threshold (common examples include tricyclics, ciprofloxacin, and phenothiazines). Think about over-the-counter drugs (e.g., Sudafed, phenylpropanolamine) and stimulants such as cocaine.
- Correct any metabolic derangement (especially glucose, sodium, sepsis).
- Advise about driving restrictions—don't assume that the patient doesn't drive.
- Detect and treat complications, e.g., aspiration, trauma, pressure injuries.

## Driving regulations and epilepsy

You have a duty to inform the patient that they should notify the Department of Motor Vehicles (although regulations vary from state to state). Patients have at least a 3-month ban on driving for a first seizure. Patients must also refrain from driving for 3 months after withdrawing epilepsy medication[1] (see also Chapter 30, The older driver, p. 727).

### Box 7.1 Epilepsy and stroke

**Onset seizures** (within a week, most commonly within 24 hours) occur in 2%–5% of strokes. They are more common with hemorrhages, large cortical strokes, and venous infarction. Consider also alcohol or drug (especially benzodiazepine) withdrawal for early seizures. Long-term anticonvulsants are not usually prescribed unless seizures recur.

**After the first week** stroke remains a risk factor for new epilepsy—the first year there is a 5% risk, subsequently a 1.5% annual incidence. Many such patients develop transient neurological worsening (Todd's paresis) or permanent worsening without MRI evidence of a new stroke. In these patients it is usually worth considering long-term anticonvulsants.

Epilepsy may occur secondary to clinically "silent" cerebral ischemia and 3% of patients with stroke have a past history off it, most instances occurring in the preceding year. Some epilepsy experts suggest that aspirin is prescribed for new-onset seizures in an elderly patient once structural lesions have been excluded.

1. Krauss GL, Ampaw L, Krumholz A (2001). Individual state driving restrictions for people with epilepsy in the US. *Neurology* **57**:1780–1785.

# Epilepsy: drug treatment

## Acute treatment
- Start with benzodiazepines (5–10 mg rectal diazepam or 2–10 mg diazepam IV or 0.5–2 mg lorazepam IV or IM).
- If seizure continues, consider setting up loading dose (1 g/kg) infusion of phenytoin (use a cardiac monitor) until oral medication can be taken.
- Rarely the patient may need intubating and phenobarbital or a general anesthetic to stabilize them or to allow an urgent CT scan.

## Chronic treatment
Because of side effects and the long duration of treatment, most doctors will resist starting anticonvulsants until after a second seizure, especially if the diagnosis is unclear or if there is a reversible precipitant. Presence of underlying structural abnormality or wishing to return to driving may tip the balance in favor of treatment.

In older adults, the risk of a second seizure is higher after a first unprovoked seizure than in a younger patient, so many epilepsy experts will treat after a first seizure in older adults.

In the past, phenytoin (200–400 mg/day) and carbamazepine (200 mg twice daily gradually increasing to 200 mg three times a day) were considered the drugs of choice for seizures in older adults, but today lamictal (25 mg twice a day slowly titrating up to 100 mg twice a day) or Keppra 500 mg twice a day) are considered the drugs of choice in the elderly because of better side-effect profile. Lamictal can cause severe skin reactions if not titrated up slowly and should be stopped for any evidence of skin reaction. Keppra can also cause irritability.

All anticonvulsants have significant side effects, e.g., sedation, confusion, rash, tremor, and ataxia. Serious liver, blood, and pulmonary side effects can also occur; ongoing monitoring to optimize dose and minimize side effects is necessary.

Many anticonvulsants interact with each other as well as with other drugs, which can increase toxicity or reduce effectiveness. If in doubt, consult a pharmacist. Gabapentin and Pregabalin do not interact at all with other drugs and are useful in this situation.

Avoid abrupt withdrawal of antiepileptics—seizures may be provoked.

Partial seizures (e.g., face or arm twitching) are rarely dangerous and often distress bystanders more than the patient, but they can progress to secondary generalized seizures. The same drugs can be employed. Partial seizures often indicate structural lesions and an early CT scan is advisable.

Sometimes a trial of anticonvulsants in patients with recurrent unexplained collapse can be revealing.

Refer to an epilepsy specialist if control is proving difficult and multiple drugs are required.

# Neuroleptic malignant syndrome (NMS)

This rare but important syndrome occurs in patients taking neuroleptics (e.g., haloperidol, chlorpromazine, risperidone), with a triad of
- Fever
- Rigidity and tremor
- Rhabdomyolysis with secondary renal failure (p. 527)

NMS can be fatal (up to 30%) and early recognition is important.

## Diagnosis

NMS may arise at any time during treatment, i.e., the patient may have recently
- Started (most common) or stopped neuroleptics.
- Increased the dose or been stable on them for a long time.
- Added a second drug, e.g., tricyclic antidepressant, lithium.

Reintroduction of the offending drug at a later date may not reproduce symptoms. Contributing factors such as intercurrent illness and metabolic derangement may be important in the etiology.

## Clinical features

- The patient looks ill with fever, severe lead-pipe rigidity, bradykinesia, occasionally tremor, and decreased conscious level.
- Time course: onset is usually over 1–3 days, starts with rigidity and altered mental state.
- Seizures and abnormal neurological signs can occur.
- Autonomic dysfunction causes sweating, tachycardia, and hypertension.
- Multiorgan failure can occur and there is a leukocytosis, and creatinine kinase levels may be over 1000 IU/L.
- Lumbar puncture, CT scan, and EEG are often required to exclude other diagnoses such as CNS infection.

The most common cause of a similar presentation is sepsis in a patient with pre-existing cerebrovascular disease.

## Management

Stop all neuroleptics. Use acetaminophen and cooling with fans and damp sponging. Provide IV fluids, with careful monitoring of electrolytes and renal function. Dantrolene (direct muscle relaxant; 1–3 mg/kg IV initial followed by 10 mg/kg/day in divided doses) can speed recovery. Short-term dialysis is sometimes required. Bromocriptine is also used in some cases, although data that it is effective are lacking.

Early transfer to an intensive care unit (ICU) is usually wise. Death most commonly occurs by hypoventilation/pneumonia or renal failure. There are sometimes persisting neurological sequelae.

## Serotonin syndrome

This similar syndrome to NMS occurs in patients taking serotonin reuptake inhibitors (SSRIs), especially if combined with tramadol or a tricyclic or monoamine oxidase inhibitor. Patients tend to be agitated and delirious rather than unconscious. Gastrointestinal symptoms (diarrhea and vomiting) occur. Onset may be within 2 hours; resolution is usually quicker than that of NMS.

# Motor neuron disease

This is a progressive idiopathic disease with selective degeneration of motor neurons causing weakness and wasting. There are a variety of manifestations depending on the site of damage; the most common site for lesions is in the anterior horn cells of spinal cord (LMN), but descending motor pathway (UMN) may be affected in the corticospinal tracts, brain stem, and motor cranial nuclei. Interestingly, extraocular muscles and motorneurons are not ever involved.

- Onset rises steeply with age, with peak incidence in the late 50s to early 60s. It is very rare before age 40. Overall prevalence is 7 per 100,000, but incidence is 1 per 10,000 for age 65–85.
- It is underdiagnosed in the elderly (it is confused with cerebrovascular disease, myasthenia, especially bulbar-onset forms, cervical myelopathy, motor neuropathy, syringomyelia, and paraneoplastic syndromes).
- It is slightly more common in males.
- 5% will have a family history (autosomal dominant is most common but it can be recessive or X-linked).

## History

- Weakness, cramps, and fatigue in limbs. Weakness usually begins in a focal area and spreads to contiguous muscles; onset in upper limbs is most common.
- Palatal and vocal cord paralysis can cause stridor, dysarthria, dysphagia, and aspiration pneumonia.
- Paresis of respiratory muscles can cause respiratory failure (may present to chest physicians or in the ICU).
- Intellect, sensation, and continence are usually retained. Some forms are associated with frontotemporal dementia (<5%). Depression is common.

## Examination

- Look for wasting of muscles with fasciculation (LMN), especially in the tongue, shoulders, and legs.
- Head drop or droop can occur.
- Brisk reflexes, clonus, and upgoing plantars can occur (UMN).
- Atrophy and weakness are less specific signs.
- Dysarthria and dysphagia are common.
- Sensory changes should make you question the diagnosis.

## Investigations

- Creatine kinase (CK) is usually modestly elevated.
- CT and MRI of brain and spine are usually normal but should be done in most cases.
- Electromyography (EMG) shows widespread denervation of muscles caused by anterior horn cell degeneration and can be diagnostic.

## Clinical pictures

There are diverse presentations and rates of progression. Amyotrophic lateral sclerosis (ALS) is the most common form, with a classical picture of mixed UMN and LMN. This term is used commonly in the U.S.

- Progressive pseudobulbar or bulbar palsy: speech and swallow are predominantly affected.
- Primary lateral sclerosis: upper motor neurons are predominantly affected.
- Progressive muscular atrophy: lower motor neurons are predominantly affected.

## Treatment

### Riluzole

This is a sodium channel blocker, taken 50 mg twice a day. It prolongs survival by a few months, but not function. Riluzole is expensive and should be supervised by a specialist. Monitor liver function and check for neutropenia if there is febrile illness.

### Supportive

- *Chest:* antibiotics and physiotherapy, noninvasive nocturnal ventilation (for diaphragmatic palsy, sleep apnea)
- *Speech:* early referral to speech therapy for communication aids
- *Nutrition:* initially pureed food and thickened fluids. Malnutrition and aspiration are indications for considering artificial feeding.
- *Muscle spasm:* baclofen, physiotherapy
- *Mobility/independence:* occupational therapy (OT) for wheelchairs and adaptations
- *Pain/distress:* opiates or benzodiazepines (but beware of respiratory suppression)

### Other

- This is a devastating diagnosis to give to a patient, as it means a life expectancy of 2–5 years. Matters are often made worse by a considerable delay between symptoms and a concrete diagnosis being made (sometimes the initial diagnosis was incorrect).
- Emphasize the retention of cognition and aspects of supportive care available. Offer regular follow-up appointments.
- Specialist referral is needed in almost all cases.
- Consider enduring power of attorney (POA) and advance directives. It is rare that patients with ALS are placed on long-term ventilators.

## Further reading

www.mndassociation.org

# Peripheral neuropathies

Some minor degree of sensory loss in the feet and reduced or absent ankle jerks are so common in older people (in up to 50% of those over 85 years old) that some classify this as a normal aging change. However, remember the following:

- Even mild, asymptomatic neuropathies can contribute to postural instability and falls.
- The diagnosis is often missed because of nonspecific symptoms and insidious onset with slow progression.

## Clinical features

- There are signs of lower motor neuron weakness with wasting and loss of reflexes.
- Sensory loss occurs, often with joint position, and vibration loss before touch and pain.
- Neuralgia-type pain may be present (especially with diabetes and alcohol).
- Autonomic failure and cranial nerve involvement can also occur.
- Severe cases may affect respiration.

## Classification

Try to determine if the signs are focal or generalized and whether they are predominantly sensory or motor because this can help identify the likely underlying pathology. Further classification by pathology (axonal or demyelinating) requires nerve conduction studies or biopsy.

The most common pattern produces widespread symmetrical sensory loss (typically glove and stocking). This may be combined with distal muscle weakness (mixed motor and sensory neuropathy). Where signs are focal or asymmetric, consider mononeuritis multiplex.

## Causes

The causes are legion and often multiple in elderly patients. Idiopathic neuropathies are very common (25% defy diagnosis in most studies). The following list is not exhaustive but is in order of common to rare:

- Idiopathic
- Diabetes mellitus
- Familial
- Alcoholism (often combined with vitamin deficiency)
- Renal failure
- B$_{12}$ or folate deficiency
- Paraneoplastic syndromes (e.g., small cell lung cancer)
- Drugs (e.g., isoniazid, nitrofurantoin, vincristine, amiodarone)
- Paraproteinemias and amyloid
- Chronic inflammatory demyelinating polyradiculoneuropathy (rare autoimmune neuropathy)
- Guillain–Barré syndrome (acute onset)
- Hypothyrodism
- Vasculitides (e.g., Wegener's granulomatosis)—actually multiple mononeuropathy

### Investigations

- Always check $B_{12}$, glucose, thyroid function, serum and urine immunoglobulins, ESR, and C-reactive protein (CRP) before labeling a neuropathy idiopathic.
- Look carefully for an occult tumor (e.g., breast examination and CXR).
- Family history
- Nerve conduction studies will confirm nerve damage and distinguish demyelination from axonal damage (which sometimes helps with differential diagnosis), but they are not always required in straightforward cases.
- Further specialist tests include immunology, tumor markers, lumbar puncture, molecular genetics tests, and nerve biopsy.

### Treatment

The important thing is to identify reversible causes quickly, especially diabetic neuropathy and immune-based neuropathies such as chronic inflammatory demyelinating polyradiculoneuropathy (CIDP). CIDP is treated by steroids, plasma exchange, and intravenous immunoglobulin (IVIG), but most other chronic neuropathies have no specific treatment. Supportive and symptomatic treatment (e.g., appropriate footwear, analgesia, environmental adaptation) is important.

Acute neuropathy due to Guillain–Barré syndrome is a medical emergency that responds to IVIG or plasma pheresis. These patients can deteriorate rapidly and should be managed in conjunction with specialist neurology units. Even patients that look well should have their vital capacity measured daily to warn of impending respiratory failure.

# Subdural hematoma

This condition is much more common in old age because as the brain shrinks, the veins that lie between it and the skull are much more likely to get torn following trauma (even minor injury). Older people are also more likely to have falls and head injuries and are more commonly on predisposing drugs (e.g., aspirin, warfarin). Other risk factors include alcoholism, epilepsy, and hemodialysis.

### Features

Subdurals frequently present with very nonspecific symptoms in a frail, confused patient. A high index of suspicion is required.

- Subdurals can occur acutely (and present within hours of an accident) or more slowly as the classical "chronic subdural hematoma," although this distinction doesn't help guide management.
- A history of head injury occurs in only about half of patients.
- Common features include drowsiness and confusion (rarely fluctuant), postural instability, progressive focal neurology (e.g., hemiparesis, unequal pupils), headache, and blurred vision.
- Rarely transient neurology (mimicking TIA) or Parkinsonism can occur.
- Some patients are asymptomatic and large collections can be incidental findings.
- Examine for papilledema, focal neurology, and long tract signs.

### Diagnosis

On a CT head scan look for crescent-shaped hematoma compressing sulci (hypodense or black is old blood, hyperdense or white indicates recent bleeding) and midline shift. All patients who have new confusion and or drowsiness without another explanation should be scanned. Have an especially low threshold for scanning patients on aspirin or warfarin and for those who have evidence of falls, particularly facial bruising.

MRI is slightly superior and useful when CT changes are subtle (an isodense phase occurs on CT in transition between hyperdense and hypotense changes) or very small hematomas are suspected.

### Management

Decisions are usually made in conjunction with the local neurosurgical team (although in practice only about one-third of patients will end up having surgery). Stop aspirin and reverse warfarin therapy, if possible. Observation is frequently used in the following patients:

- Asymptomatic patients
- Those with small bleeds who are stable and improving
- Those not fit for transfer or surgery

When conservative management is adopted, record conscious level (Glasgow coma scale [GCS]—see Appendix) and any focal neurology at least daily or if there is any change. Any deterioration should prompt a repeat CT scan and reconsideration of surgery.

# Sleep and insomnia

With increasing age, less sleep is needed (approximately 1 hour less than for young adults), circadian rhythm is less marked, and sleep becomes more fragmented with greater difficulty getting to sleep. Deep (stages 3 and 4) sleep is reduced, but dreaming sleep/REM (rapid eye movement) is preserved.

Insomnia is a symptom that correlates poorly with observed actual sleep time (i.e., patients who complain of poor sleep may be observed by nurses and family members to sleep well, whereas those who sleep very little do not necessarily complain). It can be very distressing and is associated with increased morbidity and mortality. Around 25% of older people suffer chronic insomnia—even higher rates are found with psychiatric and medical conditions.

Insomnia is a particular problem in an unfamiliar, noisy ward environment and doctors are often under considerable pressure to prescribe sedatives.

## Treatment of insomnia

First ensure that underlying causes are looked for and treated. For example:
- Pain at night—consider using analgesics
- Comorbidities, e.g., orthopnea, nocturia, esophageal reflux, Parkinson's disease
- Depression and anxiety are very common—use of an antidepressant will improve sleep much better than a hypnotic.
- Alcohol dependence
- Drugs—corticosteroids, omeprazole, phenytoin, amiodarone, sulfasalazine, atorvastatin, ramipril, as well as psychiatric drugs, e.g., paroxetine, haloperidol, and chlorpromazine can cause insomnia. Beta-blockers and levodopa cause nightmares.

The following **nonpharmacological interventions** (sleep hygiene) should be the first step for most patients:
- Reduce or stop daytime "catnapping."
- Avoid caffeine, heavy meals, and alcohol in the evening (alcohol helps you fall asleep but reduces sleep quality).
- Use a bedtime routine.
- Ensure that the environment is dark, quiet, and comfortable.
- Relaxation and cognitive-behavioral techniques can be useful.
- Try warm milky drinks.

### Drugs

Drugs are rarely justified and highly dangerous. They may be justified for short-term use in limited circumstances (e.g., acute grief where acute insomnia is stressful.)
- Benzodiazepines (e.g., temazepam 10 mg) are licensed for short-term (<4 weeks) management of insomnia and anxiety. They may have a limited role for short-term symptom relief, though risks of falls and confusion are high in frail or cognitively impaired patients.

- The newer Z-drugs (e.g., zopiclone, zolpidem, and zeleplon) are only for insomnia. They have shorter half-lives and fewer side effects (although zopiclone is still a cause of daytime drowsiness). Overall, they are probably slightly superior to benzodiazepines but the same cautions about dependence apply.
- Other hypnotics (e.g., chloral hydrate, chlormethiazole, antihistamines) can be toxic especially in overdose and provide no advantages over the above two examples.
- A new class of drugs such as ramelteon (Rozerem) for insomnia, which act on melatonin pathways, may prove beneficial but lack a proven record of safety in older adults.

# Other sleep disorders

### Hypersomnolence
This is excessive daytime sleepiness despite a normal night of sleep. Causes include brain disease (e.g., dementia, stroke), cardiopulmonary disease (e.g., cardiac failure, COPD), obstructive sleep apnea, hypothyroidism, narcolepsy, and sedative drugs. This complaint should provoke a sleep study.

### Restless legs syndrome
This is a common (10% of older people), unpleasant sensation in limbs that increases with drowsiness and recumbancy and is eradicated by movement. It can be associated with limb jerking during sleep with sleep disturbance. Both symptoms respond to benzodiazepines. Dopamine agonists are also used with some success.

### Circadian rhythm disorders
Jet-lag is the best known of these disorders, but advanced–sleep phase syndrome (sleepiness occurs too early in evening, but there is early morning wakening) and delayed sleep phase (sleepiness comes too late at night) can occur without such a precipitant. Treat by gradually altering bedtime and bright-light therapy when wakefulness is desired.

### Sleep apnea in the older adults
Obstructive sleep apnea (OSA) and central sleep apnea are very common in elderly people and can cause daytime sleepiness, accidents, and heart failure. Unfortunately, periods of apnea are less likely to be symptomatic in older people than in the young, and where symptoms do exist they are often multifactorial, so diagnosis and compliance with therapy (noninvasive positive pressure ventilation) can be problematic.

### Further reading
Harbison J. (2002). Sleep disorder in older people. *Age Ageing* **31**:6–9.

# Stroke

**Rafael Llinas**

# Definition and classification

## Definition

**Stroke** is the sudden onset of a focal neurological deficit of vascular origin due to either infarction or hemorrhage.

- *Infarction:* emboli, arterial thrombosis, or arterial hypoperfusion of the brain or spinal cord
- *Hemorrhage:* spontaneous (not associated with trauma). Excludes subdural and epidural hematomas, but includes spontaneous sub-arachnoid hemorrhage

Use of the term *cerebrovascular accident* is now discouraged. They are not always cerebral, they are not always primarily vascular, and they are NEVER an accident.

**Transient ischemic attack (TIA)** is a brief episode of neurological dysfunction caused by focal brain or retinal ischemia, with clinical symptoms typically lasting less than 1 hour, and without evidence of acute infarction.

Infarction and TIAs have the same pathogenesis, and the distinction is likely to become less helpful with time. Urgent evaluation and treatment is indicated.

The term *brain attack* is being used to describe the full spectrum of disease severity from TIA to fatal stroke. With early evaluation there are interventions to save brain tissue that have parallels with approaches to myocardial salvage in coronary syndromes.

## Stroke burden

- The incidence of first stroke is about 500,000 per year and patients suffering from recurrent stroke is about 200,000 in the United States.
- Prevalence among adults 20 and older in 2004 was 5,700,000–2,400,000 men and 3,300,00 women.
- African Americans have twice the risk of first-ever stroke. The risk is 6.6 per 1000 vs. 3.6 per 1000 for Black men vs. White men. This is true for women also, with 4.9 per 1000 vs. 2.3 per 1000 for Black vs. White women, respectively. Globally it is the third most common cause of death (after coronary heart disease and all cancers).
- In the United States, stroke accounts for 1 out of every 16 deaths.

## Classification

*Various methods*

- *Infarct or hemorrhage* (also hemorrhagic infarcts)
- *Pathogenesis:* large vessel, small vessel, cardioembolic (AF or LV mural thrombus), valve disease, infective endocarditis, non-atheromatous arterial disease (vasculitis, dissection), blood disorders, etc.
- *Vessel affected:* anterior circulation (anterior cerebral artery and middle cerebral artery), lacunar (deep small subcortical vessels), posterior circulation (posterior cerebral artery, vertebral and basilar arteries)
- *Bamford classification:* clinical features to define likely stroke territory; used in major trials giving prognostic information about each group (see Table 8.1)

**Table 8.1** Bamford classification

### Total anterior circulation stroke (TACS)

| | |
|---|---|
| *Features* | 1. Hemiparesis and hemisensory loss |
| | 2. Homonymous hemianopia |
| | 3. Cortical dysfunction (dysphasia, visiospatial or perceptual problems) |
| Infarction (TACI) | 85% |
| Hemorrhage (TACH) | 15% |
| *Causes* | Occlusion in ICA, MCA, or ACA |
| | Emboli from heart, aortic arch, or carotids, in situ thrombosis |
| *Prognosis at 1 year* | Dead 60% |
| | Dependent 35% |
| | Independent 5% |

### Partial anterior circulation stroke (PACS)

| | |
|---|---|
| *Features* | Two of the three listed above *or* cortical dysfunction alone |
| Infarction (PACI) | 85% |
| Hemorrhage (PACH) | 15% |
| *Causes* | As for TACS |
| *Prognosis at 1 year* | Dead 15% |
| | Dependent 30% |
| | Independent 55% |

### Lacunar stroke (LACS)

| | |
|---|---|
| *Features* | Hemiparesis |
| | *or* Hemisensory loss |
| | *or* Hemisensorymotor loss |
| | *or* Ataxic hemiparesis |
| | (with NO cortical dysfunction) |
| Infarction (LACI) | 95% |
| Hemorrhage (LACH) | 5% |
| *Causes* | Small perforating arteries, microatheroma |
| | Hypertensive small vessel disease |
| *Prognosis at 1 year* | Dead 10% |
| | Dependent 30% |
| | Independent 60% |

### Posterior circulation stroke (POCS)

| | |
|---|---|
| *Features* | Brain stem symptoms and signs (diplopia, vertigo, ataxia, bilateral limb problems, hemianopia, cortical blindness, etc.) |
| Infarction (POCI) | 85% |
| Hemorrhage (POCH) | 15% |
| *Causes* | Occlusion of vertebral, basilar, or posterior cerebral artery |
| | Emboli from heart, aortic arch, or vertebrobasilar artery |
| *Prognosis at 1 year* | Dead 20% |
| | Dependent 20% |
| | Independent 60% |

## How to assess risk of a major stroke after TIA Statistics

- Risk of stroke after TIA varies from 1.0% to 8.1% risk within 48 hours of a Transient Ischemic Attack
- The ABCD score can predict those that are at a high risk of stroke within a short period of time.
- Age greater than 60 = 1 point
- Blood pressure greater than 140/90 = 1 point
- Neurological deficit is unilateral weakness = 2 point
- Speech Impairment without weakness = 1 point
- Duration of deficit 10–59 minutes = 1 point
- Duration greater than one hour = 2 points
- Diabetes = 1 point

### Risk assessment

- Score 6–7. High risk. 8.1% risk in 2 days
- Score 4–5. Moderate risk. 4.1%
- Score 0–3. Low risk. 1.0%

# Predisposing factors

### Fixed

- *Age:* Stroke risk increases with increasing age (strongest risk factor).
- *Sex:* Males > females
- *Ethnicity:* Higher in Blacks and Asians than in Whites living in the West. This is due to lack of access to health care and to increased incidence of obesity, hypertension, and diabetes.
- *Family history:* Positive family history increases risk. Not simple inheritance; there is a complex genetic–environmental interaction.
- *Previous stroke or TIA:* Risk of recurrence is about 10%–16% in the first year, being highest in the acute phase.
- *Other vascular disease:* Presence of any atheromatous disease (peripheral vascular disease, ischemic heart disease, renovascular disease) increases risk of stroke, as atheroma is rarely organ specific.

### Modifiable by lifestyle change

- *Smoking* is a causal, dose-related risk factor. Risk diminishes 5 years after quitting.
- *Alcohol intake:* There is a J-shaped relationship, where heavy drinking is a risk factor, but moderate intake is protective.
- *Obesity* increases the risk of all vascular events; it is confounded by an increase in other risk factors (hypertension, diabetes) but is probably a weak independent factor, especially central obesity.
- *Physical inactivity:* Increased risk of stroke in less active persons. Again, it is confounded by the presence of other risk factors in the inert; to date there is limited evidence that increased activity lowers risk.
- *Diet:* Healthy eaters have lower risk, but such individuals often have healthier lifestyles in general. Low-salt, high-antioxidant diets with lots of fruit, vegetables, and fish are likely to be protective, but trials have failed to show an effect.
- *Estrogens:* The oral contraceptive pill confers a slightly increased risk of stroke and should be avoided in the presence of other risk factors. Postmenopausal hormone replacement therapy has recently been shown to increase risk of ischemic stroke, but not of TIA or hemorrhagic stroke.

### Medically modifiable

- *Hypertension:* There is a clear association between increasing blood pressure (BP) and increased stroke risk across all population groups. Risk doubles with each 5–7 mmHg increase in diastolic BP. It also increases with systolic rises and even isolated systolic hypertension.
- *Diabetes:* Risk factor for stroke independent of increased hypertension.
- *High cholesterol:* This is a weaker risk factor than in heart disease, likely due to diversity of stroke etiologies.
- *Atrial fibrillation:* Risk of stroke is increased in AF (p. 284).
- *Carotid stenosis:* Risk increases with increasing stenosis and with the occurrence of symptoms attributable to the stenosis.
- *Other comorbidity:* Increased stroke risk in some conditions, such as sickle-cell anemia, blood diseases causing hyperviscosity, and vasculitides.

# Acute assessment

### History

- Is it a focal neurological deficit?
- Did it come on acutely and maximal at onset or is there a hint of progression? (Simple stroke may worsen over several days, but think of alternative diagnoses, e.g., tumor.)
- Is there headache, vomiting, nausea, or drowsiness? (Hemorrhage or posterior circulation stroke is more likely.)
- Was there a fall or other head trauma? Think subdural or epidural hemorrhages and obtain urgent CT scan and possibly neurosurgical evaluation.
- What are the vascular risk factors?
- What was the premorbid state?
- What are the comorbidities? (They increase chance of poor outcome.)
- What are the medications?
- Where does the patient live, and with whom? Who are the significant family members? Who is making decisions for the patient if he or she is not competent? What is the code status?

### Examination

*Glasgow coma scale (GCS)* (see Appendix)

Designed for use in head injury, the GCS is used as a standardized measure to assess neurological deterioration. A GCS score indicating unconsciousness or deterioration suggests hemorrhage, a large infarct with edema, or a brain stem event.

*National Institutes of Health (NIH) stroke scale*

This clinical evaluation instrument has documented reliability and validity. It is used increasingly to assess neurological outcome and degree of recovery in stroke. It is used to grade the following areas: consciousness, orientation, obeying commands, gaze, visual fields, facial weakness, motor function in the arm and leg, limb ataxia, sensory, language, dysarthria, and inattention. The scale is not useful in diagnosing stroke but in giving an assessment of severity of deficits and size of infarct.

*General examination*

- Vital signs: Airway, breathing, circulation (ABC) is always first.
- Temperature (especially after a long period on the floor)
- Cardiovascular examination (pulse rate and rhythm, blood pressure, cardiac examination for atrial fibrillation, evidence of dilated cardiomyopathy, endocarditis, and carotid bruits)
- Respiratory examination (aspiration pneumonia or pre-existing respiratory conditions)
- Abdominal examination (palpable bladder, organomegaly)

*Neurological examination*

This may need to be adapted if the patient is drowsy.

- Level of arousal and orientation, inattention
- *Speech:* dysarthria (trouble enunciating because of, e.g., facial weakness or posterior circulation stroke) or aphasia (cortical disruption of speech—may be receptive and/or expressive)

- *Expressive dysphasia*: Problems producing speech—patient may be fluent (lots of words that make no sense) or nonfluent. Nominal dysphasia is part of an expressive dysphasia and is tested by asking the patient to name increasingly rare objects (e.g., watch, hand, second hand).
- *Receptive dysphasia* is an inability to understand language. Test with one-stage commands: "Close your eyes," and progress to more complex tasks: "Put your left hand on your right ear." Use language only; do not mime the task. If comprehension is intact, reassure the patient that you know they can understand but are having difficulty finding the right words.
- *Cranial nerves:* Assess especially visual fields and visual inattention (if difficulty with compliance, test blink response to threat, and look for a gaze preference, which may occur with hemianopia or neglect), test swallow (not gag).
- *Motor strength:* Assess tone (may be diminished acutely), for any weakness (grade power for later comparison. Is the distribution pyramidal—i.e., arm flexors are stronger than extensors, leg extensors are stronger than flexors? If weakness is subtle, assess for pyramidal drift and fine movements of both hands; dominant should be better), and coordination (limited if power is diminished).
- *Coordination:* Conduct basic testing of finger to nose and heel to shin, looking for ataxia. Weakness itself with can present with a form of ataxia. A patient describing clumsiness without weakness should have special attention paid to the coordination examination.
- *Sensation:* There are easy bedside tests for fine touch and proprioception. If sensation is intact there are also tests for sensory inattention.
- *Gait:* Assess in a less severe stroke—is it safe?
- *Reflexes* may initially be absent, and then become brisker with time. Test plantar extensors on affected side.

## How to assess for neglects

Neglect occurs with parietal cortex damage, where there are errors in awareness of self—the patient's "automatic pilot" has gone wrong.

In extreme cases, the patient will not recognize their own arm and only wash half of their body. Lesser degrees are more common and complicate the rehabilitation process, as the patient must constantly be reminded of the existence of the affected side.

### To test

1. Establish that sensory input is present bilaterally—i.e., check that the patient can feel a touch to each hand individually and does not have a hemianopia (it may be hard to establish where extreme gaze preference exists).
2. Provide two stimuli at once (touch both hands together, or move fingers in both sides of the visual field) and see if the patient preferentially notices the sensory input on the good side. If so, there is inattention of the bad side.
3. Severe neglects can be diagnosed by asking the neglectful patient to clap. A severely neglectful patient will clap with the normal hand expecting to meet the other hand respecting the midline. The clap will be only the good hand and respecting the midline. Those without neglect will reach across the midline to clap with the normal and hemiplegic hand. This is referred to as the Eastchester clap sign.

Even if formal testing does not reveal neglect, sometimes it will become apparent during rehabilitation, often noted by therapists.

# Investigations

See Table 8.2.

**Table 8.2** Investigations for stroke

| Test | Rationale |
| --- | --- |
| Full blood count | • Anemic or polycythemic<br>• Elevated/depressed white count suggestive of sepsis<br>• High or low platelet count |
| Urea and electrolytes | • Look for evidence of dehydration, and assess fluid replacement<br>• Aim for electrolyte normalization |
| Liver function tests | • Baseline assessment<br>• Evidence of comorbidity |
| Creatine kinase | Evidence of muscle breakdown (if prolonged, lie on floor) |
| Glucose | • Diabetic—old or new diagnosis (elevated sugars initially may represent hyperglycemic stress response)<br>• Hypoglycemia may mimic stroke |
| Cholesterol | Vascular risk factor |
| ESR | Elevation in vasculitis or sepsis (including endocarditis) |
| CRP | Any evidence of sepsis (e.g., aspiration pneumonia, etc.) |
| Blood cultures | Consider if sepsis possible or new heart murmur heard (endocarditis) |
| Urinalysis | • Diabetic<br>• Vasculitis<br>• Urinary infection |
| ECG | • Assess rhythm<br>• Evidence of ischemic heart disease/myocardial infarction or previous hypertension |
| Chest X-ray | Useful in elderly—look for any sign of aspiration, the size of the heart size, etc. |

**Table 8.2** Investigations for stroke (*continued*)

| Test | Rationale |
| --- | --- |
| CT brain | • Guidelines advise CT as soon as possible, especially when considering CNS bleed in a patient on warfarin, or with a sudden drop in GCS, suggesting possible hydrocephalus.<br><br>• CT may distinguish stroke from non-stroke diagnoses such as tumor, identify whether this is a bleed or an infarct, facilitating antiplatelet therapy, and identify the likely cause of the event—carotid territory infarcts from stenosis, multiple infarcts from cardiac emboli, etc.<br><br>• Blood appears white in early CT; infarcts may not show acutely (6–24 hr), developing low-density areas ± surrounding edema after a few days.<br><br>• Small infarcts may never be seen, and the diagnosis is made clinically.<br><br>• A normal CT does not exclude a stroke.<br><br>• MRI can often see a small stroke missed by CT scanning.<br><br>• MRI is indicated for evaluation intracranial circulation. MRI diffusion-weighted imaging can detect stroke immediately and detect small strokes missed by CT scans. |
| Carotid Doppler | Request in carotid territory events with good recovery when the patient is a candidate for endarterectomy |
| Echocardiogram | Consider for multiple (?cardioembolic) infarcts, in atrial fibrillation, after a recent MI (looking for thrombus, or when there is a murmur. |

# Acute management

In 2007, the American Heart Association published guidelines for acute care.

## Diagnosis

- Care should occur on an acute stroke unit or an inpatient unit familiar with stroke care.
- Diagnosis should be made clinically (including assessment of likely cerebral area affected), confirmed with imaging and reviewed by a clinician with knowledge in stroke diagnosis and treatment.
- CT scan should be performed as soon as possible unless there is a good clinical reason for not doing so (e.g., dying patient for terminal care). MRI can be done for confirmation or elucidation when diagnosis is unclear and to screen intra- and extracranial vessels.

## Medical interventions

- Aspirin (81–325 mg) should be given as soon as possible after the onset of stroke symptoms if the diagnosis of hemorrhage is considered unlikely (usually after a scan—can be given via nasogastric [NG] tube or PR if swallowing has not yet been evaluated).
- Neurosurgical opinion should be sought for all cases of subdural, epidural hematomas and hydrocephalus (due to bleeds).
- Centrally acting drugs should be avoided (e.g., sedatives).
- There is a debate about optimal blood pressure in the acute phase: high blood pressure is harmful long term, but may be required to provide perfusion pressure with altered cerebral autoregulation acutely. Trials are ongoing. Guidelines state that blood pressure should not be lowered acutely in general, but that existing antihypertensives be continued.
- Oxygen supplementation should be given to hypoxic patients.
- Hydration should be maintained to ensure euvolemia and biochemical normality and monitored appropriately. This usually means giving 2 liters of normal saline intravenously (without dextrose) in the first 24 hours (unless the patient is alert and swallowing normally). This would be altered if admission electrolytes were deranged (e.g., hypokalemia) and reviewed after a repeat electrolyte measurement on day 2.
- Glucose should be measured and euglycemia maintained. The patient is likely to improve recovery of ischemic penumbral tissue.
- Hyperpyrexia should be lowered with treatment of the underlying cause and/or with use of acetaminophen or cooling blanket. High temperatures are associated with poorer outcomes, but the causal nature of this association is unknown.
- TED stockings or compressive devices should be used and subcutaneous (SC) heparin or low molecular weight heparinoids given to reduce deep venous thrombosis (DVT) and pulmonary embolus (PE).
- Seizures may occur (p. 152).
- Thrombolysis with tissue plasminogen activator for acute stroke should only be given in stroke centers with appropriate experience and expertise (see Stroke units, p. 182).

## Multidisciplinary acute input

- Protocols should be developed for early management, including monitoring consciousness level, assessing swallow (not gag), risk assessment for pressure sores (including nutritional status), cognitive impairment, bowel and bladder care (avoiding catheterization, if possible), and moving and handling requirements.
- Early speech and language therapy assessment should be done for all patients with swallow or language difficulties.
- Early mobilization with the physiotherapist is advised, and the therapist should have expertise in stroke rehabilitation.

### How to perform a bedside swallowing assessment

*General examination*
- Is the patient conscious and cooperative? If not, reassess later.
- If there is facial weakness, dysarthria, dysphasia, drooling, or respiratory symptoms, the likelihood of swallow impairment is higher.

*Preparation*
- Sit the patient upright.
- Listen to the chest to establish baseline.
- Ask the patient to cough, and note the strength and effectiveness.
- Conduct a water swallow evaluation.

*Why water?*
Use water for convenience—this is a screening test to establish whether the patient should have further assessments. A small volume is used to minimize the consequences of aspiration.

*Assessment*
1. Ask the patient to drink water from cup or straw.
2. Look for leakage of water from the closed mouth.
3. Ask the patient to swallow the water.
4. Watch for signs of aspiration—coughing and spluttering. Ask the patient to say their name and listen for gurgling or a "wet voice" that is different from before swallow. These signs may not occur for several minutes. Do not leave the bedside immediately.

*What next?*
*If the patient swallows without difficulty*
- Try 6 oz of water (drunk slowly).
- If they manage this safely, then allow them to eat and drink. This does not rule out silent aspirations.
- Reassess if concerns arise later. Consider speech and language pathology evaluation

*If there are problems*
- Ask the patient to remain NPO and inform the nursing staff.
- Alternative means of hydration will be required at once—an IV drip or NG tube is common (the latter also allows medication to be given).
- Further assessment will be needed by a speech and language pathology evaluation that can stratify the swallow impairment and make a plan for safe oral intake, reviewing patient at regular intervals.
- Nutrition will need to be considered if the swallow is not safe—consider NG feeding and involvement of a dietician.

# Stroke units

### Definition
This is a geographically defined unit staffed by a coordinated multidisciplinary team with expertise in stroke The gold standard is probably to admit strokes directly and continue care through to discharge; this unit is known as a comprehensive stroke unit.

Resource limitations may mean that not all stroke patients pass through the unit, or that the length of stay is cut short. Some units deal with acute admissions only, others with the post-acute rehabilitation phase only. Coordinated stroke care can also be provided on a general rehabilitation ward or by roving stroke teams who visit all stroke patients on general wards.

### Benefits
Compared with general hospital, stroke units have lower rates of death, dependency, and institutional care, without lengthening hospital stay. The number needed to treat in a stroke unit to prevent one death or dependency is 18.

### Rationale
Most of the improvement seems to occur in the first 4 weeks; the reason for this is unclear.

Key components of stroke units include the following:
- Meticulous attention to physiological homeostasis
- Attention to prevention of complications (such as thromboembolic disease and pressure sores)
- Early mobilization
- Coordinated multidisciplinary team care
- Interest, expertise, and motivation of staff

The individual impact of each of these is unknown, but combined they confer significant benefits to the stroke patient.

# Thrombolysis

### Rationale

In acute ischemic stroke, an artery becomes occluded by thrombus in situ or embolus, and blood supply is compromised. Death of surrounding brain tissue results in deficits in function associated with that part of the brain. Early recanalization of the vessel by lysing thrombus may limit the extent of brain injury.

### Agents

The most frequently used agent is intravenous recombinant tissue plasminogen activator (rt-PA).

### Risks

Treatment with thrombolysis leads to a higher rate of death in hospital due to intracranial hemorrhage (a 5-fold increase over placebo).

### Benefits

Despite early excess of deaths due to hemorrhage, treatment with thrombolysis leads on average to 44 fewer dead or dependent patients per 1000 treated with r-tPA within 6 hours, and 126 fewer dead or dependent patients per 1000 treated with rt-PA within 3 hours.

### Imaging

This should be done prior to giving thrombolysis to exclude hemorrhage. Perfusion and diffusion-weighted MRI scans may give more information than that with CT. Both need to be interpreted by someone with the appropriate experience, prior to thrombolysis.

### Use

Overall, use of thrmobolysis is recommended in specialist centers with sufficient expertise in stroke and with facilities to deal with complications. In these centers, intravenous rt-PA is considered in all patients with definite ischemic stroke who present within 3 hours of the onset of symptoms.

Careful discussion with the patient and family of risks and benefits is recommended.

# Ongoing management

This should involve all of the multidisciplinary team.

**Dieticians** calculate food and fluid requirements for each individual patient and adapt the patient's diet for specific needs (e.g., diabetic, weight loss). The dietician can also develop regimens for NG or percutaneous endoscopic gastrostomy (PEG) feeds (see Box 8.1), advise on the provision of modified diets for stages of swallow recovery (thickened, pureed, etc.), and review nutrition as recovery alters needs.

**Doctors** confirm diagnosis, manage medical complications, and establish therapies.

**Nurses** monitor the patient continuously and assist with basic care (physiological and physical), including ongoing bowel and bladder management and ongoing skin care. Nurses also facilitate practice of skills acquired in therapy, promote functional independence, and are the first point of call for relatives.

**Occupational therapists** optimize functional ability (usually beginning with upper-limb work, coordinating with the physiotherapist) and perform specific assessments of certain tasks (washing and dressing, kitchen safety, occupational tasks, etc.) as recovery continues. They also assess adaptation to the home environment through a series of home visits, with and without the patient, supply aids (rails, bed levers, toilet raises, bath boards, etc.), and provide wheelchairs where needed.

**Pharmacists** review charts and promote safe prescribing.

**Physiotherapists** assess muscle tone, movement, and mobility, and maximize functional independence through education and exercise. They monitor respiratory function and initial bed mobility, then help the patient work on sitting balance, transfers, and, finally, standing and stepping. Physiotherapists help prevent complications such as shoulder pain, contractures and immobility-associated problems (pressure sores, DVT/PE).

**Psychologists** assess the psychological impact of stroke on the patient and family, and allow the patient to talk about the impact of the illness. They monitor for depression and other mood disorders, highlighting the need for medication. Psychologists document cognitive impairment and assist in retraining when neglect is prominent.

**Social workers** provide psychosocial assessment of the patient and family and support with financial matters (accessing pension, arranging power of attorney, financing placement, etc.). They offer advice and support for the patient and family on accommodation needs, especially finding a care-home placement, and are a link to community services (care package, community rehabilitation, day centers, etc.)

**Speech and language pathologists** assess the patient's ability to swallow (bedside ± video swallow testing) and establish a plan for safe oral intake. They reassess and plan the nutritional route during recovery and provide language screening (dysarthria, aphasia, and cognitive dysfunction) with interventions to improve deficits.

## Box 8.1 Feeding and stroke

Many patients will have acute impairment of the ability to swallow, and early identification is necessary to prevent aspiration. Hydration is essential at this time, but if the problem persists beyond 24 hours or so (research has not showed significant advantages in feeding in the very acute phase), nutritional support should be given unless the patient is terminal.

Passing a NG tube allows medication to be given as usual as well as feeding, but it is uncomfortable and may become dislodged. If the patient continues to have swallowing problems, a PEG feeding tube may be inserted, especially if the feeding issues are likely to resolve as the deficits from the stroke improve.

The need for this should be regularly reviewed. A feeding tube can fairly easily be removed, making it appropriate for both medium- and long-term feeding. See Chapter 12, The ethics of artificial feeding (p. 370) for discussion of the ethics of feeding.

## How to protect your patient from another stroke

Ensure that the following are addressed:
- Smoking, diet, and exercise
- Antiplatelet therapy
  - Aspirin reduces the relative risk of a further event by about 25%. The dose is probably not important—generally, use 81–325 mg.
  - Stroke events that occur on aspirin ("aspirin failures") do not necessarily imply that aspirin is inadequate, but there may be an argument for increasing the dose (there may be dose-dependent aspirin resistance), adding another antiplatelet agent (e.g., dipyridamole), or, rarely, changing the agent (e.g., to clopidogrel).
  - While adding clopidogrel to aspirin increases antiplatelet activity, it has been shown to increase the risk of cerebral hemorrhage and is no longer recommended for secondary prevention of stroke.
- Lower blood pressure: the choice of agent is debated. The important thing is probably just to lower the blood pressure, but there is growing evidence for the use of ACE inhibitors and thiazide diuretics as first-line treatment. If there are no contraindications, lowering blood pressure per se is likely to be beneficial, but aim for <130/85.
- Lower cholesterol: It has been known for some time that lowering cholesterol is useful secondary prevention in coronary disease, but only recently has the Heart Protection Study shown that there is benefit also in preventing stroke, and specifically in older patients. Probably the lower the cholesterol the better, as long as no medication side effects occur.
- Anticoagulation for AF: see Chapter 10, Atrial fibrillation: anticoagulation (p. 290). With infarction, it is likely safe to start warfarin after 2 weeks. With hemorrhage, judge each case individually (probably wait several months for hemorrhagic transformation; anticoagulation may never be appropriate in primary bleed).
- Carotid endarterectomy (CEA): >70% symptomatic stenosis carries a stroke risk of about 15% per year and is an indication for endarterectomy when there is good recovery and the patient is fit for surgery. If the patient is not a surgical candidate consider carotid stenting. Perform CEA early for greater benefit.

# Complications

During a prolonged admission for a large stroke, a number of problems occur frequently.

### Contractures

These are a longer-term complication.

### Fecal incontinence

This may be due to immobility, cognitive problems, or neurological impairment. Regulate the patient's bowel habit, when possible, with a high-fiber diet and good fluid intake and toilet regularly. If all else fails, deliberately constipating the patient with codeine and using regular enemas can work. See Chapter 12, Constipation (p. 380).

### Infection

Commonly infection occurs in the chest or urinary tract. Think of it early if a patient becomes drowsy, confused, or appears to deteriorate neurologically. Prompt septic screening and treatment with antibiotics, oxygen, and hydration are indicated in most patients in the acute phase (stroke outcome is very unclear initially) but may be withheld in a more established stroke where the prognosis can more confidently be assessed as dismal (this decision is made with the family).

### Muscle spasm

This is very common on the affected side. Arthritic joints are exacerbated by spasm, and antispasmodics may need to be used alongside analgesia for effective pain relief. Consider baclofen 5 mg (initially twice a day), or tizanidine 2 mg daily (increased slowly after a few days if needed, up to a maximum of 24 mg daily). Watch out for drowsiness and loss of tone in the affected side, which can hinder therapy.

### Pain

Commonly there is shoulder pain in a paralyzed arm. It is usually multifactorial—e.g., joint subluxation (treat with physiotherapy to strengthen muscles and arm support) interacting with muscle spasm and shoulder arthritis. Central post-stroke pain tends to afflict all of the affected side and can be treated with amitriptyline (start low, e.g., 10 mg at night).

### Pressure sores

These should be avoidable in the majority of patients; see Chapter 18, Pressure sores (p. 522).

### Psychological problems

Low mood is extremely common post-stroke (at 4 months, a quarter of patients will be depressed, and over half of these remain depressed 1 year after the stroke). This is unrelated to stroke type, but is associated with a worse outcome (perhaps because of less motivation to participate in therapy).

It should be actively sought in the patient (the screening question "Do you think you are depressed?" is quick and effective). Low mood may also be noticed by nurses, therapists, or family members. Tools such as the

Geriatric Depression Scale can also be used, but may be confounded by dysphasia.

Treatment is with psychosocial support and antidepressants (e.g., citalopram 20 mg). Anxiety is also very common and often responds well to explanation of this reaction and empowerment of the patient.

## Thromboembolism

This is very common post-stroke, especially if the patient is very immobile. Mobilize the patient early and use full-length compression stockings and aspirin to prevent occurrence. Low-dose heparin (5000 IU every 8 hours SC for high-risk patients) or low-molecular-weight heparinoids may have a role in bed-bound patients, but there is some evidence against it (there is increased risk of hemorrhage when all doses are considered). Have a low threshold for investigating a leg that becomes swollen or painful.

---

### How to manage urinary incontinence after stroke

This is very common, even more so after severe stroke. It does, however, improve over time, and a flexible approach is required to ensure that a patient does not get catheterized and remain so.
- Initially, try to manage incontinence with pads and regular toileting.
- If the skin starts to break down, or if the burden on caregivers is heavy, then a catheter can be inserted *for a limited time span.*
- Once mobility improves, try removing the catheter—ensure that this is seen by all as a positive and exciting step toward independence, as removal can cause considerable anxiety.
- If this fails, check for and treat urinary tract infection, then try again.
- If this fails, then replace the catheter and use bladder-stabilizing agents for about 2 weeks (e.g., tolterodine 2–4 mg/day) before removing it again.
- The need for a permanent catheter post-stroke should be reviewed regularly, as the condition is likely to improve. See also Chapter 20, Catheters (p. 560).

# Longer-term issues

## Return to the community

This is best coordinated by the stroke multidisciplinary team. Early discharge may be useful if the patient can transfer and there is a specialist community stroke team available. Later discharges are planned by the team, usually after careful assessment of the patient's needs (home alterations, care packages, etc.).

The general practitioner should be alerted to continue medical monitoring, in particular, optimizing secondary prevention. Community teams (district nurses, community rehabilitation teams, home care, etc.) should be aware of the patient's needs (continence, diabetic monitoring, ongoing therapy needs) and ideally be involved in the discharge planning.

The patient and family should have adequate information and training, as well as a contact point in case of problems (stroke coordinators often take this role). Voluntary agencies (e.g., the Stroke Association: www.stroke.org.) are often helpful and the patient should be alerted to them.

Ensure that the patient is aware of driving restrictions before discharge.

## Driving regulations with cerebrovascular disease

These vary from state to state (also see Chapter 30, The older driver). In general, restrictions apply to
- Patients with visual field cuts
- Significant cognitive deficits
- Loss of consciousness

## Follow-up

Some follow-up should be offered to all stroke survivors (see Box 8.2). The intensity and duration of inpatient care can contrast sharply with home. The realities of living with disability begin to sink in, and many questions and anxieties arise. Even minor strokes or TIAs require a further point of contact, as patients will have been committed to lifelong medication and will need monitoring of risk factors.

In addition, stroke recovery continues (albeit at a slower pace) for up to 2 years (or even longer) and management plans made at discharge may need to be adapted.

## Box 8.2 Checklist for follow-up after discharge

### Secondary prevention
- Check drugs, blood pressure, diabetic control, and cardiac rhythm.

### Continence
- Are there continence problems?
- If a catheter is in situ, has mobility improved to a point at which trial removal can be done?
- If the patient was discharged on bladder-stabilizing drugs and has remained continent, can these be tailed off?

### Nutrition
- Is nutrition adequate? If not, refer to dietician.
- If a PEG tube is in place is it still required?
- Does the patient warrant another assessment of swallowing to allow oral nutrition to begin?

### Communication and speech
- Are there still problems?
- Is there a need for a speech and language therapy review?

### Mood
- Is the patient depressed?
- Do they need referral to a psychologist or (rarely) psychiatrist?
- If discharged on an antidepressant, can it be discontinued?

### Physical progress
- Is there ongoing physical therapy?
- If not, is there continued improvement? If the patient has deteriorated, refer them for assessment for further therapy (AMA guidelines).

### Contractures
- Are any contractures developing? If so, refer to physiotherapy.

### Muscle spasms
- Have these developed or lessened since discharge?
- Review need for antispasmodic medication—titrate down if no longer required.

### Pain
- Commonly in shoulder, or post-stroke pain
- Has this developed or lessened?
- Review need for medications.

### Daily living
- Are there any issues in managing day-to-day life?
- Is all the necessary equipment in place? (And is it still needed, e.g., a commode can be returned when the patient is able to mobilize to the toilet alone.)
- Is there anything they would like to be able to do that they cannot? (e.g., read a book, take a bath)

### Support
- Are they in contact with a community stroke coordinator?
- Are they aware of voluntary organizations?

# Rapid TIA evaluation

Rapid outpatient assessment of TIA and minor stroke is needed to establish diagnosis, commence secondary prevention, and lower risk of a subsequent event.

## How fast?

Guidelines suggest as soon as possible and certainly less than 7 days. New data suggest that the risk of a second event after TIA or minor stroke is 8%–12% at 1 week, making earlier assessment seem sensible. Daily clinics or specialist services based in emergency departments may not be easily achieved, but may prove to be optimal as stroke medicine evolves.

Currently, early antiplatelet agents and early endarterectomy are known to be beneficial. The timing of blood pressure lowering and statin use has yet to be quantified. New therapies are being developed that are aimed at limiting the ischemic penumbra, where timing is likely to be crucial. The concept of "brain attack" in which "time is brain" (analogous to "heart attack") is quickly evolving.

## Function

### Confirm diagnosis

Diagnosis can be very variable, but up to a third of referrals for TIA are non-cerebrovascular. The main alternatives are cardiac dysrhythmias, orthostatic hypotension, other systemic disease (infection, endocrine), or, rarely, brain tumor or demyelination.

### Arrange investigations

These serve to aid diagnosis (e.g., CT brain, MRI or MRA head and neck) or investigate risk factors (e.g., full blood count, ESR, glucose, cholesterol, ECG, carotid Doppler, possibly chest X-ray, and echocardiogram). Carotid imaging is probably of greatest importance to do quickly, as carotid disease is a surgically treatable disorder with a high rate of recurrent events.

### Modify risk factors

Set targets for blood pressure and glucose control. Advise the patient about use of antiplatelet agents and anticoagulation in AF and about statin use, refer them for carotid endarterectomy, and advise about smoking cessation.

### Rehabilitation

If the patient has truly had a TIA then this should not be necessary. If this is required, the patient probably had a stroke. Provide point of referral for physiotherapy, occupational therapy, and speech and language therapy as outpatient or inpatient, as required.

### Education

Education of patients, relatives, and primary care doctors needs to be provided. Discuss stroke disease and its modification, time frame for recovery, psychological aspects of stroke, and driving restrictions.

### Time for explanation

Many patients will feel overwhelmed by the amount of information they are being given. The specialist nurse can be very helpful in clarifying things, and through leaflets the information can be revisited at home. Remember, we are often prescribing several new tablets, or even suggesting surgery for a patient who feels well. Comprehension is vital for adherence.

### Rapid access to investigations

Rapid access is particularly necessary for carotid Doppler imaging, CT scanning, and echocardiography. Many clinics run a "one-stop" service, where all assessments, investigations, and conclusions are completed at a single visit. Other clinics have dedicated time slots that give priority to the patients attending that day.

### Prompt communication to general practitioner

Advice about risk reduction must be relayed promptly to the primary care doctor for maximum benefit. Ideally, this information is delivered the same day by fax or by the patient.

## Further reading

Adams HP Jr, del Zoppo G, Alberts MJ, et al. (2007). Guidelines for the early management of adults with ischemic stroke. *Stroke*; **38**:1655–1711.

Albers GW, Caplan LR, Easton JD, Fayad PB, Mohr JP, Saver JL, Sherman DG (2002). TIA Working Group. Transient ischemic attack—proposal for a new definition. *N Engl J Med* **347** (21):1713–1716.

Johnston SC, Rothwell PM, Nguyen-Huynh MN, Giles MF, Elkins JS, Bernstein AL, Sidney S (2007). Validation and refinement of scores to predict very early stroke risk after transient ischaemic attack. *Lancet* **369**(9558):283–292.

# Chapter 9

# Psychiatry

**Cynthia Fields**
**Constantine Lyketsos**

# Delirium: overview

*Delirium* is a neuropsychiatric syndrome characterized by a disturbance in consciousness and cognition. It typically presents as an acute confusional state, with inattention as its core symptom. Confusion is not specific to delirium; it may be found in other psychiatric disorders, such as dementia or depression.

The acute onset and fluctuating course of delirium help to distinguish it from other disorders. It is important to note that while delirium typically develops over hours or days (e.g., during a hospitalization), it may also be more slowly evolving (e.g., during the weeks leading up to presentation). Acute confusion in an older person should be considered delirium until proven otherwise.

Because delirium may be secondary to a life-threatening illness, it is important to recognize delirium and to initiate treatment early. For an older patient who is unable to mount fever, for example, delirium may be the first sign that an infection is present. In addition, delirium itself can be life threatening. Potential dangers of delirium are numerous: dehydration from decreased PO intake, injury from pulling out IV lines and falling out of bed, consequences of agitation, etc.

Unfortunately, the diagnosis of delirium is often delayed or missed, especially the hypoactive form that is common in older persons. The syndrome of delirium is a clinical (i.e., bedside) diagnosis, and a high index of suspicion may be required.

Delirium may be viewed as a cascade of events. General medical conditions (e.g., infection) and substances (e.g., medications), often in an additive fashion, may precipitate delirium in a predisposed individual. Persons with dementia are particularly vulnerable to the development of delirium.

Although the pathogenesis is poorly understood, delirium is thought to involve cholinergic deficiency and dopaminergic excess. Delirium is often reversible with treatment of the underlying condition(s). Perhaps even more importantly, delirium is potentially preventable (e.g., by minimizing medication use and ensuring adequate hydration).

Delirium is common in hospital settings. Though estimates vary, it is widely accepted that at least 15%–30% of hospitalizations are complicated by delirium. Delirium prolongs hospital stays and results in increased morbidity and mortality.

The symptoms of delirium may persist long after the precipitant has been removed. The presence of comorbid dementia in particular delays recovery from delirium by weeks to months. In delirious patients whose functional status declines significantly during hospitalization, the making of irreversible decisions (e.g., home vs. residential care) should be postponed until they have a chance to fully recover from delirium so that their final functional level is established.

Delirium is a medical emergency. Initiate treatment early.

# Delirium: diagnosis

While delirium is a recognizable syndrome, its presentation is variable both within and between patients. Besides fluctuating day to day or hour to hour, delirium manifests distinctly in different patients.

### Key features of delirium[1]

#### 1. Disturbance of consciousness

Awareness of the environment is impaired, referred to as "clouded." Sensorium is not clear. Inattention is the core symptom, with decreased ability to focus, shift, or sustain attention. The patient may be easily distracted, may repeat questions or perseverate, and may be unable to follow commands. Often the patient cannot sustain attention enough to fully participate in a conversation. After recovery, memory for the period will be poor.

#### 2. Change in cognition

Cognitive changes are typically global, with disorientation (especially to time), memory impairment (recent memory in particular), and language disturbance (e.g., dysgraphia, dysnomia). Perceptual disturbances may occur, such as hallucinations (typically visual) and illusions (misinterpretation of an external stimulus, e.g., slamming door = gunshot). If delusions occur, they are usually persecutory in nature, transient, and not well-formed. Thinking is disorganized. Speech may be rambling.

#### 3. Acute onset, and fluctuating course

The usual onset of delirium is over hours or a few days. Sometimes changes are subacute (weeks to a few months) and may be misdiagnosed as dementia or depression. Severity of symptoms varies during the course of a day, and symptoms typically will worsen at night. "Lucid intervals" are characteristic. A classic example is a patient who was cooperative and AAOX3 (awake, alert, and oriented x3 [person, place, and time]) on morning rounds becomes confused in the evening, attempting to pull out IV lines and get out of bed.

### Other associated features of delirium

#### Change in psychomotor behavior

Patients may have psychomotor agitation ("hyperactive"), psychomotor slowing ("hypoactive"), or a mix of features ("mixed delirium").

- *Hyperactive:* oversensitive to stimuli, agitated, restless, picking at bedclothes, repeatedly getting out of bed, wandering, noisy (e.g., may call out, scream, or moan), vigilant and aggressive, typically with psychotic symptoms. *Symptoms are often obvious.*
- *Hypoactive:* lethargic, slow, immobile, excessively sleepy or somnolent (but arousable), quiet, with occasional incoherent speech, not drinking or eating, with few or no psychotic symptoms. *This presentation is much more subtle and therefore more often missed.*

One-third of elderly patients have **hypoactive delirium**. In addition to the above, they are withdrawn, are quiet and passive, and sleep a lot. Such patients may answer brief questions but then drift off as if the interaction did not happen. This interaction can be mistaken for passivity or disinterest.

Hypoactive delirium is easy to miss, especially if the patient cooperates with basic hospital routines.

### Emotional disturbances

The full range of mental status abnormalities can be seen in delirium. Patients may exhibit anxiety, fear, irritability, anger, depression, or euphoria, with sudden shifts in emotion. Acute paranoia and aggression may occur in response to hallucinations or delusions. Apathy and with-drawal are other common presentations. These mental status examination (MSE) abnormalities are often what prompt a psychiatric consultation (e.g., to evaluate for depression, dementia, or psychotic disorder).

### Alteration of the sleep–wake cycle

Sleep is fragmented. Patients are typically drowsy during the day and have insomnia at night. A complete reversal of the sleep–wake cycle may occur.

### Poor insight

Poor insight is typical in delirium. Patients are not aware of their deficits and will not attempt to cover them up.

## Screening tests for delirium

Making the diagnosis of delirium can be difficult. Screening tests (typi-cally the MMSE or the CAM) are valuable and may be easily administered. Screening tests should be performed in all older persons upon admission, and serially during the hospitalization. Unlike some aspects of the physical examination, it is necessary to fully wake up the patient to assess cognition. This will alert the clinician if changes in the clinical condition occur. Both tests can be reliably administered by nursing staff.

- *Mini-Mental State Exam (MMSE)*[2] may be used to detect cognitive impairments. Items most often missed in delirium are orientation (time), calculation, and three-item recall at 5 minutes; registration and naming are likely to be intact. This exam is less sensitive and not specific for delirium.
- *Confusion Assessment Method (CAM)*[3] operationalizes the *Diagnostic and Statistical Manual of Mental Disorders (DSM)* criteria in an algorithm format. Diagnosis of delirium requires the following: acute onset and fluctuating course, inattention, and EITHER disorganized thinking OR altered level of consciousness. Sensitivity and specificity are >90%. It is available for free download at: www.hartfordign.org.

**1.** American Psychiatric Association. (2000). *Diagnostic and Statistical Manual of Mental Disorders, fourth edition, Text Revision.* Arlington, VA: American Psychiatric Association,

**2.** Folstein MF, Folstein SE, McHugh PR (1975). Mini-Mental State: a practical method for grading the cognitive state of patients for the clinician. *J Psychiatr Res* **12**:189–198.

**3.** Inouye S, van Dyck CH, Alessi CA, et al. (1990). Clarifying confusion: the Confusion Assessment Method. A new method for detection of delirium. *Ann Intern Med* **113**:941–948.

### How to distinguish delirium from dementia

The most common challenge in diagnosing the older patient with confusion is whether the patient has delirium, dementia, or both (i.e., delirium is often superimposed on a pre-existing dementia). The history, particularly the duration of symptoms, is key to making the diagnosis. Information from medical records and reliable informants, such as family members, will help determine whether dementia was present before the onset of delirium.

| Feature | Delirium | Dementia |
|---|---|---|
| Mode of onset | Acute or subacute | Chronic or subacute |
| Fluctuation | Diurnal or hour-to-hour fluctuation common | Generally little diurnal variation*, although some worsening later in the day ("sundowning") |
| Poor attention | Yes (but may fluctuate) | In more severe disease |
| Consciousness | Usually impaired (but may fluctuate); can be subtle | Normal; patient accessible and engageable |
| Hallucinations and misinterpretations | Common | In more severe disease* |
| Fear, agitation, aggression | Common | In more severe disease |
| Disorganized thought, unreal ideas | Common | In more severe disease |
| Motor signs | Tremor, myoclonus, asterixis common | More severe or in certain forms (e.g., vascular or Lewy body disease) |
| Speech | May be dysarthric, dysnomic | Normal, unless associated with certain brain diseases. |
| Dysgraphia | Often present | Usually late |
| Short- (STM) and long-term memory (LTM) | Both are poor | STM is poor. LTM may be normal until more severe disease |
| Reversibility | Often reversible | Rarely reversible |

\* Note: Lewy body dementia is characterized by fluctuating consciousness, alertness, and cognition, as well as prominent visual hallucinations.

# Delirium: causes

A particular case of delirium is often **multifactorial**. One or more precipitating factors combine to push a predisposed patient across his or her threshold to delirium. Even more minor acute illnesses (classically, a urinary tract infection [UTI]) can cause delirium in an older person who is predisposed (e.g., has dementia). In this context, think of dementia as the equivalent of ischemic cardiomyopathy, and delirium as the equivalent of superimposed acute congestive heart failure.

Usually there is evidence of the general medical condition and/or substance that has led to delirium. Although this is not necessary to make the diagnosis of delirium, it is necessary to treat the delirium effectively. Delirium is generally reversible and will resolve with treatment of the underlying medical condition(s). All contributing factors need to be addressed.

## Predisposing factors

- **Dementia** or other cognitive disorder
- Advanced age (i.e., 65 and older), male gender
- Physically frail or immobile
- Sensory impairment (i.e., hearing or vision)
- Malnutrition or dehydration
- Polypharmacy, especially multiple psychoactive drugs
- History of excessive alcohol intake
- Severe illness or multiple medical comorbidities

## Precipitating factors

- **Medications:** most commonly, anticholinergic drugs, psychotropics (especially sedative hypnotics), and opiates. Effects of polypharmacy, e.g., additive side effects, elevated lithium level secondary to hydrochlorothiazide (HCTZ). See Box 9.1.
- Infection: viral or bacterial, not necessarily severe. Common sources are urine (UTI/catheter), chest (lower respiratory tract or pneumonia), and skin. Also central nervous system (CNS), abdomen, etc. bacteremia, early sepsis, septicemia
- Metabolic disorder, e.g., hypo- or hyperglycemia, dehydration, electrolyte imbalance (Na, K, Ca), acid–base disturbance, uremia, renal encephalopathy, hepatic encephalopathy, hypoalbuminemia, thyroid dysfunction
- CNS pathology, e.g., CNS infection, stroke, seizure (ictal or postictal), head trauma, subdural hematoma, mass or lesion
- Cardiopulmonary disorder, e.g., myocardial infarction (MI) (may be silent), arrythmia, congestive heart failure (CHF), acute blood loss, anemia, hypoxia or hypercarbia, respiratory failure
- Alcohol or drugs. Alcohol and benzodiazepine withdrawal can be life threatening. A classic sign of withdrawal is tremulousness. Monitor for progression to alcohol withdrawal delirium (i.e., delirium tremens). Avoid precipitating Wernicke's encephalopathy—always give thiamine before glucose. Intoxication of illicit drugs can mimic delirium.

- Surgery and trauma. Delirium in the postoperative state is particularly common in older people status post (S/P) hip fracture repair, coronary artery bypass graft (CABG) surgery, or vascular surgery.
- Fever or hypothermia
- Constipation or urinary retention
- Unrecognized or inadequately treated pain
- Environmental factors, e.g., moves within the hospital, sensory deprivation, sleep deprivation, use of restraints

---

### Box 9.1 Drugs causing delirium

- **Anticholinergics**: diphenhydramine
- **Anxiolytics**: benzodiazepines, e.g., lorazepam
- **Sedative hypnotics**: barbiturates, benzodiazepines, zolpidem
- **Antipsychotic drugs**: chlorpromazine, thioridazine
- **Tricyclic antidepressants**: amitrityline, imipramine
- **Lithium**
- **Anticonvulsant drugs**: phenytoin, carbamazepine
- **Opioid analgesics**: meperidine, codeine, tramadol
- **Alcohol and Illicit drugs**: marijuana, LSD, amphetamines, cocaine, opiates, and inhalants may cause delirium
- **Antihistamines**: hydroxyzine, diphenhydramine.
- **H2 receptor blockers**: cimetidine, ranitidine
- **Corticosteroids**: prednisone/prednisolone
- **Antiparkinsonian**: L-dopa, dopamine agonists, benztropine
- **Cardiovascular drugs**: digoxin/digitalis, antihypertensives
- **Diuretics**

Both newly added and long-standing medications can be associated with delirium. Any drug may be the "final straw" that leads to overt delirium. For example, a septic patient who has previously tolerated Tylenol with codeine may become delirious when it is again administered in the hospital. Or in the summer, mild dehydration might compound polypharmacy, leading to delirium.

# Delirium: assessment

Remember that delirium is a clinical diagnosis. Thorough chart review is essential in making a proper diagnosis. Because symptoms wax and wane, a delirious patient may be clear during any one examination. Therefore, 24-hour documentation, such as nursing notes, can be particularly helpful.

Once the diagnosis of delirium has been made, the cause(s) of the delirium needs to be determined. Most contributing factors (e.g., medications) can be identified by doing the H&P and by reviewing available labs.

### History and physical examination (H&P)

- Attempt the history even if the patient appears confused or forgetful. They will likely report ongoing symptoms (e.g., pain) if asked.
- **Obtain history from an informant in all cases.** Include the acuity of any cognitive changes, medication history, and any recent symptoms (e.g., cough).
- Inquire about alcohol and sedative (benzodiazepine) use. Carefully review the medical history for occult substance use.
- Focus the physical examination. Pay particular attention to signs of infection (including skin), new focal neurological deficits, and hydration status.
- Check vital signs regularly, especially temperature. Obtain pulse oximetry. Monitor fluid intake and output.
- Always assess cognition objectively, e.g., using the MMSE or the CAM. Establish a baseline. Serial testing may be used to track the condition.
- If a patient is noncompliant with any part of the examination, use distraction (such as chatting) or complete the examination in parts.

### Investigation

- One contributing factor may be obvious (e.g., UTI), but do not assume that this is the sole, or even the most important, factor until others have been excluded.
- All patients should have some baseline tests. These will vary according to the clinical picture, the availability of tests, and whether a clear cause is already apparent. See Box 9.2.
- If the cause remains unclear despite a careful history, thorough examination, and routine labs, it is best to repeat the clinical assessment. Consider less common causes and obtain more advanced tests such as CT/MRI brain or cerebrospinal fluid (CSF) examination.

## Box 9.2 Laboratory workup for delirium

*Basic laboratory tests*
- Complete blood count (CBC)
- Electrolytes, including Ca, Mg, phosphate
- Glucose (although hypo- or hyperglycemia may have normalized)
- BUN/Cr ratio
- Liver function tests (LFT) and albumin
- Chest X-ray
- Electrocardiogram (ECG)
- Urinalysis. Asymptomatic bacteriuria is common and may not explain a patient's delirium. Look for additional causes.

*Additional laboratory tests as indicated*
- Arterial blood gas (ABG). Even mild hypoxemia may indicate important cardiopulmonary pathology. *Pulse oximetry may be inadequate.*
- Blood cultures
- Thyroid function tests. Thyroid dysfunction may be contributing.
- Other blood tests, e.g., ammonia, $B_{12}$ and folate, VDRL, HIV, ESR
- Urine culture and sensitivity
- Urine drug screen
- Drug levels, e.g., digoxin, theophylline, lithium
- Lumbar puncture (LP)
- Head CT or MRI
- Electroencephalogram (EEG). In this context, EEG is used to differentiate delirium from depression or a psychotic disorder. Delirium will be evidenced by diffuse slowing of cortical background activity.

# Delirium: treatment

Prevention of delirium is the best strategy. Modify risk factors whenever possible. Examples include adequate nutrition and hydration, and the use of eyeglasses and hearing aids. Several of the "treatments" for delirium, such as frequent reorientation and appropriate pain management, can also be used to prevent the development of delirium. These techniques should be used routinely in all older patients.

In the case of routine or elective surgery or procedures (e.g., cataract repair, colonoscopy, hip fracture repair) in predisposed patients with dementia, delirium can be prevented by minimizing exposure to anesthetics and augmenting agents, anticipating its possible occurrence, and making sure familiar faces are around in recovery.

## Nonpharmacologic management

- Identify and treat all underlying causes. Provide supportive care, e.g., fluid, nutrition, supplemental oxygen. Discontinue all unnecessary medications. Limit the use of bladder catheters.
- Create a calm, comfortable environment with appropriate lighting and orienting influences (e.g., clock, calendar, items familiar to the patient). Keep the environment consistent by limiting staff and room changes.
- Optimize visual and auditory acuity with glasses and hearing aids.
- Reorient and reassure the patient frequently. Explain all procedures. Enlist the help of family members to reorient and reassure the patient.
- Normalize the sleep–wake cycle. During the day, use bright lights and open the blinds. Encourage activity, with early mobilization as tolerated. Darken the room and minimize interruptions to sleep at night.
- *Avoid the use of physical restraints.* A "sitter" is preferred and might be a family member. Restraints may increase agitation and result in injury. In cases of severe aggression, where parenteral drugs are required, brief immobilization of the patient using the minimum force necessary may be in the patient's best interests. Document the necessity clearly in the medical record and re-evaluate often.
- *Patients with delirium often lack decisional capacity.* If a delirious patient attempts to leave against medical advice, consider executing a Physician's Emergency Certificate (PEC) to hold the patient in the hospital for continued evaluation and treatment.

## Pharmacologic treatments

Use medications judiciously. Drugs are needed only when the agitation that accompanies delirium is causing significant patient distress, is threatening the safety of the patient or others, and/or is interfering with medical evaluation or treatment.

Drugs should complement, not replace, non-drug approaches. It is preferable to use only one drug, starting at a low dose. The correct dose is the minimum effective dose. The patient's response (adverse and beneficial) should be evaluated regularly and the medication adjusted accordingly. Once the behavioral symptoms have improved, consider step-wise dose reduction. Aim to stop the drug as soon as possible without prompting relapse.

In general, medical teams should attempt one drug, typically haloperidol, and obtain psychiatric consultation if that is not successful. In the absence of alcohol or benzodiazepine withdrawal, the use of benzodiazepines is no longer considered first line as several trials have shown them to be inferior to antipsychotics, haloperidol in particular.

## Further reading

Inouye S (2006). Delirium in older persons. *N Engl J Med* **354**: 1157–1165.
Young J, Inouye S (2007). Delirium in older people. *BMJ* **334**: 842–846.

## How to prescribe medications for delirium

### High-potency typical antipsychotics

- Haloperidol is considered first line. Compared to low-potency antipsychotics, there are fewer side effects of relevance (e.g., less anticholinergic, sedation, hypotension).
- Administer haloperidol 0.5–1 mg orally twice daily. Depending on the clinical condition, consider starting at a smaller dose (i.e., 0.25 mg). Peak effect is at 4–6 hr. Repeat every 4–6 hr as needed and as tolerated. Total daily dose is usually 0.5–3 mg.
- In the very agitated patient you may administer haloperidol 0.5–1 mg IM. Depending on the clinical condition, consider starting at a smaller dose (i.e., 0.25 mg). Peak effect is at 20–40 min. Repeat after 30–60 min if needed. Haloperidol IV may also be used, but the duration of action is shorter.
- In older people, the half-life of haloperidol may be as long as 60 hr. Dosing can be cumulative. Failure to titrate may overly sedate.
- The incidence of extrapyramidal side effects (EPS) is high, especially at daily doses of 3 mg or greater. Avoid in dementia with Lewy bodies, Parkinson's disease, and neuroleptic malignant syndrome (NMS).
- These antipsychotics may prolong the corrected QT interval. Monitor ECG. If corrected QT interval is >450 msec or 25% above baseline, consider obtaining cardiology consult and decreasing or discontinuing the medication.

### Atypical antipsychotics

- Evidence is lacking for the use of atypical antipsychotics in delirium. Small, usually uncontrolled studies have shown benefit from risperidone 0.5 mg, olanzapine 2.5–5 mg, and quetiapine 25 mg orally twice daily.
- Adverse effects of EPS and prolonged corrected QT interval are similar to that of the typical antipsychotics (i.e., haloperidol).
- These should be considered when response to other strategies is poor.

### Short-acting benzodiazepines

- Use mainly to treat withdrawal delirium (e.g., alcohol withdrawal or delirium tremens). Short-acting benzodiazepines without active metabolites (e.g., lorazepam) are preferred.
- Lorazepam may be monotherapy for the treatment of delirium caused by alcohol or benzodiazepine withdrawal.
- May administer lorazepam 0.5 mg orally or IM. Repeat as needed and as tolerated to maximum 3 mg/day. In emergency cases only, consider giving a small IV dose. Respiratory depression is the major risk.
- Lorazepam may be used in combination with a typical antipsychotic. It is for treatment of refractory symptoms, severe anxiety, or agitation, or in a patient who cannot tolerate an adequate dose of haloperidol.
- Adverse effects include excitation or disinhibition, respiratory depression, and oversedation. These agents may prolong or worsen delirium.

### Cholinergic agents

- In cases of delirium caused by a centrally acting anticholinergic agent, physostigmine 2 mg IM/PO or donepezil 5–10 mg/day may be administered. The offending anticholinergic agent must also be stopped.

# Cognitive aging

Normal aging affects cognition. Expected changes with advancing age include slowed information-processing speed and declines in working memory. Mild deficits in recent memory (as tested by 5-minute delayed recall of items) are also common. Hence, older individuals exhibit a slower pace of learning, as well as mild forgetfulness that can be helped by clues or prompts.

In contrast, intelligence (e.g., vocabulary) and language (e.g., syntax) remain relatively stable with age, with an overall increase in one's fund of knowledge.

Three factors support a diagnosis of normal aging rather than disease:
• Gradual decline, i.e., over 10–30 years
• Relative decline, i.e., relative to young adults
• The ability to maintain function in day-to-day living through aids (e.g., lists) or adaptations (of one's environment or of one's expectations)

Normal age-related changes do *not* cause a significant reduction in functional level.

## Age-related cognitive decline

*Age-related cognitive decline* refers to the development of mild cognitive changes, such as those noted above, that are considered to be the result of normal aging. The deficits can be objectively measured, but they fall within normal limits for age (i.e., they are age-appropriate). Examples include forgetting of names or appointments, or occasionally losing things around the house. Age-related cognitive decline is a focus of clinical attention, rather than a disorder per se.

### Activities of daily living (ADLs)
• Toileting, personal hygiene, grooming, bathing, dressing, transferring, feeding

### Instrumental activities of daily living (IADLs)
• Working, keeping house, driving, using the telephone, shopping, cooking, managing medications, managing money

# Cognitive impairment not dementia, and mild cognitive impairment

## Diagnosis

Cognitive impairments are present, but full criteria for a diagnosis of dementia are not met. Deficits may be broader than memory alone, but overall function remains unimpaired. With time, many patients do develop dementia, but many do not, and some patients revert back to normal cognition.

*Cognitive impairment not dementia (CIND)* is a broad term referring to all such conditions where cognitive impairment is beyond what would be expected for age and education. *Mild cognitive impairment (MCI)* refers to a condition that resembles a dementia prodrome, typically that of early Alzheimer's disease.

MCI can be divided into subtypes: amnestic MCI (prominent memory deficits) and nonamnestic MCI (e.g., problem-solving or word-finding difficulties, in the absence of memory complaints). Patients may have deficits in a single domain or in multiple domains. Patients with the amnestic subtype of MCI are at greatest risk of progressing to Alzheimer's dementia (AD).

Although widely agreed-upon criteria do not exist, distinguishing features of MCI include the following:

- Subjective complaints of memory loss by the patient and/or memory problems noted by an informant
- Objective memory deficits when compared to age and education peers and past abilities
- No significant functional impairment: functioning well overall (i.e., ADLs are preserved), with minimal (if any) change in IADLs
- Progression to dementia at a rate as high as 10%–15% per year

## Cognitive testing

Most patients with MCI score normally on the Mini-Mental State Exam (MMSE), primarily because of MMSE's ceiling effects and limited ability to assess executive cognition, and hence low sensitivity for CIND/MCI. The modified MMSE (100-point MMSE) may be more sensitive to CIND/MCI.

The Trail Making Test (or its verbal form, the Mental Alternation Test) or clock-drawing tests may detect early executive dysfunction or visuoconstructional changes and, as such, can be useful adjuncts to the MMSE. Neuropsychological testing is more sensitive for CIND/MCI; however, it is not definitive.

## Treatment

- Reassure the patient by distinguishing CIND/MCI from dementia.
- Carefully look for late-life depression, often presenting with unusual features (e.g., easy frustration, irritability, anhedonia, social withdrawal, but not sadness, crying, or self-deprecation).
- Educate patients and families. Valuable resources include the following:
  - Alzheimer's Association (www.alz.org)
  - National Institute on Aging (www.nia.nih.gov/Alzheimers)

- Modify risk factors for progression:
  - Control cardiovascular conditions (hypertension, diabetes mellitus [DM], hyperlipidemia)
  - Moderate exercise of at least 30 minutes, 3 times per week
  - Cognitively stimulating activities and increased social engagement may also be of benefit.
- There is no proven treatment to date: acetylcholinesterase inhibitors, rofecoxib (an NSAID), and vitamin E have not been shown in randomized clinical trials to prevent the progression of MCI to dementia.
- Donepezil may reduce the rate of progression to Alzheimer's disease during the first year of treatment, i.e., transiently. At this time, treatment of MCI with donepezil is not the standard of care.

Patients with CIND/MCI should be monitored every 6–12 months, with prompt intervention if progression occurs. Evaluate for comorbid psychiatric conditions, such as depression, anxiety, or sleep disturbance, at each visit. Depression (both major and minor) puts patients at higher risk for developing dementia. If depression is present, it should be treated. Refer to subsequent pages for diagnosis and treatment of depression in older adults.

# Dementia: overview

*Dementia* is an acquired decline in memory and other cognitive function(s) in an alert (i.e., nondelirious) person that is sufficiently severe to affect daily life (home, work, or social function). Each of the elements within the definition—i.e., functional impairment, a decline from baseline, and the absence of delirium—must be present to make the diagnosis of dementia.

Prevalence increases dramatically with age. Specifically, Alzheimer's disease (AD) affects 5% to 7% of persons aged 65 and older, and rises to 40% to 50% of those 90 years and older. Two-thirds of assisted living and the majority of nursing home residents have a dementia syndrome.

## Major dementia syndromes

- Dementia of the Alzheimer's type (60%–70%)
- Vascular dementia (10%–20%)
- Other neurodegenerative dementias (5%–10%): dementia with Lewy bodies, Parkinson's disease with dementia, frontotemporal dementia
- Dementia of late-life depression—see How to distinguish dementia due to depression from other causes of cognitive impairment (p. 218)
- Other dementias (<5%)

Mixed pathology (especially Alzheimer's with vascular) is common.

Diagnostically, there are many false-positive and false-negative cases in primary care. Mild to moderate dementia is easy to miss on a cursory, unstructured assessment. Patients labeled incorrectly as having dementia may be deaf, dysphasic, delirious, or under the influence of drugs or alcohol.

## Common features of dementia syndromes

### Cognitive features

- Impaired retention of new information. Short-term memory loss is often severe, with repetitive questioning.
- Language impairment. Word-finding difficulties with circumlocution are common. Speech may be vague or empty. The patient may be unable to hold a conversation.
- Visuospatial dysfunction (e.g., getting lost in familiar places)
- Loss of executive control (e.g., unable to plan and organize, may be socially inappropriate, disinhibited, or disinterested). Management of complex tasks is impaired (e.g., paying bills, cooking a meal for family).
- Patients require assistance with IADLs, and eventually basic ADLs. In more severe dementia, inability to perform self-care is seen.
- Poor insight and judgment (e.g., irrational, may insist on driving)
- Prone to the development of delirium

### Associated motor features of dementia

- These typically occur in more severe dementia or in certain conditions such as normal-pressure hydrocephalus, vascular dementia, and disseminated Lewy body disease.
- Gait disorders, postural instability, and falls are seen.
- Less commonly there are focal findings and Parkinsonism.

Neuropsychiatric symptoms affect the vast majority of dementia patients at some point in their illness.

- Affective and related mood changes (e.g., irritability, depression, anxiety, apathy, agitation)
- Drive disturbances (e.g., sleep and sleep–wake cycle, appetite and weight loss, sexual dysfunctions or inappropriateness)
- Behavioral changes (e.g., aggression, wandering, disinhibition)
- Psychotic features, including persecutory delusions and visual hallucinations

## History

The history of present illness is the most important component of the assessment. It should be taken from both the patient and a reliable informant. Note the onset of cognitive symptoms and the speed of progression. Assess the nature and severity of symptoms (e.g., inquire about problems that have resulted from memory loss). Ask about behavioral symptoms.

In the majority of dementia cases, there is a progressive decline in cognitive function over several years, ending with complete dependency and death. Deterioration that is stepwise or abrupt suggests a vascular etiology. Rapid deterioration, i.e., over weeks to months, suggests a toxic, metabolic, or structural cause (e.g., tumor), which may be reversible. It is important to rule out causes of dementia that are potentially reversible.

In actuality, the reversibility of dementia depends on the severity of associated brain damage. While the causes listed in Box 9.3 can lead to dementia, most are detected well before they cause other symptoms (e.g., fatigue resulting from hypothyroidism). By the time dementia has onset, it is rarely reversible but may be stabilized. Also, some of these conditions may be the result of a different dementia cause (e.g., if a patient with AD forgets to take thyroid medication or does not eat well).

---

**Box 9.3 Potentially reversible causes of dementia syndromes**

- Thyroid disease (especially hypothyroidism)
- Thiamine and/or folate deficiency, pernicious anemia (vitamin B12)
- Brain tumor (primary or metastatic); chronic subdural hematoma
- Hypertension, vascular disease, cerebral ischemia or hypoxia
- Opiates; anticholinergic effects of psychopharmacologic agents
- Chronic alcohol use, as well as other drugs of abuse

---

Additional elements of the history include past medical history, a medication history (including over-the-counter medications, illicit drugs and alcohol), family history of early dementia, and personal history of psychiatric illness (especially depression).

### How to work up a patient with dementia

Cases of reversible dementia are uncommon, but their identification is important. Effective treatment may reverse the impairment and prevent its progression.

*Basic laboratory tests*

The following are generally considered useful:

- CBC
- Electrolytes, including calcium
- Complete metabolic panel (CMP)
- Vitamin $B_{12}$ and folate levels
- Thyroid function tests, TSH
- RPR (syphilis); HIV if high risk
- Random glucose
- Resting ECG
- Chest radiograph
- Urinalysis with toxicology

*Neuroimaging*

It is arguable whether every person with dementia should undergo brain imaging. Imaging is indicated where there is the following:

- Early onset (<65 years old)
- Sudden onset or brisk decline
- Focal CNS signs or symptoms
- High risk of structural pathology (e.g., infarct, subdural hematoma, normal-pressure hydrocephalus, or tumor)

In typical cases suggestive of either Alzheimer's, vascular, or mixed (Alzheimer's–vascular) dementia, the diagnostic yield is low. Thus, in most cases, imaging does not alter the clinical management. If a patient or caregiver is particularly anxious (e.g., fear of brain tumor), imaging may be indicated to allay those particular fears.

- **CT** is the usual imaging modality and can be used to rule out most causes of structural pathology.
- **MRI** has greater sensitivity for ischemia and infarction, especially involving the posterior circulation and subcortical areas. Coronal MRI also affords a close look at the hippocampus, which is shrunken in Alzheimer's disease.
- **SPECT (single photon emission computed tomography) and PET (positron emission tomography)** are used uncommonly, usually in specialty centers, to more reliably differentiate between Alzheimer's, frontotemporal, and vascular dementia.

*Additional testing as clinically indicated*

- Lumbar puncture (LP) if CNS infection is suspected
- Electroencephalogram (EEG) if seizure activity is suspected

### Physical examination

- The goal is to define whether or not a dementia syndrome is present and, if it is, to search for possible causes.
- Basic laboratory tests. See How to work up a patient with dementia.
- Complete physical examination: look for signs of vascular disease, thyroid disease, malignancy, dehydration, alcoholic liver disease, etc.
- Focused neurological examination: look for focal deficits, Parkinsonism, frontal release signs, neuropathy, etc.

**Mental status exam**

- Exclude delirium. Features of delirium include agitation, restlessness, poor attention, and fluctuating conscious level.
- Search for depression. Features include low mood, poor motivation, and negative self-statements. Administer the Patient Health Questionnaire (PHQ-9) or use the Geriatric Depression Scale (GDS) (see Appendix).
- Perform a *cognitive assessment*. This will provide objective evidence of cognitive impairment. It will serve as a baseline; serial testing may show evidence of progression. Many measurement tools are available, e.g., clock-drawing and the Mini-Cog (see Appendix), MMSE, Modified MMSE, number of four-legged animals named in 1 minute, and the Trail-Making Test Part B.
- Perform a *functional assessment*, including whether the patient can independently carry out ADLs and IADLs.
- Neuropsychological testing may be helpful, especially in cases of mild dementia.

Late-life depression can cause a full-blown dementia syndrome. The term *depressive pseudodementia* is no longer used, in preference for the term *dementia of depression*, which might be reversible with antidepressant treatment.

**How to distinguish dementia due to depression from other causes of cognitive impairment**

Severe depression may present with poor memory and concentration, as well as impaired functional capacity, e.g., for ADLs. The cognitive impairment of depression is usually distinguishable from dementia, because

- The history of cognitive impairment is short and the onset relatively abrupt.
- Patients generally complain about poor memory and are distressed by it.
- Assessment of cognition often results in "I don't know" responses, and effort in cognitive performance may be reduced.
- Memories are often accessible with hints or cues, i.e., memories have been "stored" (forgetfulness as opposed to amnesia).
- There is often a past history of depression, an identifiable precipitant, or clear timing of the onset.

The prognosis is variable. In some patients, mood and cognition respond to antidepressants. However, many of these individuals go on to develop dementia, usually of the Alzheimer's type.

*Coexistence of depression and dementia*

- Both depression and dementia are relatively common and often coexist.
- Over 20% of people with an early degenerative dementia may be depressed or apathetic. This sometimes reflects a depressive reaction to the onset of dementia.
- This is quite different from pseudodementia (where there is no actual dementia).

*General guidance*

- Treat the depression, regardless of whether a coexisiting dementia is present.
- Avoid mislabeling a depressed patient as also suffering from degenerative dementia without longitudinal information. The management and prognoses are very different.
- Always screen for depression when assessing patients with cognitive disorders, including those with short-term memory loss alone.

# Dementia: common causative diseases

## Alzheimer's disease (AD) or dementia of the Alzheimer's type (DAT)

- AD is the most common cause of a dementia. Age is the main risk factor. Family history of AD is also a risk factor.
- Insidious onset and slow progression occur over several years. The true time course can be difficult to determine. Deficits may not be apparent to others (i.e., informants) early on in the disease. This is especially true if life has been structured and routine. Deficits then become apparent in the context of a major stressor or life change that challenges the patient's ability to compensate. This may give the false impression of a new-onset rapidly progressing dementia.
- Short-term memory loss (i.e., amnesia) is the earliest symptom; uncommon first presentations with executive dysfunction (e.g., "personality change"), depression, or visuospatial loss are well documented.
- AD and DAT progress to include broad, often global, cognitive dysfunction, behavioral change, and functional impairment. A decline of 3–4 points per year on MMSE is typical.
- Diagnosis is made clinically, based on the typical history, mental status examination, and unremarkable physical examination and workup. Clinical diagnosis of AD is validated by autopsy in 70%–90% of cases. Pathology includes neurofibrillary tangles and senile plaques.
- Loss of cholinergic neurons in the basal forebrain plays a role in AD.
- Comorbid depression is common, especially in mild DAT. The presentation may be atypical (e.g., with anxiety or delusions). Apathy, i.e., loss of interest and motivation, is also common.
- Moderate to severe DAT may have psychotic features (visual hallucinations and persecutory delusions). Behavioral problems, including agitation, aggression, and wandering, often occur in more severe disease.
- Sleep may be disturbed, with sundowning (increased activity at bedtime).
- Early-onset AD (<65 years old) is uncommon, has a stronger genetic component, and is more rapidly progressive.

## Key features of DAT[1]

### 1. Memory impairment
- Retention of new information is impaired. Short-term memory loss is often severe, with repetitive questioning. Cues and prompts are of little help.
- Remembering of previously well-learned material may also become impaired at later stages of dementia.

### 2. One or more of the following:
- Aphasia (i.e., deterioration of language function, such as word-finding difficulties and circumlocution)
- Apraxia (i.e., impaired ability to execute motor activities, despite intact motor abilities; e.g., unable to mime how to comb one's hair)

- Agnosia (i.e., failure to recognize and identify objects or persons, despite intact sensory function)
- Executive dysfunction (i.e., impaired abstract thinking, and difficulty managing complex tasks, such as paying bills, cooking a family meal).

*3. Significant functional impairment from the above deficits*

## Vascular dementia (VaD)

- Thought to be etiologically related to cardiovascular disease
- DSM-IV criteria are similar to dementia of the Alzheimer's type:
  - Memory impairment
  - Aphasia, apraxia, anomia, and/or executive dysfunction
- Diagnosis requires focal neurological signs and symptoms and/or laboratory evidence of cardiovascular disease (e.g., neuroimaging).
- Suggested by cardiovascular disease and associated risk factors, e.g., hypertension, smoking, hyperlipidemia, diabetes mellitus.
- May coexist with AD ("mixed" dementia).
- Classically, deterioration is abrupt and/or stepwise; onset is often associated with stroke. It can be slowly progressive after initial onset.
- VaD may also have a more gradual onset and course, making it difficult to differentiate from AD (see Box 9.4).
- Physical examination may reveal focal neurological signs and symptoms, as well as evidence of vascular disease.
- Neuroimaging may show multiple large vessel infarcts, a single critical infarct (e.g., thalamus), small-vessel disease, or other stroke patterns.
- Cognitive deficits may be patchy, as compared to the more uniform and global impairments seen in AD.
- Depressed mood and emotional lability are common.
- Urinary incontinence, gait disturbance, and falls are often early features.

---

### Box 9.4 Differentiating between Alzheimer's disease and vascular dementia

The importance of differentiating between Alzheimer's and VaD is often overemphasized. Their presentations overlap, and the two pathologies commonly coexist. Pragmatically:

- In cases where vascular risk factors and/or signs exist, treat vascular risk factors aggressively, regardless of whether there is significant cerebrovascular pathology on brain imaging. This approach may well slow the progression of "pure" AD.
- A trial of cholinesterase inhibitors (effective in Alzheimer's but much weaker evidence in vascular dementia) is probably worthwhile where vascular risk factors and/or pathology exists, but Alzheimer's may be contributing to the presentation.

---

**1.** American Psychiatric Association. (2000). *Diagnostic and Statistical Manual of Mental Disorders, fourth edition, Text Revision.* Arlington, VA: American Psychiatric Association.

# Dementia and Parkinsonism

Dementia with Lewy bodies (DLB) and Parkinson's disease with dementia (PDD) may be considered extremes of a continuum. In DLB, cognitive and behavioral disturbance dominate the clinical picture. In PDD, motor impairments develop first and dominate the clinical picture.

The distinction may be even more complex if combined with contributions from Alzheimer's or vascular pathology.

### Dementia with Lewy bodies (DLB)

- Onset is insidious, but tends to have a faster course than PDD.
- DLB is characterized by the following:
  - Fluctuations in cognitive function and alertness
  - Prominent visual hallucinations, often with paranoia and delusions
  - Parkinsonism is commonly present, but often not severe.
- Hypersensitivity to neuroleptics:
  - Typical antipsychotics (e.g., haloperidol) are very poorly tolerated, leading to worsening confusion or exacerbation of Parkinsonism.
  - Atypical antipsychotics (especially clozapine and quetiapine) may be better tolerated, but great caution is advised in their use.
- Levodopa or dopamine agonists may worsen confusion and psychosis.

Note that several features are common to both DLB and delirium, e.g., fluctuation of symptoms, effect of drugs, and perceptual and psychotic phenomena. When comparing the two, the following is true of DLB:
- Onset is insidious and progression gradual.
- No precipitating illness (e.g., infection) is found.
- Hallucinations are complex and not the result of misperception of stimuli.
- Delusions are well-formed and may be persistent.

### Parkinson's disease with dementia (PDD)

- People with Parkinson's disease (PD) are at an increased risk of developing dementia, especially in later stages of the disease.
- Typical motor features of PD are present, and may be severe:
  - Tremor
  - Akinesia/bradykinesia
  - Rigidity
- The presentation of PDD is variable and may resemble Alzheimer's disease, vascular dementia, or DLB.
- Acute confusion and psychotic symptoms can be precipitated by antiparkinsonian medications.
- By definition, if features of PD precede dementia by more than a year, then the diagnosis is of PDD, not DLB. This applies even if the dementia syndrome is otherwise typical of DLB.

### Other conditions

Multiple-system atrophy, progressive supranuclear palsy, and corticobasal degeneration may also present with both Parkinsonism and dementia.

# Dementia: less common causative diseases

### Frontotemporal dementia (FTD), aka Pick's disease

- Insidious onset and slow (several years) progression, involving the frontal and temporal lobes. Onset is often early, by the sixth decade.
- Memory and visuospatial ability are relatively spared. Insight is lost early on in the disease.
- Personality change may be one of the earliest manifestations of FTD, including loss of social awareness and increased extroversion. Difficulty at work may be an early sign.
- Behavioral problems include disinhibition and impulsivity, restlessness and agitation, aggression, hyperorality, repetitive behaviors, impairment of executive function, decreased personal care, and sleep disturbance.
- Mental rigidity, inflexibility, and catastrophic reactions are common.
- Language dysfunction may include word-finding difficulty, problems naming or understanding words, lack of spontaneous conversation, or circumlocution.
- Later in the course of disease, impairments become more broad, similar to those in severe Alzheimer's.
- Neuroimaging usually demonstrates frontal and/or temporal atrophy.
- Commonly used assessment tools (e.g., MMSE) do not test frontal lobe function; hence, executive dysfunction may be present despite "normal" cognitive screening tests.
- Family history of FTD or a related disorder occurs in 50% of cases.
- As many as half of patients with amyotrophic lateral sclerosis (ALS) develop FTD; the condition also shares pathologies with progressive supranuclear palsy and corticobasal degeneration.

### Dementia and infection

- *HIV-associated dementia* is a subcortical dementia that generally affects younger people, reflecting the epidemiology of HIV infection. It generally occurs late in HIV. Psychomotor slowing, impaired concentration, and apathy are typical. Deficits in fine motor skills may be present. Opportunistic infections, neoplasms, stroke, and drug effects also contribute to cognitive decline.
- *Neurosyphilis should be suspected if a dementia syndrome has atypical features (e.g., seizures) or risk factors for sexually transmitted disease (STD) are present (including mental illness, history of STD, drug or alcohol abuse). If FTA-ABS is positive, sample CSF and test for VDRL. Consult infectious diseases regarding IV penicillin treatment.*
- *Creutzfeldt–Jakob disease (CJD)* is a prion-mediated, rapidly progressing cortical dementia. Psychosis occurs early. Myoclonus is found on neurological exam.

### Dementia and drugs and toxins

Alcohol-associated persisting dementia may occur after many years of heavy drinking. It presents with disproportionate short-term memory impairment. Use of alcohol itself is probably NOT the causative factor of dementia. Rather, alcoholics often have repeated traumatic brain injuries and chronic nutritional deficiencies that are most likely the causes of brain damage leading to dementia.

Psychoactive drugs may cause a dementia-like syndrome that is substantially reversible.

## Normal-pressure hydrocephalus

Normal-pressure hydrocephalus (NPH) classically presents with the triad:
- Cognitive impairment (psychomotor slowing, apathy, depressed)
- Gait disturbance (wide-based)
- Urinary incontinence

### Assessment
- Neuroimaging: shows ventricles that are enlarged disproportionately compared to the degree of cerebral atrophy.
- Lumbar puncture is both diagnostic *and* therapeutic. It is performed if clinical and radiological findings are suggestive of NPH. Before the procedure, assess baseline gait (e.g., timed walk) and cognition (e.g., MMSE, clock-drawing test). Remove 20–30 mL CSF—opening pressure will be normal. Check for improvement in gait and cognition after 1–2 hours, and again after 24 hours. Improvement in gait is most predictive of improvement after shunting.

### Treatment
- Serial lumbar punctures with large-volume CSF removal.
- Ventriculoperitoneal (V-P) shunting is effective for some patients. Gait is more likely to improve than cognition. It is a major neurosurgical procedure, and complications are common, e.g., infection and subdural hematoma. Benefit is more likely in those who had therapeutic response to LP and large-volume CSF removal.

# Dementia: overall management

- Refer to the American Association for Geriatric Psychiatry "Principles of Care for Patients with Dementia Resulting from Alzheimer Disease" (2006) for management roadmap.
- Modify reversible factors that are individually minor but have a cumulative effect (e.g., constipation, pain, low-grade sepsis, anemia, drug side effects).
- Simplify the medication regimen. Provide pillboxes to caregivers. In the later stages, some medications may be discontinued if the risk begins to outweigh the benefit.
- Create a safe, caring environment, usually in the patient's own home. Home assessments can be used to identify hazards and provide visual safety cues, etc. Organize caregivers or outside services to administer medication and assist with IADLs and ADLs as needed.
- Suggest simple interventions to improve coping with memory loss (e.g., lists, calendars, and alarms). A predictable routine is helpful to reduce a patient's confusion and frustration.
- Encourage physical and mental activity, including social activities (e.g., senior centers, day programs, taking a walk, looking at old pictures, listening to music, simple games, perhaps dancing).
- Educate patients and families about the disease and how to cope with its manifestations. This includes appropriate modifications to the home environment and learning to communicate and interact with the patient with dementia. Counseling and support may delay nursing home admission.
- Support caregivers:
  - Inquire about caregiver burden: over 50% of all caregivers suffer from depression. Refer to individual treatment when appropriate.
  - Refer caregivers to support groups if they wish (see the Alzheimer's Association for details).
  - Suggest sitting services (usually for 2–3 hours once or twice weekly), or respite care (usually in a facility, for a few days or up to 2 weeks).
- Inform patient and caregivers of legal and ethical issues:
  - Driving—see How to manage the driver who has dementia (p. 228). (Also see Chapter 30, The older driver)
  - Advance directives
  - Power of attorney and wills: National Academy of Elder Law Attorneys (www.naela.com)
  - Discussion of end-of-life issues (artificial feeding, etc.) may be appropriate.

### Disclosure of diagnosis

Each case should be considered individually, but in general, the diagnosis should be revealed. Disclosure is consistent with patient autonomy, facilitates medical, legal, financial, and long-term care planning, and allows for patients to consent to treatment, including possible participation in research studies. Arguments against disclosure include psychological distress. Such a reaction is minimized by sensitive multidisciplinary support that emphasizes the positive therapeutic solutions available. On balance, the degrees of disclosure should match the patient's insight and remaining abilities, and should be guided by input from the family.

### How to manage the driver who has dementia

The risk of having a traffic accident increases with age and with the severity of dementia. Public safety must be weighed against individual autonomy. State statutes vary with respect to specific medical conditions that must be reported to driving authorities. It is important to be familiar with state-specific motor vehicle regulations. A state-by-state reference list of reporting laws can be found through the American Medical Association (www.ama-assn.org). Also see Chapter 30, The older driver.

Assessment of driving ability during an outpatient medical visit (or inpatient stay) can be difficult. A diagnosis of dementia by itself is not sufficient for revoking driving privileges. Driving privileges should be based on the individual's actual driving ability. But, in general, the following apply:

- Mild dementia: patients may be competent and it may be safe for them to drive.
- Moderate dementia: nearly all patients should not drive.
- Severe dementia: patients are not competent and it is not safe for them to drive.

In general, patients who have MMSE <18, have already had driving problems, and whose family members would not let them drive small children alone ("the grandchild test") should be told to stop driving until they pass a driving test (unless it is clear they would not pass).

#### General assessment

- Dementia severity, including evidence of major impairment in visuospatial function, attention, or judgment. However, a combination of modest impairments may be as important.
- Presence of noncognitive impairments:
  - Vision (including visual acuity and visual fields)
  - Cognition (memory, visuospatial skills, attention, judgment)
  - Motor function (strength, range of motion, proprioception)
- Other conditions that affect driving safety (e.g., seizures or syncope)
- Medication review for any adverse effects on cognition or function.

#### Driving history obtained from an informant

- First-hand observations of the patient's driving skills and any concerns about being a passenger
- Unsafe driving behaviors (e.g., driving too fast or too slow, not noticing or obeying traffic signs)
- Driving problems (e.g., getting lost), incidents (e.g., tickets, near-misses), or accidents (may be evidenced by dents in the car)
- Changes in driving patterns (i.e., are journeys now brief, infrequent, and confined to quiet local roads?) and the reasons behind them
- Has anyone tried but failed to limit or prohibit driving by the patient?

## How to manage the driver who has dementia (cont'd.)

*Driving assessment*

- If the individual would like to continue driving, refer for a formal assessment of driving abilities. The best assessment is by a professional, in the patient's own vehicle on the public roads.
- Performance-based road testing is done through the Department of Motor Vehicles; many occupational therapists also do such testing. Such professionals can both deliver an opinion and offer useful, practical advice to the cognitively or physically impaired driver.
- Serial assessment of driving abilities should be done every 6 to 12 months, or as prompted by driving incidents.

*General management*

- It is preferable that the patient, family, and doctor agree that stopping voluntarily is advisable. Compulsory licence withdrawal by the driving authorities generates great anger and distress.
- The issue is best discussed early in the course of the disease, when the patient has the best insight and before decision-making capacity becomes impaired.
- If driving is safe for the moment, encourage the patient and family to think ahead, to a time when driving cannot be continued.
- Counsel to prepare the patient and family for eventual driving cessation. If the family will not be providing future transportation, refer patient to alternate senior-friendly methods of transportation.

*Driving cessation*

- Use sympathetic communication with the patient when it is no longer safe for them to drive.
- Give strategies to the family: have an intervention, move the car, change the locks on the car, revoke the driving license.
- Provide resources: American Society on Aging's "Drive Well" program (www.asaging.org); the Alzheimer's Association (www.alz.org); *The 36-Hour Day* (Mace and Rabins, 2006).
- Document the discussion.
- Rarely, a patient will continue to drive when it is clearly unsafe and after having been informed that they must stop. In most cases, further clear statements of this, backed up by the threat of medical reporting to the authorities (if applicable), are sufficient to prompt cessation.
- If driving continues despite recommendations to the contrary, the clinician may be ethically justified in reporting this to the authorities, and will usually have the strong support of the family.

# Dementia: risk management and abuse

Risk management is an essential part of care.
- Is there a risk of harm to the patient or to others?
- How great is the risk, how long has the patient (or other person) been exposed to it, and how severe are the consequences of the risk?

Common risks include the following:
- *Driving.* Refer to How to manage the driver who has dementia.
- *Falls.* Moving from the patient's own home to institutional care is rarely the answer. Supervision is far from continuous in any institution, the environment is less familiar, and the floors are often uncarpeted and unforgiving.
- *Wandering is usually more distressing to caregivers than risk-presenting to the patient.*
- *Aggression* by a patient toward caregivers or family is *usually* verbal, but sometimes physical or sexual. It may lead to caregivers to refuse to work with a patient.
- *Elder abuse* may be difficult to identify, as the patient may not complain (due to fear or cognitive problems). Be concerned if there are unexplained "falls" or unusual patterns of bruising.
- *Neglect of self-care* is often with poor insight. It may manifest as poor diet, poor hygiene, etc.
- *Fire risk* may be easily modifiable, through removal or modification of kitchen appliances, gas stoves, etc. Cigarette smoking may be more problematic.
- *Financial abuse.* For example, theft or fraud, modification of wills, or misuse or transfer of a patient's money.
- *Medication administration.* Skipping doses or taking extra doses of medication is common. Thereafter, medications should be administered by a caregiver. Pill boxes may be an option in some cases.

Having determined the nature and magnitude of a risk, consider if the risk can be reduced and if it should be reduced. Risk reduction should be done in cases where it will not significantly affect patients' independence or enjoyment of life. However, if reducing risk involves curtailing liberty or restricting enjoyable activity (walking, wandering, living alone), then the following should be considered:
- What is the patient's current attitude toward risk? What was his or her premorbid attitude, and what would he or she want now?
- What is the caregivers' attitude toward risk?

Commonly, discussions around risk occur when a patient is perceived by someone (i.e., caregiver, relative, hospital staff) to have become unsafe to remain at home. This should prompt multidisciplinary assessment and discussion, including whether a move to institutional care would involve a change of risk patterns rather than a reduction in overall risk. Occasionally a brief psychiatric hospitalization on a geriatric unit can help sort out these issues.

# Dementia: cholinesterase inhibitors

Cholinesterase inhibitors (ChEIs) are the first drug class proven to improve cognition in some patients with dementia.

### Effectiveness

They are far from miracle drugs, with very variable response. In general:

- ChEIs offer symptomatic benefit through stabilization of cognition. The underlying disease continues to progress at the same rate.
- Of the dementias, AD, DLB, and PDD have the greatest cholinergic deficit, and these are the dementia types known to benefit most from ChEI treatment.
- About half of patients show no benefit, a significant minority show moderate improvements ("clock turned back a few months"), and for a small minority there is substantial improvement.
- In some, there is a worsening in cognition, or onset of agitation that may be temporary or respond to a change in drug.
- Early studies focused on effects on cognitive function, and these are overall modest. However, small improvements in cognition can translate into significantly improved day-to-day function, reducing caregiver burden (by ~30 minutes daily in moderate dementia).
- There is some evidence that ChEIs can reduce the requirements for home care and can delay placement in nursing home.
- Benefit has been demonstrated for mild to moderate dementia, not in severe dementia.

### Choosing a drug

The three ChEIs currently available are the following:

- *Donepezil* starting at 5 mg daily, increased to 10 mg daily after 4–6 weeks, target dose 5–10 mg daily
- *Rivastigmine* starting at 1.5 mg bid, increased to maximum dose 6 mg bid over 3 months
- *Galantamine* starting at 4 mg bid, increased to 8 mg bid after 4 weeks, target dose 8–12 mg bid after 8 weeks.

Selecting an agent can be difficult. As a class, ChEIs are approved for use in mild to moderate AD. There is no definitive evidence from head-to-head comparisons to support one agent over another. Effectiveness seems broadly similar, and choice can be made on the basis of costs and the treatment team's experience.

Much evidence exists for donepezil in treatment of AD and for rivastigmine in Lewy body dementia and dementia in PD. Overall, the evidence for ChEIs is strongest in Alzheimer's and Lewy body dementia, and weakest in vascular dementia.

## How to treat with cholinesterase inhibitors

Introducing and monitoring ChEIs is a specialist area, usually undertaken by geropsychiatry teams, or by geriatricians or neurologists working in the setting of a memory clinic.

In general, ChEIs should not be initiated in inpatient medical or rehabilitation settings, as the effects of environmental changes, physical illness, or drugs may dominate those of the ChEI, rendering assessment of effect impossible. It is preferable to initiate treatment when the patient is physically well and living in their own home.

Where given for behavioral disturbance or noncognitive symptoms (e.g., hallucinations), ChEIs may be initiated more urgently in an institutional setting.

### Before treatment
- Consider the relative risks and benefits and discuss them with patient and caregiver.
- Explain that the drugs do not provide a cure, and may reasonably be deferred until symptoms worsen.
- Consider how concordance can be assured.

### Treatment trial
- There are significant side effects, commonly gastrointestinal (nausea, dyspepsia, diarrhea, anorexia). These occur especially during the dose titration phase at higher doses, and are often short-lived.
- A ChEI should be given for an initial treatment period of 2–3 months. If there is no effect at the maximum tolerated dose, the drug should be discontinued. There is probably little benefit from trying another ChEI if one has failed.

### Assess impact
- Use the clinician's subjective global assessment, based on the views of relative(s) or caregiver(s) and serial clinical observations.
- Use the results of cognitive tests, e.g., MMSE, clock drawing test.

### Continuing therapy
- If benefit appears to have occurred, the drug should be continued at that dosage. Benefit may be absolute, or relative: a small decline would be expected during the 2- to 3-month evaluation period, so an absence of deterioration may be attributed to drug benefit.
- ChEIs can be given indefinitely, but should be withdrawn periodically (18 months) to determine whether benefit continues. If the patient deteriorates promptly after drug withdrawal (within weeks, thus probably secondary to drug withdrawal rather than disease progression), then ChEI is restarted. The evidence for ChEIs in advanced dementia is weak, and they are sometimes withdrawn at this point, unless the patient has clearly benefited in the past.

# Dementia: other drug treatments

### Memantine
- The second class of antidementia drugs approved for use in AD
- It blocks NMDA receptors, which may reduce glutamate-mediated destruction of cholinergic neurons.
- It appears to have a small beneficial effect in moderate and severe dementia of Alzheimer's or vascular etiology. It may have small benefits in mild dementia. It is unclear whether there are important effects on quality of life, caregiver time, or institutionalization.
- It may be used alone or in combination with donepezil.
- It is well tolerated. Uncommon side effects include hallucinations and worsening confusion.
- Memantine enhances the effect of levodopa and dopamine agonists.
- Avoid it use in severe renal failure.

### Preventing progression
Although no drugs have been proven to slow or halt progression, dementia is seen as so catastrophic that the following are often used:
- *Vascular secondary prevention,* e.g., aspirin, lipid-lowering drugs, ACE-inhibitors, and other antihypertensives. For patients with vascular dementia and mixed (Alzheimer's–vascular) dementia, aggressive risk factor modification and tailored drug treatment akin to that following stroke is logical and may slow progression, although is not well evidenced.
- *Vitamin E.* High doses (e.g., 400–800 IU twice a day) are widely used by patients and have been supported by some doctors, but recent evidence is less convincing. It has not been shown to be beneficial in cardiovascular disease, and high doses may even be harmful. Therefore, high-dose vitamin E supplementation cannot be recommended.

# Dementia: managing neuropsychiatric and behavioral symptoms

These symptoms include agitation, anxiety, phobias, irritability, wandering, hoarding, aggression, socially inappropriate behavior (e.g., sexual disinhibition, inappropriate urination, attention seeking), hallucinations, and delusions.

These are common in dementia, including Alzheimer's, and may occur early in the disease. They often occur in clusters, one affective (depressive or agitated, often with delusions) and one psychotic (typically with hallucinations and psychomotor agitation). Often it is these symptoms rather than cognitive impairment that lead to institutionalization; managing them successfully may enable patients to remain in their own home.

## General

- Consider whether acute illness (e.g., sepsis), pain (e.g., urinary retention), or changes in drug treatment (e.g., anticholinergic) have contributed, especially if behavior has deteriorated rapidly.
- Consider whether agitation or aggression is a manifestation of depression (consider an SSRI) or of fear (which may respond if care is given in a non-challenging way by a familiar team).
- Symptomatic treatment may not be needed if symptoms are transient, do not cause the patient significant distress, and are not threatening care of the patient in the current environment.

## Non-drug management

These are preferred, and may alone be sufficient.
- Avoid precipitants.
- The environment should be home-like, familiar, and interesting. Effective therapies may include music, bathing, exercise, pets, art therapy, aromatherapy, etc.
- Activities and structure should be used to reduce boredom and introduce stability and predictability. They will at times reduce wandering and aggression.
- Delusions and hallucinations may be helped by distraction and reassurance. Anxiety may respond to relaxation or a discussion of worries.
- Referral to a geropsychiatry team is needed for more severe disturbances.

## Drug treatment

The best drug is that which, for that patient with that problem, has worked well previously.
- Target therapies to the most prominent neuropsychiatric syndrome evident. If there is evidence of an affective syndrome and it is most prominent, try an SSRI (typically citalopram or sertraline). Note that delusions alone are most often associated with affective syndromes in dementia and will respond to SSRIs in this context.

- Short-term use of an antipsychotic, usually an atypical, may be needed in addition to an SSRI if the patient's behavior is aggressive or if psychosis is prominent.
- A non-SSRI antidepressant, such as venlafaxine or mirtazapine, might be used as a second line, depending on the symptom profile.
- For a primary sleep disturbance, consider trazodone (a sedating antidepressant), initially 25–50 mg at bedtime, increased as needed, and maximum 300 mg daily.
- If the syndrome is primarily psychotic, especially with prominent hallucination, introduce an atypical antipsychotic (risperidone 0.5–2 mg twice a day, olanzapine 2.5–10 mg daily, quetiapine 25–200 mg daily).
- Low-dose conventional antipsychotics, such as haloperidol 0.5–2 mg daily, are a reasonable second line.
- There is an increased risk of vascular events and death with the use of both conventional and atypical antipsychotics in dementia patients. The Food and Drug Administration now requires a specific "black box warning," which should be discussed in detail with patients and their families.
- Anxiolytics such as benzodiazepines may be used for brief, anxiety-inducing situations or when agitation is acute and prominent, but should be avoided in the long term.

Review drug use regularly, being aware of potential side effects such as falls, immobility, or confusion. Behavioral problems are often periodic, so consider trials off treatment, especially in patients whose behavioral disturbance was not severe and has responded to treatment.

Beware of iatrogenic deterioration. Modest behavioral deterioration in a patient with moderate dementia at home may lead to hospital admission, with a loss of all familiar routine, physical environment, and caregivers. This will lead to further behavioral decline, administration of sedatives, and further worsened confusion. Where appropriate, manage the patient at home, with a brief but thorough outpatient attendance if there is concern about physical precipitants.

### Further reading

Rabins P, Lyketsos C, Steele C (2006). *Practical Dementia Care, second edition.* New York: Oxford University Press.

Rosenberg P, Johnston D, Lyketsos C (2006). A clinical approach to mild cognitive impairment. *Am J Psychiatry* **163**: 1884–1890.

# Depression: overview

Depression is the most common mood disorder in older adults. Geriatric depression has an estimated prevalence of 1%–3% in the community. Another 15% of older adults have depressive symptoms that do not meet full criteria for major depressive disorder. Estimates are higher for primary care and hospital settings.

**Risk factors** for depression include the following:
- Disability and illness (especially if serious)
- Nursing home residents
- Bereavement
- Social isolation
- Chronic pain
- Sensory impairment (e.g., hearing or sight)

Depression is **underdiagnosed** and **undertreated** in older people, for the following reasons:
- Social stigma of depression. Older adults in particular may not want to be diagnosed with "mental" problems.
- Atypical presentation: patients often present with somatic complaints (e.g., weight loss, decreased appetite, or low energy), rather than sadness. This is especially true in the context of dementia.
- Misattribution of symptoms to physical rather than psychiatric illness. Medical illness is the most common feature of geriatric depression, so distinguishing the two conditions is often difficult.
- Perception by physicians that geriatric depression is "understandable," when, in fact, the majority of older people are not depressed.

Have a low threshold for opportunistic screening of depression.

**Comorbidity** may mask or precipitate depression, which may be
- Medical or neurological (e.g., Parkinson's disease, cerebrovascular disease or stroke, cardiovascular disease, arthritis, diabetes, hypothyroidism, malignancy, post-acute illness).
- Psychiatric (e.g., dementia, anxiety, personality disorders, alcohol use disorders).

## Differential diagnosis of depression

### Depression due to a general medical condition
- Depression may be the direct result of the condition itself (e.g., hypothyroidism) or of its treatment (e.g., cancer chemotherapy).
- It is commonly seen in association with chronic medical illnesses, especially ischemic heart disease (post-MI), diabetes, and arthritis. Post-stroke depression is a well-documented phenomenon, as is depression in the context of Alzheimer's or vascular dementia.
- Depression may be a reaction to having a serious medical condition, but this conclusion should be reached only after other causes have been ruled out.

### Depression secondary to substance use
- Medications commonly used in the elderly can cause depressive symptoms in some patients. These medications include antihypertensives (such as beta-blockers), narcotics, NSAIDs,

antiepileptics, antipsychotics, anxiolytics and sedative-hypnotics, cancer chemotherapy, and other miscellaneous medications (e.g., digoxin). Look for onset of symptoms within 1 month of medication initiation or dose adjustment.

- Substances of abuse can lead to depression, most commonly alcohol. Sedative-hypnotic (especially benzodiazepines), narcotic, and illicit drug abuse also occur in the elderly. Physical health problems with chronic pain are frequently seen in association with substance use. Always inquire about drug and alcohol use in every patient.

*Grief and bereavement*

Up to 15% of those who experience the loss of a loved one experience an episode of major depression. Normal bereavement symptoms overlap with depressive symptoms (e.g., sleep disturbance, excessive crying, psychomotor agitation or retardation). Symptoms generally last for 2 months or less, and most individuals are trending toward their baseline by about 1 year after the loss.

Active suicidality is never consistent with "normal" grief and should be regarded as a psychiatric emergency.

## Depression and dementia

In the elderly, depression itself can cause cognitive impairment or even dementia. Even if dementia remits with treatment, it can be a harbinger of decline years later. As the cognitive impairments of depression are very real, the term *pseudodementia of depression* has been replaced with the term *dementia of depression*.

# Depression: diagnosis

Depression often presents differently in the elderly than in younger persons. Rather than a report of sadness, multiple somatic and functional complaints (such as insomnia or anorexia) may dominate the clinical picture; memory problems are another common presentation. These complaints may be linked to a stressful life event (such as a loss or humiliation) that precipitated the change in mood.

It is important to note that psychotic features, i.e., delusions, hallucinations, or both, are present in up to one-quarter of elderly individuals with major depression. The presence of prominent psychotic features, such as persecutory delusions, can make the diagnosis more challenging.

## Common clinical features

### Sadness

Sadness is commonly denied, and tearfulness is less often seen than in younger adults. Likewise, mood may not be described as "depressed." Neither sadness nor depressed mood is necessary for the diagnosis of depression.

Anhedonia (inability to enjoy—ask, "What do you enjoy or look forward to?") and depressive thoughts (guilt, worthlessness, low self-esteem, self-blame, suicidal thoughts, hopelessness and helplessness) are frequently seen. Depressive thoughts may be of delusional proportions (e.g., belief of having caused a catastrophic event).

### Somatization

The expression of emotional distress as physical symptoms is common in the elderly. The term *masked depression* has been used to describe a depression that presents with somatic complaints rather than complaints of depressed mood. Hypochondriasis (disproportionate concern over health) is also common in the elderly.

In the patient presenting with somatization or hypochondriasis, the risks are of failing to investigate and treat when a true physical illness is present, or conversely, of failing to appreciate that antidepressant treatment is actually what is needed. Somatic concerns may be of delusional proportions (e.g., belief of being unable to swallow, rotting from the inside, having an infectious disease).

### Sleep disturbance

Early-morning awakening is typical; in conjunction with diurnal mood variation, it may indicate a melancholic subtype of depression. Obtain a full sleep history, as waking up early may be appropriate, e.g., if the person is going to bed very early or if sleeping during the day. Others may have difficulty initiating or maintaining sleep.

Some older people do sleep much less than when they were younger—the key is whether they wake up refreshed. Good sleep hygiene (e.g., avoidance of caffeine) should be encouraged.

### Anorexia and weight loss

Anorexia and weight loss are common to both depression and to serious physical illness. In the patient who presents in this way, a medical work-up is necessary. If there is no evidence of a physical cause, whether antidepressants should be initiated is a matter of judgment, as is whether more invasive tests should be delayed pending the results of that therapeutic trial. Monitor weights to help follow progress of treatment.

### Cognitive impairment

Poor attention and decreased concentration may result in impairments in several cognitive domains, typically short-term memory. Executive dysfunction (e.g., difficulty with planning and decision-making) is commonly seen in depression. If severe, this may manifest as "dementia of depression." See How to distinguish dementia due to depression from other causes of cognitive impairment (p. 218).

### Psychomotor retardation

Exclude physical causes, including Parkinsonism, cerebrovascular disease, and hypothyroidism. Psychomotor retardation may manifest as increased dependence or "failure to cope." It may be severe, with very reduced mobility or total immobility—the depressed, anorexic, near-catatonic patient must be treated as an emergency.

### Behavioral disturbance

Behaviors may include attention seeking, cries for help (e.g., intentional falls), aggression, irritability, self-neglect, malnutrition, and social withdrawal. Behavioral symptoms are commonly seen in depression with psychotic features, e.g., agitation in the context of persecutory delusions (such as the belief of being watched or monitored).

### Suicidal ideation and self-harm

Suicidal thoughts should always be taken seriously. Twenty percent of completed suicides occur in older adults, especially those with physical illness. Self-harm, even if medically trivial, should mandate psychiatric referral, as parasuicidal behaviors (i.e., "cry for help") are rare in this population. Most older people who self-harm are at least moderately depressed.

## How to assess depression

### Depression rating scales

- The Geriatric Depression Scale (GDS) is a 30-item self-report that has been validated in community and hospital settings. It may be used in the setting of comorbid physical illness. The Short Form of the GDS contains only 15 items and is more commonly used (see Appendix). A score of >5 points suggests depression and should warrant further assessment; 10 points or greater is indicative of depression.
- Hamilton-D (Ham-D) is an observer-rated scale; 16 points (out of 21) indicates depression. It may be used in combination with self-report.
- Patient Health Questionnaire (PHQ-9) is a 9-item self-report validated for use in primary care settings. Forms are available for download in English or Spanish at www.depression-primarycare.org. Scoring instructions are also available at that site.
- The Cornell Scale for depression is a 19-item clinician-administered scale using information from both the patient and caregiver. It has been validated for use in demented and nondemented geriatric patients.
- Two simple questions can be an effective screening tool: "Over the past 2 weeks, have you felt down, depressed, or hopeless?" "Have you experienced a loss of interest or pleasure in most things?" These have reasonable sensitivity and specificity for depression.

### Psychiatric history and examination

### Physical history and examination

Target evidence of physical illness contributing to or mimicking depression, and contraindications to drug treatments.

### Cognitive assessment screen

For example, use the Mini-Mental State Examination or clock-drawing test. Is coexisting cognitive impairment present? If so, does it improve with treatment for depression (as in a dementia of depression)?

### Blood tests

- CBC with differential (anemia, macrocytosis reflecting alcohol use)
- Thyroid function tests (hypothyroidism)
- Cortisol levels
- $B_{12}$ and folate levels (low levels may contribute to depression or result from anorexia)
- Electrolytes, including calcium (hypercalcemia)
- Complete metabolic panel (uremia, dehydration, alcohol use)
- Urinalysis
- CT or MRI if tumor, stroke, or structural pathology is suspected
- ESVR (malignancy, vasculitis)

# Depression: non-drug management

In addition to being underdiagnosed, depression is frequently under-treated in the elderly. Treatment should be started promptly, its intensity (e.g., medication dose) increased as needed for remission, and continued until the likelihood of relapse off treatment is low.

## Supportive treatment

- Includes counseling and relief of loneliness
- Treat physical symptoms and pain.
- Address anxieties, e.g., financial, housing, physical dependency.
- Consider stopping contributory drugs when feasible.

## Psychotherapy

Psychotherapy is as effective as antidepressants for mild to moderate depression, and may be preferred by some patients and providers. It is often used in combination with antidepressants, especially for severe depression. Both cognitive-behavioral therapy (CBT) and interpersonal therapy (IPT) have good supporting evidence. Problem-solving therapy (PST) may be used for major depression with executive dysfunction.

Formats for psychotherapy include individual, group, and family therapy. Access to psychotherapy may be limited (provider availability, affordability, transportation, etc.).

## Electroconvulsive therapy (ECT)

ECT is a highly effective treatment for moderate to severe depression in older adults. ECT is used in the following cases:
- Depression has psychotic features (considered first-line treatment).
- The patient is catatonic or with other severe functional impairment.
- Rapid response is necessary (e.g., suicidality, food or fluid refusal).
- Antidepressant medications are not tolerated or are contraindicated.
- The patient has failed psychopharmacologic treatment.

ECT is relatively safe, and can be safer than a complex medication regimen in the elderly. A brief seizure is induced under general anesthesia. Risks include those associated with general anesthesia use. Side effects are limited to transient memory impairment (less with unilateral ECT to the nondominant hemisphere). There are few relative contraindications.

In geriatric patients, ECT is generally performed 3 times per week as tolerated. The average number of treatments for improvement of symptoms in a given depressive episode is 6–10.

Because depression is a chronic condition and relapse is common, maintenance ECT is usually given. Continuation or maintenance ECT typically consists of once-weekly treatments, gradually reduced to one treatment every 4–8 weeks, depending on the patient's depressive symptom severity. Pharmacological management is often initiated while a patient is undergoing maintenance ECT.

# Depression: drug treatments

Drug treatment is generally effective and well tolerated. There is significant stigma associated with taking antidepressants, and this should be explored and addressed with the patient. Response by a first-degree relative to a particular antidepressant may guide choice of medication.

## Starting a medication

As with other medications in elderly patients, "start low and go slow." Typical starting dose is one-half the usual adult starting dose. Inform the patient that side effects appear early on (i.e., before the therapeutic effects), are usually transient, and may reappear each time the dosage is increased. Choice of antidepressant is often based on side effect profile, as the various first-line antidepressants have similar efficacy.

## Continuing a medication

Clinical response may take several weeks, and the patient should be informed of this. As long as the patient's depressive symptoms are responding to a given medication, continue to titrate the dose as tolerated. Despite the need to proceed slowly, elderly patients may still require a significant dose of medication.

The goal of treatment should be remission of symptoms, and treatment should be continued for up to a year. Thereafter, if depression has been severe and/or recurrent, consider continuing indefinitely as maintenance treatment.

Many elderly patients are undertreated for depression when "keep low" is inadvertently added to the rule—e.g., a patient is started on citalopram 10 mg daily and the medication is never increased despite the continued presence of depressive symptoms.

## Stopping and switching

Withdrawal reactions (e.g., headache, light-headedness, flu-like symptoms) may occur if drugs are stopped abruptly after having been taken for 8 weeks or more. Therefore, reduce the dose gradually, over 2–4 weeks. If switching medications, gradual "cross-tapering" is generally advised, i.e., tapering the old drug while titrating the new one. Rarely, a washout period between drugs is required (e.g., before or after MAOIs).

### Selective serotonin reuptake inhibitors (SSRIs)

These include, e.g., citalopram or sertraline.

- SSRIs are considered first-line treatment.
- Compared to tricyclic antidepressants, they are less sedating, have fewer anticholinergic and cardiotoxic side effects, fewer drug interactions, and are much safer in overdose. Paroxetine tends to be the most anticholinergic of the SSRIs.
- Common side effects include gastrointestinal symptoms (nausea and diarrhoea), orthostatic hypotension, anxiety and restlessness, and hyponatremia. Hyponatremia is usually moderate (Na >125 mM) and asymptomatic, and especially common in combination with diuretics.
- Start at low doses to minimize side effects, and increase as needed to give a therapeutic response. Response may take up to 8 weeks.

- If there is no response to an adequate trial of one SSRI, or if the side effects of a particular SSRI are intolerable, try another one. Switching to another class of antidepressant (e.g., to mirtazipine or venlafaxine) may also be advisable. Partial response may justify augmentation with another agent, such as buproprion.

### Serotonin and norepinephrine reuptake inhibitors (SNRIs)

These include, e.g., venlafaxine desvenlafaxine, and duloxetine.

- SNRIs are commonly used for severe depression, or when there has been a poor response to SSRIs after 6 weeks.
- They may cause less orthostatic hypotension than the SSRIs, but other side effects are similar. There are few, if any, cytochrome P450 interactions.

### Mirtazapine

- Mirtazapine is an atypical antidepressant.
- It has fewer anticholinergic side effects. Sedation and weight gain are the most common side effects. It is given at bedtime because of sedation.

### Buproprion

- Buproprion is an atypical antidepressant.
- It has fewer anticholinergic side effects. Because it tends to be activating, buproprion is usually given in the morning.
- It is often used as an augmentation agent (in conjunction with SSRI).

### Tricyclic antidepressants (TCAs)

These include, e.g., amitriptyline, nortriptyline, and desipramine. TCAs are second-line agents due to orthostatic hypotension, anticholinergic side effects, and drug–drug interactions.

Uses of TCAs include the following:

- When anticholinergic effects are desirable (e.g., urge incontinence)
- When there is neuropathic or other pain that may respond to its analgesic effect
- When insomnia is present, TCAs are given at bedtime to aid in sleep initiation.

The secondary amines (e.g., nortriptyline and desipramine) are preferred, as they cause less orthostatic hypotension than other TCAs. Anticholinergic side effects are less troublesome if doses start low and are increased gradually.

- Follow drug levels in the serum.
- Monitor ECG for widening of QT interval.
- They are lethal in overdose of as little as 3x the daily dose of the drug.

### Mononamine oxidase inhibitors (MAOIs)

Phenelzine and tranylcypromine are MAOIs.

MAOIs are occasionally used, under expert guidance. Dietary (tyramine) and drug interactions are problematic. Hypertensive crisis can be life threatening.

*Stimulants*

These include, e.g., methylphenidate and d-amphetamine.

- Stimulants increase central release of norepinephrine, dopamine, and serotonin.
- They are used in cases of prominent apathy or withdrawal, treatment failure with more than two drugs, or for augmentation of an antidepressant. Stimulants may be used for depression in the setting of dementia.
- Side effects are generally related to excess stimulation of CNS and cardiovascular systems. Stimulants may increase blood levels of other medications metabolized by the cytochrome P450 system.
- Atomoxetine is a nonstimulant medication used for similar purposes. The side-effect profile is more benign than that of the stimulants.

## Specialist referral

Consider referral to a geriatric psychiatrist if the following occur:
- Treatment is unsuccessful after 6–8 weeks at an adequate dose.
- Depression is severe, e.g., with delusions or suicidal ideation.
- The diagnosis is unclear, e.g., when depression and significant cognitive impairment coexist.
- A patient is refusing treatment or otherwise threatening self-harm.
- There are questions of decisional capacity or competency.

# Suicide and attempted suicide

Older people, especially men, have a higher risk of completed (rather than attempted) suicide. Following an attempted suicide, further attempts—and successful suicide—are common.

Risk factors include being male, single (i.e., unmarried, divorced, separated, or widowed), socially isolated, having financial problems, having made previous attempts, and suffering recent bereavement. The presence of physical illness, chronic pain, and psychiatric illness, such as mood disorder, anxiety, and alcohol and drug use, also increase suicide risk.

The substantial majority of older people who attempt suicide are psychiatrically unwell at the time of the attempt; most are depressed. Many seek contact with medical services prior to the attempt, although they may not express depressive or suicidal thoughts at that visit.

Suicidal behaviors may be overt or covert.

**Overt behaviors** include the following:
- Intentional drug overdoses (opiates, antidepressants, benzodiazepines; more common in women)
- Self-injury (shooting, hanging, jumping, drowning; more common in men). Firearms are the most common means.

**Covert suicide** is relatively more common in older people and includes
- Social withdrawal
- Severe self-neglect
- Refusal of food, fluid, or medication

This may manifest in subtle ways that encourage extensive investigation to exclude physical illness, leaving the psychiatric illness unrecognized and untreated.

Suicidal ideation is more common in institutional settings (hospital wards, rehabilitation centers, and nursing homes) and in people with acute or chronic physical illness. At their mildest, suicidal ideas manifest as common and relatively benign doubts about whether life is worth living. More severely, they are carefully considered, well formulated, and strongly held beliefs that death is preferable to life, and how that could be achieved. In the elderly, hopelessness in the context of depressive symptoms may predict the presence of suicidal ideation.

Assessment of the severity of an attempt requires an effort to determine perceived risk from the patient's perspective at the time of the attempt. This may not parallel the medical seriousness. Consider the following:
- Degree of planning vs. impulsivity
- Likelihood of interruption during attempt
- Reaction to interruption to attempt (disappointment or relief?)
- Suicide note and its contents
- Planning for future (e.g., making of will, contents of suicide note)
- Personal view of suicide as a reasonable "life choice"

## Specialist referral

All cases of attempted suicide, suicidal ideation, or covert suicide should be referred to a specialist. Referral is probably not necessary in cases of nonpersistent or poorly formulated views that life is not worth living.

# Psychosis

Psychotic symptoms, e.g., delusions and hallucinations, are common in older people, particularly those who are acutely unwell, hospitalized, or in nursing homes. These symptoms are distressing to the patient, cause anxiety for caregivers, and often indicate important, treatable disease.

## What is psychosis?

Psychosis is a state of severe impairment in reality testing. Manifestations include the following:

- Distortions of perception, e.g., hallucinations (perception in the absence of an external stimulus, commonly referred to as "hearing voices" or "seeing things"), and illusions (distortion of an actual stimulus, e.g., the back-firing of a car is perceived to be a gunshot)
- Distortions of thought content, i.e., delusions—beliefs held with great conviction despite contrary evidence. These are usually secondary, i.e., a response to perceptual disturbance or low mood.

## Causes of psychotic symptoms in older people

- Delirium
- Dementia
- Depression
- Parkinson's disease
- Medications, e.g., levodopa, anticholinergic, incontinence treatments
- Other brain diseases, e.g., cerebrovascular disease, brain tumor
- Persistence into late life of chronic schizophrenia
- Delusional disorder of later life ("late paraphrenia")
- Feature of bipolar disorder (manic or depressive episode)

## Treatment of patients with psychotic symptoms

- Referral to geriatric psychiatry or psychiatry consult service is advised.
- Avoid reinforcing a patient's paranoid beliefs: don't avoid contact with the patient, don't arrange rapid transfer from the ward, etc.
- Directly challenging the patient's beliefs may lead to increased agitation. Calm, reassuring communication is best.
- Make a diagnosis and treat the underlying cause, e.g., stop drugs leading to delirium.
- Attend to hearing and visual impairments.
- Treat underlying mood disorder, if present.
- In dementia, especially Alzheimer's and DLB, consider ChEIs.
- If symptoms are distressing and persistent, consider the use of antipsychotics, e.g., haloperidol, risperidone, olanzapine, usually after specialist advice. Be cautious in patients who may have dementia with Lewy bodies.
- On discharge, offer opportunities for social interaction and practical home support.

## Further reading

American Psychiatric Association. (2000). *Diagnostic and Statistical Manual of Mental Disorders, fourth edition, Text Revision.* Arlington, VA: American Psychiatric Association.
Alexopoulos G (2005). Depression in the elderly. *Lancet* **365**: 1961–1970.

# Cardiovascular medicine

**Susan Zieman**

# The aging cardiovascular system

Advanced age is the *most potent* risk factor for cardiovascular disease (CVD). This increased vulnerability stems from (a) cumulative exposure to lifestyle and environmental factors (diet, lack of exercise, stress, smoking), (b) higher rates and longer impact of traditional risk factors (hypertension, hyperlipidemia, diabetes), (c) impact of comorbidites (chronic lung disease, anemia, renal disease), and (d) age-associated alterations in cardiovascular structure and function.

An understanding of the physiological alterations is important as they affect the vulnerability to CVD development, presentation, hemodynamic response, treatment, and prevention. The changes described in Table 10.1 accompany "normative aging" (in the absence of disease), but occur in individuals at different rates and are additionally influenced by superimposed disease.

Table 10.1 addresses the three important questions:
• What are the common changes with age?
• How do these changes have an impact on function?
• What are the clinical implications?

**Table 10.1** Age-related changes and their impact on function

| Age-related change | Impact on function | Clinical implications |
|---|---|---|
| *Arterial* ↑ Central arterial stiffness, ↑ proximal aortic diameter, ↑ peripheral vascular resistance, ↓ endothelial function, ↑ intima-medial thickness, fibrosis and smooth muscle hypertrophy | ↑SBP,↓DBP, ↑PP, ↑pulse wave velocity – reflected aortic wave returns to ventricle prematurely (in systole rather than in diastole), which ↑ ventricular afterload and ↓ coronary perfusion | Isolated systolic hypertension very common |
| | | ↑ afterload causes LVH |
| | | Sluggish coronary flow ↓ ischemia threshold (esp. with LVH) even in absence of CAD |
| | Stiff arteries cause labile BP to intravascular volume shifts (↑↑ pressure/↑ volume and ↓↓ pressure/ ↓ volume) | Postprandial and orthostatic hypotension |
| | | Labile BP to IV fluids and diuretics |
| | | Vascular changes ↑ atheroma formation |
| | | CXR may show enlarged aortic knob and arch unfolding |

**Table 10.1** Age-related changes and their impact on function (*continued*)

| Age-related change | Impact on function | Clinical implications |
|---|---|---|
| *Ventricular*<br>Myocyte hypertophy, collagen-cross-linking, ↑ fibrosis<br><br>Resting LV end diastolic volume same | ↑ Intraventricular pressure, ↓ LV filling in early diastole (~30% in elderly vs. ~70% in young), ↑ dependence on atrial systole for LV diastole filing (70% in elderly and ~30% in young)<br>↑ preload dependence | ↓ Ischemia threshold (↑ myocardium to perfuse), ↑ dyspnea and pulmonary edema with tachycardia, hypertension, physical exertion and/or ischemia (heart failure with normal EF); ↑ heart size on CXR; ↑ dyspnea, ↓ BP in AF; LVH may impact ECG evaluation in illness |
| *Atrial*<br>↑ Atrial size (from ↑ intraventrcular pressure) | | Predisposes to atrial fibrillation |
| *β-adrenergic response* to stress (physical, exertional/emotional) ↓ inotropic, lusitropic, chronotropic responses despite ↑ circulating catecholamines | ↓ Maximal HR and cardiac output (CO) response to exercise and stress, ↓ cardiac reserve. Resting HR, CO, and EF unchanged | Tachycardic response to acute illness less reliable. ↓ threshold for DOE and with stress. Hemodynamic instability to illness |
| *Conduction system*<br>↓ Pacemaker cells, ↑fibrosis, calcification and fat infiltration of SA node and conducting system | Susceptible to sinus arrest, delayed conduction | Primary AVB, ↑ PR, QRS, RBBB, left axis deviation can be seen; LBBB not due to aging alone; tachy–brady rhythms. Sick sinus syndrome, junctional rhythms, sinus pauses; ↑ susceptible to blocks and bradycardia from beta and calcium blockers; baseline ECG may obscure disease evaluation |
| *Volume-regulating hormones*<br>↓ Renin, angiotensin, aldosterone, vasopressin. ↑ atrial natriuretic peptide | With ↓ renal handling of salt and fluid and ↓thirst, add to ↑ fluid shifts, ↑ salt sensitivity | BP lability, ↑ peripheral edema to salt and fluids, ↑ susceptible to dehydration |
| *Baroreflex*<br>↓ sensitivity | | Orthostatic hypotension |
| *Exercise*<br>↓ maximum oxygen consumption | ↓ maximal HR and CO, ↓ muscle oxygen extraction from sarcopenia | Contributes to ↓ cardiovascular reserve to stress |

For abbreviations see Abbreviations and Symbols.

# Chest pain

Chest pain is a common and worrisome symptom in all settings. It may be a primary complaint, mentioned only in response to direct questioning, or it may occur with other conditions (e.g., pneumonia).

Chest pain always warrants a thorough and sensible evaluation, beginning with a careful and efficient history and physical examination. While many instances are benign, some are serious and life threatening. This is especially true in older adults, who often have atypical presentation of disease and may downplay symptoms, and who have a high likelihood of coronary artery disease.

Common conditions not to be missed include cardiac pain; pleuritic pain due to pulmonary infarction or infection; peptic pain (including bleeding ulcers); pain from dissecting aortic aneurysm; and pneumothorax (especially in COPD).

Other possibilities include muscular pain (e.g., after unaccustomed exertion); costochondritis (local tenderness at sternal joint); pericarditis; pain from injury (e.g., after a fall); rib fracture; early herpes zoster infection (shingles); referred pain from the back and neck (e.g., osteoarthritis or osteoporosis); and referred pain from the abdomen.

Differentiating these conditions depends on accurate history and careful examination, both of which can be more challenging in older patients. Because presentation may be atypical and the patient may have many other problems, teasing out the important symptoms can be difficult (although experience improves the ability to "feel" your way around the history).

## History

- Is this a new symptom? (e.g., patient may suffer from chronic angina)
- If not, is it different from the usual pain? (e.g., intensity, pattern)
- What is the nature of the pain? (e.g., pleuritic, heavy, tight, etc.) This is often hard for patients to describe, and hand gestures can help—a clenched fist for a heavy pain, a stabbing action for a sharp, pleuritic pain.
- Where is the pain located? (e.g., size of area; radiation to neck, arm, jaw)
- How acute is the onset and what is the duration? (Pain that is constant for days without signs of distress or ECG changes is rarely cardiac.)
- What makes it better or worse? (e.g., positional, eating, exertion, movement, effect of medications)
- Are there any associated symptoms? (nausea, dizziness, diaphoresis, fever, chills, dyspnea)

Patients with cognitive impairment can be particularly difficult to assess, but free conversation may reveal symptoms, followed by closed questions that may prompt appropriate answers. Family members may have noted signs or symptoms, e.g., clutching the chest after walking, and are an invaluable aid to assessment.

Remember that cardiac symptoms may differ for each patient. Allow patients to use their own language for discomfort, as many older adults with angina or myocardial infarction will deny overt "chest pain." Some will simply experience dyspnea, weakness, or nausea.

## Examination

- How does the patient look? A sweaty, clammy patient needs urgent and exhaustive assessment, whereas a patient watching television and chatting is less likely to have a devastating condition.
- What are the basic observations? (blood pressure [BP], pulse, heart rhythm, respiratory rate and pattern, presence of pulsus paradoxus, position of patient)
- Signs of shock alert to a serious condition (ischemic heart disease, pulmonary infarction, dissection, sepsis, blood loss), but remember that these may be late signs and are less useful in older patients. The patient may usually be hypertensive, so a BP of 120/80 may be very low for them; they may be on a beta-blocker and thus unable to mount tachycardia.
- Different blood pressures in the arms may indicate dissection (but can also be due to atheroma).
- Is the jugular venous pressure elevated (heart failure)?
- Are there signs of shingles (vesicular lesions), bruising, or reproducible tenderness (fracture, costochondritis)?
- Listen to the heart—are there new murmurs (dissection, infarction, papillary rupture, endocarditis) or a rub (pericarditis is best heard with diaphragm of stethoscope at left sternal border during expiration while patient is sitting), or an $S_3$?
- Listen to the lungs—is there consolidation (sepsis) or a pleural rub (consolidation or infarction)?
- Look at the legs—is there any clinical deep vein thrombosis (DVT)?

## Investigations

Some tests can be less useful in older patients and should be individually tailored to the patient. Sending off every single test on all patients with chest pain will only lead to confusion.

### Electrocardiogram (ECG)

An ECG should be done as a priority on most patients with chest pain. Remember, the baseline ECG may be abnormal or paced in an older person, thus comparison with old tracings is extremely useful. If your patient has a very abnormal ECG (e.g., left bundle branch block [LBBB]), it is useful to give them a copy to carry with them.

### Chest X-ray

Look for lung abnormalities and widening of the mediastinum. Remember that the aorta often "unfolds," so a careful look at the contours of the aortic arch and/or comparison with old films is needed to assess possible dissection. A patient can look fairly well in the early stages of aortic dissection. Look for rib fractures as well. Is the cardiac silhouette large (e.g., pericardial effusion, aortic dissection, dilated heart)?

### Blood tests

Basic complete blood count (CBC) and biochemistry are often useful. Remember that in acute blood loss, the hemoglobin may not drop immediately, and an elderly septic patient may take a day or two to develop an elevated white cell count.

### Troponin

This is useful in a patient with suspected cardiac chest pain (for risk stratification). It is NOT a useful test if you do not think this is cardiac pain—there are many false positives that will only cause confusion. Troponin may be slightly elevated in the setting of hypotension, supply–demand ischemia, and does not always equate an acute coronary syndrome.

### D-dimer

D-dimer testing is only useful if it is negative in cases of suspected thromboembolism. There are many causes of a positive D-dimer (including old age itself), thus a positive result does not imply the diagnosis of pulmonary embolism (PE).

### Further tests

These include transesophageal echocardiogram (TEE), chest CT or MRI for suspected dissection, exercise testing for angina, VQ scans or spiral CT for thromboembolism, echocardiogram for pericardial effusion, heart and valve function evaluation depending on clinical factors.

Always attempt to explain a chest pain—both for the patient and future clinicians. A "diagnosis" of "ruled out for MI" or "noncardiac chest pain" is not a diagnoses and is not helpful. Patients without elevated cardiac enzymes may still have a cardiac etiology.

# Coronary artery disease

Coronary artery disease (CAD) is the greatest cause of mortality and the second greatest cause of morbidity (next to arthritis) of older adults. Coronary events can be "silent," especially in patients with diabetes mellitus (DM). Silent infarctions may be discovered inadvertently on routine ECG (pathologic Q waves) or on echocardiogram (wall motion abnormalities).

The diagnoses of peripheral vascular disease, atherosclerotic stroke or carotid disease, and/or diabetes mandate aggressive risk factor control and are considered coronary heart disease (CHD) equivalents.

## Presentation

CAD may present as stable exertional symptoms (stable angina or dyspnea, p. 326) or as an acute coronary syndrome (which includes unstable angina and myocardial infarction, p. 266). The presentation of CAD may be atypical and/or downplayed by the patient. Symptoms and treatments may also be altered by comorbid illnesses. Early diagnosis and aggressive risk factor management are the cornerstones of therapy.

## Risk factor reduction

Therapeutic goals are listed below. The Framingham Risk Score Calculator (http://hp2010.nhlbihin.net/atpiii/calculator) is a popular tool to calculate CVD risk, but is less predictive in those >80 years of age.

### Primary prevention

- **Hypertension management:** Vigilant blood pressure control reduces the primary CVD risk.
- **Cholesterol lowering:** With increasing age, elevated total cholesterol is less associated with primary events. Lifestyle and diet are the initial strategies to lower cholesterol, followed by medications. Primary prevention in those over 80 with drug therapy has not been shown to be effective.
- **Smoking cessation** at any age is strongly associated with CVD risk reduction.
- **Exercise:** Regular aerobic exercise (recommended for 30 minutes/day, 5 days a week) is associated with CVD risk reduction.
- **Diabetes** raises the risk of CVD, thus risk factors should be targeted more aggressively if compatible with the patient's goals and health status.

### Secondary prevention

The risk of recurrent CVD events is high in older adults, thus risk factor reduction should be aggressive when consistent with the patient's health status and goals. The 10-year risk for myocardial infarction (MI) can be calculated using an interactive tool available at: http://hp2010.nhlbihin.net/atpiii/calculator.asp

- Goals for Risk Factor Reduction: National Cholesterol Education Program—ATP-3 updated guidelines available at: http://www.nhlbi.nih.gov/guidelines/cholesterol/
- JNC-7 blood pressure targets (see Hypertension, p. 274)

## Further reading

Grundy SM, Cleeman JI, Merz CN, et al. (2004). Implications of recent clinical trials for the National Cholesterol Education Program Adult Treatment Panel III Guidelines. *Circulation* **110**:227–239.

Williams MA, Fleg JL, Ades PA, et al. (2002). Secondary prevention of coronary heart disease in the elderly (with emphasis on patients ≥75 years of age). *Circulation* **105**:1735–1743.

# Angina

Recognizing angina can be difficult because it is often an atypical presentation (dyspnea on exertion [DOE] may be thought to be primarily of pulmonary rather than cardiac etiology) and there is the tendency for some to downplay symptoms.

The term *angina* is often used by older patients to refer to any type of chest discomfort. It is important to ensure that what the patient is calling "angina" is truly of cardiac etiology. Conversely, angina may elicit unique symptoms in different patients (only jaw or arm pain, dyspnea or indigestion without chest symptoms). Clarify whether the patient's symptoms are similar to their previous "heart symptoms."

Often anginal symptoms may be relieved by addressing a mismatch between the myocardial blood or oxygen supply and myocardial energy demands rather than by mechanical intervention (see Aggravating conditions, p. 263).

Maximizing medical therapy and ongoing risk factor reduction (managing hypertension and hyperlipidemia, smoking cessation, and diabetes management) are the cornerstones of therapy. Invasive intervention such as percutaneous coronary intervention (PCI) or coronary artery bypass grafting (CABG) may improve symptoms and quality of life (QOL) in appropriately selected patients.

This section will deal with the management of new-onset or recurrent stable angina. Unstable angina (USA) will be addressed in the next section (Acute coronary syndromes). Patients should be instructed to alert their physicians if their anginal symptoms ever change quality (become more frequent or occur at rest), in which case they are considered USA.

## Stable angina

### Risk factor reduction

- Cholesterol and blood pressure are less likely to be lowered to recommended targets in older patients, especially those with CAD, but the risk reduction is equal if not greater than for younger subjects.
- Life style advice (exercise, smoking, and diet) is also highly effective but commonly avoided by older patients or their careproviders.

### Medication

- Medication is underused, particularly aspirin (concerns about bleeding) and beta-blockade, despite evidence that they are both equally useful in treating symptoms and reducing risk of recurrent events.
- First-line therapies for stable angina include aspirin, beta-blocker, and a statin, if not contraindicated. These may be introduced one or two treatments at a time to minimize the risk of side effects.
- Start on low doses, and titrate upward (e.g., atenolol 25mg).
- Long-acting agents reduce adherence problems.
- If angina is resistant to these medications, consider additional therapy, e.g., nitrates (patch or long-acting oral), dihydropyridine calcium channel blockers (amlodipine, felodipine), diuretic for BP control, ACE inhibitor if there is poor left ventricular (LV) function, and oxygen if hypoxia is a factor.

- Choice of medication should be pragmatic—if a patient has bradycardia, for example, a non-negatively chronotropic drug is most appropriate (e.g., amlodipine 5–10 mg). If the patient also has COPD, it may be wise to avoid beta-blockade. If a patient has cardiac dysfunction, a cardioselective beta-blocker (e.g., carvedilol, metoprolol, bisoprolol) is a better choice than a calcium channel blocker.
- Short-acting nitroglycerin may result in significant hypotension, so instruction on correct use is essential. It should be first tried sitting down. If hypotension occurs with sublingual pills, they can be spat out once the pain starts to settle. Nitroglycerin oral spray is often easier to use and can be taken prophylactically before significant exertion.

### Aggravating conditions

Always look for correctable factors impacting the supply–demand balance of myocardial energy. Such imbalance may result in a small increase in troponin, and treatment should be focused on the cause of the mismatch.

- **Myocardial supply:** anemia, blood loss, hypoxia, fever, aortic stenosis, isolated systolic hypertension or hypotension (results in decreased coronary blood flow)
- **Myocardial demand:** heart failure, aortic stenosis, severe or acute mitral regurgitation, hyperthyroidism, tachycardia, fever, tachyarrhythmias (atrial fibrillation), hypertension

### Revascularization

This should be considered with specific anatomy or if angina is resistant to maximal medical therapy (see Box 10.1). The success rate of PCI is similar in older and younger patients, but procedural risks are higher in older patients. In chronic angina, PCI reduces symptoms and readmission but does not reduce mortality in older adults.

Similarly, the risk from CABG is greater in older than in younger patients but can reduce symptoms and mortality in certain patients (see p. 264).

### Palliation

Consider this for diffuse disease not amenable to revascularization with ongoing symptoms (e.g., home oxygen therapy, opiates for pain control).

### Box 10.1 Revascularization procedures

These include percutaneous coronary angiography and intervention (PCI) and coronary artery bypass grafting (CABG).

*When?*
- These procedures are used when stable symptoms persist despite maximal medical therapy, or when unstable symptoms fail to settle.
- Risk stratify with exercise testing and troponin measurements. Older patients may be unable to exercise, but consider bicycle exercise, stress echocardiography, or an isotope myocardial perfusion scan to look for evidence of reversible ischemia.

*What are the risks?*
PCI
- Higher risk of death, renal failure, and infarction in the elderly. Age is an independent predictor of increased complication, as are diabetes, cardiac failure, and chronic renal impairment.

CABG
- Increased early mortality and stroke in older patients.
- Increased morbidity and mortality risks: advanced age, female, MI <30 days, higher New York Heart Association (NYHA) class, ejection fraction (EF) <20%, chronic renal insufficiency (CRI), COPD, peripheral arterial disease (PAD) or stroke, left main or triple-vessel (3V) disease, or emergent, urgent, or re-do.

*What are the benefits?*
PCI
- Success rate appears same as in young, but increased risk. Increased QOL and less readmission in chronic angina but no decrease in mortality. Primary PCI preferred in ST-elevation MI (STEMI) and early invasive in non-STEMI (NSETMI). There is variable evidence from studies—all show more early complications, but longer-term benefits in older patients are equivalent or even better.

CABG
- Preferred with left main, 3V CAD, poor exercise tolerance, poor LV function, and diabetes. It is generally well tolerated in the elderly, with similar long-term improvements in symptoms and QOL to those of younger patients. New minimally invasive techniques that do not require bypass are likely to reduce the early complications without impairing outcome.

*Overall recommendations*
Consider all patients who fail medical treatment for revascularization procedures. The decision will be driven by comorbidities, patient preference, dedication to improve postoperatively (rehab), and functional status. The early complication rate is higher in older patients, but the eventual benefit is equal if not better than for younger patients.

Approach a cardiologist and cardiac surgeon with a record of treating older patients.

It is crucial to include the patient in the decision, with a frank and individualized discussion about risks and benefits.

# Acute coronary syndromes and myocardial infarction

*Acute coronary syndromes (ACS)* describe a clinical scenario in which myocardial cells are not receiving enough blood and oxygen to meet their demands. ACS comprises a spectrum from unstable angina (USA) to non-ST-elevation myocardial infarction (NSTEMI) and ST elevation infarction (STEMI), defined in Table 10.2. ACS may be the primary reason for presentation, or it may occur during hospitalization (illness or surgery) or in the setting or trauma or accident.

**Table 10.2** Definitions of acute coronary syndromes (ACS)

|  | USA | NSTEMI | STEMI |
|---|---|---|---|
| **Symptoms** | ± chest discomfort, arm, neck, jaw pain, dyspnea, confusion, diaphoresis, nausea/vomiting, light-headedness | | |
| **Symptom time course** | Change in usual angina pattern, ↑ frequency, occurring with less exertion, new pain at rest | Constant or intermittent | Usually constant |
| **ECG** | Nonspecific changes, may be without changes | Nonspecific ST or T wave changes, may be unchanged | 1–2 mm ST elevation in 2+ territorial leads with reciprocal changes (ST depression in opposite territory) |
| **Cardiac enzymes** | − | + | + |
| **Pathophysiology** | Fixed coronary lesion, supply–demand mismatch | Partially occluding, thrombus and/or supply–demand mismatch (usually with fixed lesion) | Acute thrombus or embolus occluding blood supply |
| **Initial therapy** | Medical— invasive if persistent | Medical or invasive if persistent | Thrombolytic, invasive preferred, medical if contraindicated |

Because therapy is directed at reestablishing myocardial energy supply, it is important to determine whether the lack of energy delivery is caused by an acute coronary blockage or by an alteration in the myocardial supply–demand balance (see Aggravating conditions, p. 263), as the therapeutic approach can differ significantly.

The initial ACS assessment and management is shown in the next section. ACS management is the same as for older as for younger patients, but there are some points relating to older patients in particular.

- **Atypical presentation:** Older patients are more likely to present with atypical or vague symptoms (e.g., intense dyspnea, weakness, confusion, nausea, abdominal pain), which may not include chest pain or discomfort. Symptoms may be obscured by comorbidities. ECG may be difficult to interpret due to underlying changes, pre-existing LBBB, or pacing. Typical ischemia or infarction ECG changes may be absent in up to one-third of older adults with MI. Vital signs or symptoms may be obscured by medications (beta- or calcium blockers, pain meds).
- **Different pathology:** There is more pre-existing CAD with more multivessel disease; NSTEMI is more likely than STEMI. Patients are more likely to develop heart failure, atrioventricular (AV) block, atrial fibrillation (AF), or cardiogenic shock after a coronary event.
- **Later presentation:** There is increased prevalence of angina, so be less alarmed by chest pains. Patients may modify lifestyle to avoid symptoms (if an activity gives them angina they may stop doing it). "Silent ischemia" occurs more often (especially in diabetics) and there are more social and attitudinal factors ("I didn't want to bother the doctor"). A third of patients over 65 with MI will present >6 hours after symptom onset.
- **Increased comorbidity** makes diagnosis difficult (e.g., a patient with COPD who has DOE) and therapy less well tolerated (e.g., aspirin and gastritis). As comorbidities add up, so does frailty; medications are generally less well tolerated (e.g., symptomatic hypotension from anti-anginals).
- Higher inpatient **mortality** occurs from ACS, so prioritize older patients for intensive monitoring. All patients ≥70 years old are at intermediate to high risk for short-term death and recurrent MI.
- Patients may have comorbidities that exclude them from **aggressive acute therapy** (e.g., less thrombolysis, angiography and PCI, CABG, and maximal medical treatment) or patients may refuse procedures.
- Older patients are often less likely to have received or been discharged on **full secondary prevention**, even without contraindications.

## Acute coronary syndromes: initial assessment and therapy

Rapid and efficient assessment is critically important to prevent myocardial damage or spare jeopardized myocardial tissue. This is particularly true of STEMI, for which the rapid reperfusion (PCI or thrombolytics) reduces myocardial damage and lowers the risk of mortality.

Accordingly, parts of the assessment may be done simultaneously with the initiation of some of the therapies (see Table 10.3). The goal of initial therapy is to relieve symptoms and signs of ischemia and infarction. Initial management of USA and NSTEMI is the same, since diagnosis is not confirmed until cardiac enzymes results return.

These factors, along with age-related changes in physiology and pharmacology, make management of the older ACS patients challenging and contribute to their increased mortality and morbidity. Adults over age 65 comprise 13% of the U.S. population but make up >65% of hospital admissions for ACS and account for >80% of the related deaths. Lack of clinical trial data is often cited for the underuse of therapies in this cohort. Yet, lack of evidence does not necessarily equate to lack of benefit; rather, it has not been evaluated in this complex and heterogeneous population.

Patient-centered care dictates when to use an aggressive approach, considering the patient as a whole:
• Patient preference where possible
• Comorbidities (alter risk profile)
• Current medication
• Frailty and likely life expectancy

Recent guidelines address the nuances of ACS care in older adults and should be used as a resource (see Further reading, p. 272).

**Table 10.3** Assessment and treatment

| Assessment | Therapy |
| --- | --- |
| • Vital signs (BP, HR, O$_2$ sat, weight) | • Aspirin 325 mg |
| • ECG—ASA | • Oxygen—regardless of sat, low dose if history of chronic lung diabetes |
|   • If STEMI, target therapy, cath lab activation, consider lytics if no contraindications and cath lab <3 hours | • Telemetry |
| | • IV access |
| • Brief, targeted history can be taken while ECG performed. Consider Aggravating conditions (p. 263) | • Nitroglycerin—sublingual to start if adequate BP. If no relief, consider paste or IV if BP permits |
| • Physical exam (signs of heart failure, right ventricular [RV] infarct—hypotension without rales and ↑ jugular venous pressure [JVP], murmurs, shock) | • Beta-blockers |
| |   • Avoid if bradycardia or suspect RV infarct |
|   • Can be performed during ECG |   • IV metoprolol 5 mg IV push x3 doses if BP permits |
| • Blood (cardiac enzymes, CBC, basic metabolic profile—creatinine) | • Unfractionated heparin (UFH) IV if no signs of active bleeding |
| • Chest X-ray |   • Weight-based bolus and infusion |
|   • Consider if dissection, or pulmonary disease in differential diagnosis. Usually not necessary in initial workup | • Morphine IV for pain if BP permits |
| | • Diuresis |
| • Echocardiogram |   • For heart failure |
|   • If suspected pericardial effusion, valve rupture, severe hypotension or shock |   • Avoid if evidence of RV infarct (in which case, fluids may be warranted) |
| | • Low-molecular-weight heparin (LMWH) is renally cleared and has inconsistent results vs. UFH |
| | • Glycoprotein (GP)IIb/IIIa inhibitors |
| |   • Beneficial in high risk, especially + enzymes |
| |   • With ASA and UFH |
| |   • Abciximab if PCI planned |
| |   • Tirofiban or eptifibatide if no PCI but high risk |
| |   • **Dose must be based on CrCl** |
| |   • ↑ Bleeding in older adults, especially when not dosed by CrCl |
| | • Clopidogrel |
| |   • If ASA intolerant |
| |   • Loading dose usually given in cath lab if needed |

### STEMI management in older adults

Older adults have the highest risk of death (usually mechanical or electrical complications) and a 50% likelihood of developing heart failure in the setting of an STEMI (see Table 10.4). Time to treatment is critical, recognizing the following:

Primary PCI is generally favored over thrombolytic therapy as below (↓ death, recurrent MI and stroke). Data are limited for those >80 years old. Primary PCI is favored in the following situations:
- When skilled lab is available with surgical backup
- Door-to-balloon time <90 minutes
- Killip 3–4, or cardiogenic shock
- When thrombolytics are contraindicated
- If STEMI diagnosis in doubt
- If symptom onset is >3 hours, unless shock or hemodynamic instability
- Within 36 hours of failed thrombolytic therapy if shock develops

Thrombolytic therapy is favored if there are no contraindications and under the following circumstances:
- Presentation <3 hours and invasive strategy not available
- Invasive strategy not an option
- Delay to invasive strategy—long transport time
- **Do not administer** if presentation >12 hours after onset (unless ongoing symptoms and ST elevation is within 24 hours).
- Renally dose UFH or LMWH medications to decrease bleeding risk
- Avoid GPIIb/IIIa inhibitor cotreatment in those ≥75 years old

Urgent CABG is performed when PCI fails, the patient is hemodynamically unstable, in shock or ongoing ischemia is present.

**Table 10.4** Management of STEMI in older adults

| Therapy | Evidence |
|---|---|
| Aspirin | Equivalent risk reduction in older population |
| Primary PCI | **USA/NSTEMI:** Early invasive strategy (within 48 hours) shown to decrease death and recurrent MI over conservative strategy. Bleeding risk is higher with invasive than with conservative strategy. Role of PCI for those >80 and with multiple comorbidities has not been well studied. |
| | **STEMI:** PCI is preferred over lytics if presentation <3 hours of onset, with experienced lab with surgical backup, and door-to-balloon time <90 minutes. It is also used for patients in shock, with Killip 3–4, after failed lytics, with ongoing ischemia, or with contraindications to lytics. |
| Thrombolysis | **USA/NSTEMI:** NOT indicated |
| | **STEMI:** Use thrombolysis if there are no contraindications, primary PCI is not available or requires long transit time, if presentation <12 hours, there is ↓ bleeding risk by renal dosing adjuvant heparin, ↑ risk bleeding if hypertensive, low body weight, previous stroke, or patient is on warfarin. |

**Table 10.4** Management of STEMI in older adults (*continued*)

| Therapy | Evidence |
|---------|----------|
| Low-molecular-weight heparin (LMWH) | Controversial benefit over UFH. ↑ bleeding if not renally dosed. For USA/NSTEMI, some studies suggest a beneficial role in older patients if properly dosed. |
| GP IIb/IIIa inhibitors | Trials using this therapy in unstable angina and NSTEMI show benefit that is equal in older patients but there is ↑ bleeding if patient is not renally dosed (by CrCl). |

## Prior to discharge

Regardless of the intervention and hospital course, all patients admitted with or who experience an acute coronary syndrome should be considered for the following to reduce their risk of recurrent events and to improve their level of functioning and independence.

### Medications
Use medications unless they are absolutely contraindicated. Also remember to reconcile them with home medication.
- Aspirin: 325 mg unless on another antiplatelet agent or warfarin (81 mg). If new coronary stent, 325 mg/day for 30 days, then 81 mg/day. Clopidrogrel if ASA intolerant.
- Beta-blocker if tolerated. Long-acting agent will improve adherence.
- ACE inhibitor if decreased LV function and/or diabetic. If normal cardiac function, use if BP tolerates use.
- Nitroglycerin: Prescription and instructions for sublingual or spray
- HMG CoA reductase inhibitor (statin): Higher doses are more likely to ↑ LFTs in older adults. Avoid pravastatin in CrCl <30. Watch for drug interactions with cytochrome P450 34a (pravastatin avoids this).
- Clopidogrel (or ticlodpidine if clopidogrel is not tolerated) if coronary stent (1 month for bare metal, >1 year for drug-eluting). May be required for longer with smaller stents, multiple stents, or stents crossing branch points. Patients should be instructed NOT to stop antiplatelet drugs without a doctor's approval.

### Education
- Diet, nutrition, cholesterol control
- Smoking cessation
- Activity restriction
- Emergency activation for recurrent symptoms
- Follow-up appointment, stent cards if applicable

### *Cardiac rehabilitation referral*
See Box 10.2.

## Box 10.2 Cardiac rehabilitation

Older adults benefit greatly from a formal phase II cardiac rehabilitation program, which is currently reimbursed by Medicare following PCI, myocardial infarction, CABG, or valve surgery.
- Involves structured exercise program
- Proven to improve exercise tolerance and decrease readmission
- Under-prescribed for older cardiac patients despite Medicare reimbursement
- Older people adhere well to programs and seem to suffer no complications.
- Some adaptations are needed (more time to warm up and cool down, longer breaks, avoidance of high-impact activity, lower intensity for a longer time).
- Benefits include improved cardiovascular fitness, decreased blood pressure and cholesterol values, increased bone mineral density, improved mood, decreased depression scores, maintained independence, and fewer falls.

## Further reading

Alexander KP, Newby LK, Cannon CP, et al. (2007). Acute coronary care in the elderly. Part I: Non–ST-segment–elevation acute coronary syndromes: a scientific statement for healthcare professionals from the American Heart Association Council on Clinical Cardiology: in collaboration with the Society of Geriatric Cardiology, *Circulation* **115**:2549–2569.

Alexander KP, Newby LK, Armstrong PW, et al. (2007). Acute coronary care in the elderly. Part II: ST-segment–elevation myocardial infarction: a scientific statement for healthcare professionals from the American Heart Association Council on Clinical Cardiology: in collaboration with the Society of Geriatric Cardiology. *Circulation* **115**:2570–2589.

# Hypertension

Hypertension is the most significant and prevalent risk factor for cardio-vascular disease in older adults. Yet, in those over 60 years old, at least 30% are unaware that they have hypertension, and only 44% of those being treated have BP at or below treatment goals (see Table 10.5).

The incidence of hypertension rises exponentially after age 50, reaching a prevalence of 60%–80% beyond age 65. With advancing age, systolic blood pressure (SBP) rises steeply while diastolic blood pressure (DBP) falls, leading to widening of the pulse pressure (PP) and relative frequency of isolated systolic hypertension (ISH).

Although ISH is a manifestation of age-associated arterial stiffening (p. 254), elevated PP and ISH are independent risk factors for stroke, CAD, peripheral vascular disease, heart failure, renal failure, dementia, and total mortality. In this age group, elevated SBP and PP portends a greater risk than elevated DBP. Accordingly, a meta-analysis of multiple clinical trials shows that treatment of ISH in older adults results in a 30% reduction in stroke, 23% reduction in CAD, and a 26% decrease in all CVD events. More recently, clinical trials of various agents suggest that it is the effective lowering of BP, rather than the specific agent used, that consistently lowers CVD and other comorbid risks.

**Table 10.5** JNC-9 blood pressure targets

| Classification | Systolic | Diastolic |
|---|---|---|
| Normal | <120 | <80 |
| Prehypertensive | 120–139 | 80–89 |
| Stage 1 | 140–159 | 90–99 |
| Stage 2 | ≥160 | ≥100 |

The goals of hypertension therapy are the same for older as for younger patients. Because antihypertensives were not specifically designed to increase central arterial distensibility, it is often challenging to control ISH with currently available medications. Often a combination is needed.

## Assessment

- **Ask about** symptoms (including orthostatic hypotension), comorbidities, alcohol use, smoking and medications. See Table 10.6.
- **Measure** blood pressure with a well-maintained, calibrated device, with an appropriate-sized cuff.
  - Check supine and standing blood pressure (orthostatic hypotension can cause symptoms when treatment is initiated).
  - Take at least two measurements in a single visit.
  - Measure the BP in both arms on the first visit to evaluate for coarctation, atherosclerosis and for future monitoring.

- Never initiate treatment based on a single reading.
- Consider ambulatory measurements if there is drug resistance, variable BP, white-coat hypertension, or postural symptoms.
- Engage the patient in home BP monitoring once the device has been calibrated and the patient demonstrates correct use.
- **Examine** for causes (drugs and renal disease are most common) and evidence of target organ damage (stroke, dementia, carotid bruits, cardiac enlargement, ischemic heart disease, peripheral vascular disease, renal disease, retinal changes).
- **Investigations** are used to assess target organs (urinalysis, blood urea and electrolytes, ECG) and for risk factor analysis (glucose, lipids).

**Table 10.6** Secondary causes of hypertension

| Comorbidities | Medications, etc. |
|---|---|
| Cushing syndrome | NSAIDs and COX-2, COX-I |
| Sleep apnea | Steroids |
| Primary aldosteronism | Some SSRIs |
| Renovascular disease | Cyclosporin |
| Pheochromocytoma | Erythropoietin |
| Coarctation of aorta | Sympathomimetics |
| Thyroid/parathyroid | Tobacco |
| | Dietary supplements |
| | Alcohol |
| | OTC cold medicine |

### Treatment thresholds and goals
- Attempt to reach goals, but you may need to accept a higher BP target if lowering produces weakness, dizziness, or other symptoms, and in setting of recent CVA. Gradual lowering over weeks and months is often necessary.
- A target of ≤130/85 is proposed for patients with diabetes, renal disease, active CAD, or evidence of other end-organ damage, but some patients may not tolerate this.
- Advancing age is associated with increased salt-sensitivity; counsel patients on eating a low-sodium diet.
- Labile blood pressure is characteristic of aging (stiff vasculature), thus BP may drop rapidly with loop diuretics or dehydration, or may increase dramatically with IV fluids, salt intake, or medications that promote fluid or salt retention.
- Educate patients to get up slowly from lying or sitting, as their BP/HR reflexes may be blunted by aging and/or medications.
- There is a paucity of data for very elderly (>85 years) people, and a pragmatic approach based symptoms and risk is appropriate.

# Hypertension: treatment

The approach used is similar to that used in younger patients, but it is important to bear the following in mind:

- Side effects are more common and debilitating in older patients (due to more sluggish baroreceptors and reduced cerebral autoregulation).
- There is a greater risk of drug interactions as older patients are more often victims of polypharmacy.
- Comorbidity is common and should direct the choice of antihypertensive agents (see How to use antihypertensives in a patient with comorbid conditions, p. 277).
- Hypertension should be seen as a risk factor, and the decision to treat should be weighed along with other risk factors. In a very frail older person with a limited life expectancy, the side effects suffered may far outweigh any future benefits from risk factor modification. This, however, should be an active decision reached with the patient, if possible, and not be a simple omission.
- Begin with lower doses and titrate up slowly to minimize adverse reactions. It is better to be on a drug at a low dose than nothing at all.
- Patient home-monitoring can assist in medication titration and involve patients in their own care.

## Nonpharmacological measures

Lifestyle modifications are as important and effective in reducing blood pressure in older patients as they are in the young. Salt restriction, weight reduction, and regular exercise are particularly effective. With aging, there is increased fluid retention associated with salt consumption.

It is sometimes difficult for older patients, especially those without transportation or those living in a care facility, to control their salt intake, but education on reduction of processed foods can be helpful. Moderate alcohol intake is advised. Smoking cessation and decreasing saturated fat intake help with overall risk reduction.

## Choice of medication

There have been many large trials comparing the different classes of antihypertensive, with little consistency in results. Overall, it seems that lowering the blood pressure is the important factor, and this benefit continues up until at least age 84 (possibly beyond—evidence is pending).

In older patients with much comorbidity there may be compelling reasons for using or not using certain agents (see How to use antihypertensives in a patient with comorbid conditions). Use a drug that will treat both blood pressure and a coexisting disease, to limit polypharmacy.

- Thiazide diuretics are effective in ISH as they reduce the intravascular volume and may decrease vascular fibrosis (hydrochlorothiazide or chorthaladone). Generic forms are inexpensive.
- Dihydroyridine calcium channel blockers (CCB) (amlodipine, felodipine) have been shown to decrease central arterial pressure associated with improved CVD outcomes.
- Non-dihydropyridine CCBs (verapamil, diltiazem) are effective in ISH with normal cardiac function. Verapamil has been shown to reduce ventricular and vascular stiffness, improving myocardial efficiency.

- Beta-blockers have been effective as a secondary agent in ISH, but have not been suggested as first line unless there is prior CAD.

## How to use antihypertensives in a patient with comorbid conditions

### Calcium channel blockers (CCBs)

For example, diltiazem sustained release (SR) 90 mg (rate limiting)
- Helpful to slow HR with atrial fibrillation or reduce angina with normal LV function
- May make cardiac failure worse
- Dihydropyridine calcium channel blockers (e.g., amlodipine, felodipine) are effective in ISH and for angina.
- Watch for constipation, peripheral edema.

### Thiazide diuretics

For example, hydrochlorothiazide (25 mg/day)
- Useful first-line therapy in most older patients—may help with ankle swelling and cardiac failure symptoms
- Avoid if severe history of gout, renal impairment
- May worsen urinary incontinence

### Beta-blockers

For example, atenolol 25 mg/day
- Useful with angina, atrial fibrillation, MI history, and cardiac failure
- Avoid with COPD, asthma, heart block

### ACE inhibitors

Fore example, ramipril 2.5–10 mg/day
- Use for secondary prevention after vascular event (stroke, TIA, heart attack) in diabetes, heart failure, and chronic renal impairment
- Avoid in renal artery stenosis and aortic stenosis
- Monitor potassium and renal function

### Angiotension receptor blockers

For example, losartan 50 mg/day
- Use when ACE intolerant (usually cough) where an ACE is indicated
- May cause less orthostatic symptoms than ACE inhibitors
- Monitor potassium and renal function

### Alpha-blockers

For example, doxazosin 1 mg/day
- Helpful for resistant hypertension in older patients
- Use if prostatic hypertrophy
- May provoke othostatic hypotension

## Further reading

Dahlöf B, et al. (2000). STOP hypertension 1 and 2 (1st and 2nd Swedish Trial in Old People with hypertension). *Heart* **84** (Suppl I):i2–i4.

Perry HM, Davis BR, Price TR, et al. (2000). Effect of treating isolated systolic hypertension on the risk of developing various types and subtypes of stroke: the Systolic Hypertension in the Elderly Program (SHEP). *JAMA* **284**(4):465–471.

# Arrhythmias: presentation

Arrhythmias are very common in older people, but are not commonly a presenting complaint. A patient with recurrent presyncope preceded by palpitations should be worked up for an arrhythmia. A greater diagnostic challenge occurs when an older patient presents with vague symptoms and arrhythmia must be considered:

• Recurrent falls
• Patient covered in bruises who has been explaining them away as clumsiness
• General fatigue
• Dizzy spells
• Light-headedness
• Increased DOE
• Blackouts
• Worsening or new angina or cardiac failure

## History

It is important to ask about palpitations with any of these problems (indeed it should form part of the systems review in all older people), but be aware of the following points:

• Clarify carefully what you mean—many people do not understand what we mean by "palpitations" and may be describing an ectopic heart beat followed by a compensatory pause, or even just an awareness of the normal heart beat, e.g., when lying in bed at night.
• Do not exclude the possibility of an arrhythmia just because the patient does not complain of palpitations—especially with confused patients. Also remember that atrial fibrillation is often asymptomatic in older adults.
• For palpitations and light-headedness, establish an order whenever possible. Postural drop is also very common in older patients and can produce a similar set of symptoms (falling BP causing light-headedness, then a compensatory tachycardia)—in theory the palpitations should come first in an arrhythmia.
• Are there any constant features of the symptoms? For example, dizziness occurring on standing is more likely to be postural drop. Dizziness on exertion may have an ischemic component. Dizziness on turning the head may be due to vestibular problems, or carotid sinus hypersensitivity (see p. 100). Dizziness that can occur anywhere or at any time is much more likely to be due to an arrhythmia.
• A history of injury with a blackout increases the chances of finding particularly a bradycardia requiring pacing or a tachyarrhythmia.
• Always take a full drug history—antiarrhythmics can be pro-arrhythmogenic, many drugs cause bradyarrhythmias (commonly beta-blockers, digoxin, or non-dihydropyridine CCBs such as diltiazem), and antidepressants (especially the tricyclics) may predispose to arrhythmias. Similarly, medications containing ephedrine (cold medications), dietary supplements, exogenous thyroid, caffeine, and beta-agonists may cause arrhythmias.

## Examination

- This should always include orthostatic blood pressures, assessment of the baseline pulse character, rate, and rhythm, and full cardiovascular examination to look for evidence of structural cardiac disease (e.g., cardiomyopathy, heart failure, valvular lesions), all of which may predispose to arrhythmias.
- General problems require a full general examination—it is rarely appropriate to examine a single system only in an elderly patient. A rectal examination, for example, may reveal a rectal tumor or guaiac positive stool causing anemia and, hence, palpitations.
- Examine for thyroid nodules or goiter.
- It may also be appropriate to examine the vestibular system (p. 581) and central nervous system.

## Investigations

- *Blood tests:* CBC (anemia), BUN, creatinine, and electrolytes (low vitamin K predisposes to arrhythmias), thyroid function, digoxin levels
- *ECG:* Look for baseline rhythm and any evidence of conducting system disease (e.g., a bundle branch block, or any heart block). Check the QT interval. Also look for LV hypertrophy (arrhythmias are more likely) or ischemia. Obtain a long rhythm strip, if possible.
- *CXR:* Look at cardiac size.
- *Holter monitoring*—a prolonged ECG recording. This is usually done over a 24-hour period initially, which can be repeated if unrevealing. Remember this is a very small snapshot and of limited value, especially if symptoms are infrequent. It can be useful if the symptoms are experienced while the monitor is on and the ECG trace shows normal sinus rhythm. If the suspicion of arrhythmias is high, then repeat the test, or arrange for trans-telephonic event recording or even an implantable loop recorder when the symptoms are severe enough (e.g., sudden syncope).

# Arrhythmias: management

Management of arrhythmias in older patients does not differ significantly from that for other age groups. However, remember the following:
- Presentation may be atypical with confusion or falls, rather than palpitations.
- There is more likely to be underlying cardiac pathology—always check for ischemia and structural heart disease even for apparently benign arrhythmias (e.g., SVT).
- Always check for common precipitants in older patients:
  - Electrolyte abnormalities (especially hypo- or hyperkalemia, hypocalcemia)
  - Medications
  - Anemia
  - Thyroid disease
  - Myocardial ischemia or prior infarction (scar)
  - Antiarrhythmic toxicity (especially digoxin)
  - Sepsis
  - Hypothermia
  - Any other acute illness
- If the precipitant cannot be remedied immediately (commonly sepsis) then the arrhythmia is likely to be recurrent—consider cardiac monitoring during this period.
- Tachycardia may be less well tolerated than in a younger patient, causing significant hypotension, angina, or cardiac failure.
- Hypotension itself may be less well tolerated than in younger patients (risk of cerebral injury), thus prompt action is required.
- For cardiac failure due to an arrhythmia, fluids cannot be used for resuscitation, thus definitive action is required sooner rather than later. Begin by using standard treatment for acute heart failure (oxygen, IV diuretics, opiates, etc.) while organizing cardioversion or rate limitation (appropriate for atrial fibrillation—use IV digoxin or amiodarone only for emergent hypotension or if AF is < 48 hrs or clot has been ruled out by TEE.).
- Bundle branch block is common, so there may be confusion between supraventricular and ventricular arrhythmias. (Look for irregularity suggesting atrial fibrillation.) There are numerous subtle ways of distinguishing between these, but in an emergency:
  - If the patient is compromised, electrical cardioversion will treat both effectively.
  - If the patient is stable, an amiodarone infusion will treat both effectively and has the advantage of causing little myocardial depression. Anticoagulation should be started first and clot should be ruled out by TEE if stable unless arrhythmia < 48 hrs.
- Older patients are much more likely to be on an antiarrhythmic drug already. They are also more sensitive to CCBs and beta-blockers.
- Check the medication carefully before administering any therapy. See Box 10.3 for common pitfalls.
- Electrical cardioversion is well tolerated, usually more effective, and less likely to cause side effects than many medications. It should be

considered early if there is significant compromise. In complicated patients, involve anesthesia for sedation. In a setting such as sepsis where the arrhythmia is likely to recur, cardioversion is less useful.
- If the rhythm is sinus tachycardia, it will respond best to treating the underlying illness (hypotension, fever, sepsis, pain, hyperthyroidism).

---

### Box 10.3 Common pitfalls with antiarrhythmics

*Adenosine*
- Its action is prolonged by dipyridamole (sometimes prescribed with aspirin in stroke), so avoid using together.
- Exacerbates asthma and is antagonized by theophylline, so avoid in asthmatics

*Amiodarone*
- Risk of ventricular arrhythmias when used with disopyramide, procainamide, and quinidine, so avoid concomitant use
- Increases plasma half-life of flecainide, so reduce dose

*Atropine*
- Can precipitate glaucoma, so avoid in patients with this condition

*Flecainide*
- Contraindicated when there is ischemic heart disease, cardiac failure, and hemodynamic compromise
- Probably best avoided in most older patients, who may well have occult cardiac disease

*Verapamil*
- Use very cautiously in patients already on a beta-blocker (risk of asystole and hypotension)

### General guidance
Most antiarrhythmic medications used concomitantly increase the risk of myocardial depression and arrhythmias. This effect is more pronounced in older patients. Exercise caution when using more than one, and consider using sequentially rather than additively if one alone is ineffective.

---

### When to consider an ICD
Implantable cardioverter defibrillators (ICD) can be placed in the setting of a risk of a lethal arrhythmia or recurrent ventricular tachycardia. Although the indications have broadened to include ischemic and nonischemic cardiomyopathies with ejection fraction <35%, the decision to proceed with implantation in an older patient should include several important factors:
- Patient's preferences regarding resuscitation
- A clear understanding that the device may prolong life, cause debility and pain, and prevent a "natural death"
- The device will not improve QOL, but is designed to prevent sudden death.

*Indications for ICD implantation*
- Sudden cardiac death
- Ischemic or nonischemic cardiomyopathy (EF <35%). Typically, wait until several months after acute infarct to see if LV function improves.
- Recurrent or symptomatic VT refractory to medical treatment
- Right ventricular dysplasia

# Atrial fibrillation

Atrial fibrillation (AF) is the most common arrhythmia in older adults, becoming more common with age. Often associated with other disease (e.g., hypertension, coronary artery disease, mitral valve disease, thyrotoxicosis), it also occurs in otherwise healthy elderly. Unlike other arrhythmias, it is often chronic.

Atrial fibrillation may be asymptomatic in older patients, but given their reliance on atrial systole (p. 255), they often present with shortness of breath, orthopnea, fatigue, DOE, and even signs of heart failure. Atrial fibrillation carries a high risk of stroke in older patients, in part because of age-associated alterations in clotting factors. Whereas the stroke risk for a 50-year-old with AF is 1%–2% per year, the risk jumps to 8%–12% per year in a person over 80.

Disorganized atrial activity with variable conduction to the ventricles leads to an irregularly irregular pulse rate and volume. Up to a third of older patients with AF will have AV nodal disease that limits the rate to <100 bpm, often making it asymptomatic. It is therefore often noted incidentally during routine examination—but should never be ignored.

## Assessment

A complete medication history (prescription and OTC) should be taken as well as caffeine and alcohol history. The examination should focus on hypertension and valve disease, blood tests for thyroid disease, and an ECG to confirm the diagnosis (it may be sinus rhythm with ectopics). Paroxysmal AF may cause intermittent symptoms and should be looked for with Holter monitoring.

## Complications

Atrial fibrillation causes an increase in morbidity and mortality, even if there is no underlying cardiac disease.

- Pulse >120 often causes palpitations, light-headedness, or syncope.
- Rapid rate may also cause dyspnea, angina, or cardiac failure.
- General malaise may also result from a chronically suboptimal cardiac output.
- AF is rarely associated with periods of AV conduction delay ("pauses") and if >3 seconds, these may cause syncope.
- The main complication is stroke from cardiac emboli.

## Atrial flutter

- Rapid, regular atrial activity (usually 300/minute)
- Characteristic saw-tooth appearance on ECG (revealed by carotid sinus massage if rate is high)
- Rate depends on degree of AV block (150 bpm if 2:1 block, 75 bpm if 4:1 block, etc.). Always think of atrial flutter when the pulse rate is 150.
- Commonly associated with COPD or ischemic heart disease
- Estimated to be about the same embolic risk as AF, but may be higher if the patient flips in and out of flutter and fibrillation.

- Treat with rate control and stroke prophylaxis. This rhythm is usually amenable to cardioversion, but if there are significant comorbidities, structural heart disease, or valve disease, sinus rhythm is unlikely to be sustained.
- Atrial flutter ablation can be successful and curative in carefully selected older adults.

# Atrial fibrillation: treatment

### Acute AF

- Treat underlying condition, e.g., sepsis, ischemia, pneumonia, hyperthyroidism, and cardiac failure.
- If the patient is hemodynamically compromised, consider electrical cardioversion.
- If stable, begin heparin with transition to chronic anticoagulation (if not contraindicated) and rate control (usually a beta-blocker or verapamil if no contraindication e.g., heart failure, digoxin if resistant).
- It may resolve once precipitant has been dealt with.
- If it persists and is symptomatic, consider transesophageal echocardiogram (TEE) to rule out intracardiac thrombus, and proceed with cardioversion if there is no thrombus. The patient must be therapeutic on heparin for TEE and be anticoagulated for at least 3–4 weeks following the procedure.
- If symptomatic, cardioversion may be performed after therapeutic on heparin without TEE if the cardioversion can be done within <48 hours after AF onset.
- If AF persists and is asymptomatic, consider cardioversion after at least 3 weeks of therapeutic oral anticoagulation (which should continue for an additional 3–4 weeks after the procedure if successful, and indefinitely if sinus rhythm is not restored).
- DO NOT initiate antiarrhythmic medication if AF lasts >48 hours and the patient has not been anticoagulated at therapeutic levels for 3–4 consecutive weeks or thrombus is demonstrated by TEE.

### Chronic AF

- Provide rate control, if necessary, using beta-blockade (e.g., atenolol 25–50 mg) or CCBs (e.g., diltiazem), which should be considered if needed to treat comorbidities, e.g., hypertension, angina.
- Alternatives include digoxin, which slows AV conduction (see How to use digoxin, p. 288).
- Start oral anticoagulation and document therapeutic INR for 3–4 consecutive weeks before attempting cardioversion (electric or chemical).
- If oral anticoagulation is contraindicated, use aspirin 325 mg/day.
- When chemical cardioversion is considered on symptomatic grounds (after proper anticoagulation, as above) give amiodarone (initially 400 mg bid for a week, then 200 mg bid for a week, then 200 mg daily thereafter). High-dose amiodarone often causes GI distress, which will improve. You may be able to drop the dose further to 100 mg/day, or even every other day. Remember that amiodarone interacts with warfarin and regular monitoring of INR will be needed if the two are used together, as is often the case. It can also cause thyroid abnormalities; this should be monitored with thyroid function tests (TFTs). A baseline CXR and eye exam should also be performed as a baseline and a yearly eye exams to monitor side effects.(see p. 604).

- Other useful agents to maintain sinus rhythm include sotalol (should be initiated in the hospital), flecainide or propafenone (if no structural heart disease or CAD), and dofetilide (which must be started in the hospital). There is limited experience with dofetilide in older adults; use with extreme caution if the patient has reduced renal function.
- Ongoing stroke prophylaxis with aspirin or warfarin should ensue, even after cardioversion.
- Electrical cardioversion for chronic AF should only be attempted after a period of anticoagulation (minimum 3 consecutive weeks in therapeutic range). It is more likely to succeed (and less likely to recur) when fewer of the following are present:
  - Structural heart disease (hypertrophy, atrial enlargement, valvular heart disease)
  - Comorbidity (especially hypertension, cardiac failure)
  - Increasing age

Recent evidence suggests that an asymptomatic older patient with several of the above is better off being treated with rate control and anticoagulation only, without attempting cardioversion. One attempt at cardioversion is usually warranted, though.

## Paroxysmal AF

- There is equal embolic risk, so consider anticoagulation as for chronic AF.
- Remember that digoxin does not prevent AF; it just slows AV conduction.
- Amiodarone (as above) or beta-blockers (e.g., atenolol 25 mg) are useful to prevent paroxysms of AF.
- AF ablation has been performed successfully in older adults, but the rate of recurrence is higher than in younger patients. Those with paroxysmal AF without significantly enlarged atria and comorbidites may be candidates.

## How to use digoxin

### Indications
- Rate control of atrial fibrillation
- Mild positive inotrope sometimes used in cardiac failure

### Not useful for
- Paroxysmal AF prevention
- Exercise-induced fast AF

### Loading with digoxin
- 1 mg in divided doses over 24 hours

This dose is always required, regardless of renal function—modify *maintenance* doses only in renal impairment. Example:
  - Day 1: 8 AM digoxin 500 mcg orally, 8 PM digoxin 500 mcg orally
  - Day 2: 8 AM digoxin at maintenance dose

### Deciding on a maintenance dose
- The main determinant is renal function—digoxin is excreted this way, so use a low dose with renal impairment.
- Consider also body mass (e.g., start with 62.5 mcg for a small, older woman—the dose can always be increased if there is inadequate rate control).
- Dosage is determined clinically, but serum levels can be used to assess toxicity or concordance.

### Digoxin toxicity
- Hypokalemia predisposes to this, so always monitor potassium and supplement if needed. Target [K] > 4.0 mmol/L.
- Symptoms include confusion, nausea, vomiting, arrhythmias (especially nodal bradycardia and ventricular ectopics), and yellow or green visual haloes.
- ECG may show ST depression and inverted T wave in V5 and V6 (reversed tick).
- Treat by stopping medication, rehydrating, and correcting hypokalemia.
- Life-threatening poisoning can be treated with digoxin-specific antibody fragments.

# Atrial fibrillation: anticoagulation

The issue of chronic anticoagulation in older patients often provokes anxiety in providers because of fear of bleeding, falls, nonadherence, drug interactions, and/or monitoring. However, the risk of embolic stroke in atrial fibrillation rises steeply with age, and physicians tend to underestimate the stroke risk and overestimate risk of significant bleeding. Nevertheless, safe anticoagulation occurs within a narrow therapeutic window.

The cornerstone of treatment involves an open and objective conversation with the patient and/or their family to clearly understand the risks, benefits, and use of chronic anticoagulation. Such conversations are shown to improve adherence and lower risk. This takes time and patience. It is important to have a simple way of explaining the facts as they are known, perhaps writing them down for clarity, then allowing time for them to sink in before coming to a final decision.

There is no enormous urgency—the stroke risks quoted are per annum, and it is worth giving the patient time to think things over if required. Address each of the following questions.

### What is the risk of stroke in this patient with AF?

Overall, the risk is about 5 times greater than that for a person with similar health and age who does not have AF. Paroxysmal AF carries the same embolic risk. This risk may be more accurately quantified as follows.

*High risk (6%–12% chance of stroke per year)*
- Older than 65 with cardiovascular risk factors (hypertension, diabetes)
- Previous stroke or TIA
- Cardiac disease (MI, cardiac failure)
- Echocardiogram abnormalities (poor LV function on echo, atrial clot)
- Thyroid disease

*Medium risk (3%–5% chance of stroke per year)*
- Older than 65 but with none of the high-risk characteristics
- Younger than 65 with cardiovascular risk factors (hypertension, diabetes)

*Low risk (less than 1% chance of stroke per year)*
- Younger than 65 with no additional risk factors detailed above

### What is the risk of therapy?

When taken correctly and monitored carefully, warfarin has ~1.3% per year risk of major bleeding in older patients and 0.5% risk of intracranial hemorrhage. This risk can be reduced by certain strategies (see How to discuss warfarin for atrial fibrillation, p. 292) and is no more than in younger patients if the INR is kept in therapeutic range. The risk of GI bleeding can be lowered by screening for Helicobacter pylori, avoiding NSAIDs or cotreating necessary NSAID use with proton pump inhibitors or misoprostol.

## How effective is therapy at reducing risk?
- Warfarin reduces stroke risk in AF by ~60%–70% in older patients.
- Aspirin (325 mg) reduces risk by ~20%–25%.

## What are the recommendations?
If there are no contraindications, any patient with a stroke risk estimated at >4% per year should have warfarin (i.e., the high-risk and most of the moderate-risk groups above), those with a risk of 1%–4% should have aspirin and those with a risk <1% should have no treatment.

### How to discuss warfarin for atrial fibrillation

Your patient is an 86-year-old woman with hypertension, ischemic heart disease, and mild cardiac failure. She currently takes aspirin, atenolol, bendrofluazide, furosemide, and ramipril. She has newly diagnosed AF, which is rate controlled because of the atenolol.

You wish to discuss starting warfarin with her. The conversation may go as follows:

Doctor: You have a condition called atrial fibrillation—where the heart beat is irregular. It is not causing you any problems at the moment, it is common and it is not a dangerous heart condition. However, there is a risk that this irregular beat could send a clot to the brain and cause a stroke, and I would like to consider a treatment to reduce the risk of this happening.

Patient: A stroke? I'm going to have a stroke?

Doctor: If we took 100 people in your situation, in a year about 10 of them would have a stroke—but 90 would not.

Patient: I would hate to have a stroke. What can you do?

Doctor: We can thin your blood with a drug called warfarin.

Patient: I've heard of that—isn't it very dangerous?

Doctor: You would need to have regular blood tests to make sure the dosage was right. If those 100 people all took warfarin, one of them would have a serious problem with bleeding.

Patient: But it will stop me from having a stroke?

Doctor: Going back to those 100 people—if they all take the warfarin, then only 3 or 4 will have a stroke instead of the original 10. The risk is reduced by about 2/3.

Patient: Which 3 or 4 people?

Doctor: There is no way of predicting who will benefit from treatment and who will have a problem. What we do know is that overall, the risk is lower with warfarin, and so we do recommend treatment for someone like you.

Patient: Do I have to?

Doctor: No, of course not. It is your decision. I will give you an information leaflet. Why don't you think it over? We will talk again in a few weeks.

See also Chapter 6, How to initiate warfarin (p. 134).

# Bradycardia and conduction disorders

As the heart ages, the function of the cardiac pacemaker (the sinoatrial node) and the conducting system (bundle of His and Purkinje fibers) tends to decline. This is due to the following:

- Declining numbers of pacemaker cells in the sinoatrial (SA) node
- Increasing prevalence of disease (infarction or scar, amyloid and hypertension)
- Degeneration with fibrosis, calcification, and fat infiltration

This is not inevitable, but around 50% of older patients will have some ECG evidence of conduction delay (prolonged PR and QT interval, left axis deviation, etc.) and be prone to symptomatic bradycardia and conduction disorders.

## Causes

- **Medication:** digoxin, amiodarone, beta-blockers, calcium-channel blockers
- **Sick sinus syndrome:** isolated sinus node dysfunction; very common in older patients, with uncertain cause (theories include vascular insufficiency or amyloid infiltration, but often no cause is found)
- **Ischemic heart disease**
- **Systemic disease:** hypothyroidism, liver failure, hypothermia, hypoxia, hypercapnia, hypothyroidism, cerebral disease (e.g., stroke, raised intracranial pressure, hemorrhage)

## Presentation

- Bradycardia is often picked up incidentally on an ECG.
- When symptomatic, bradycardia causes low-output syndromes ranging from fatigue, dizziness, dyspnea and presyncope, syncope, and falls, to angina, cardiac failure, and shock.
- It may be intermittent (with paroxysmal bradyarrhythmias), chronic (with stable arrhythmias), or occur acutely (usually post-MI).

## Management

Not every bradycardic patient needs an urgent pacemaker. Key questions are: Is the patient symptomatic? Is there an associated block or pause? Are there secondary reversible causes? When necessary, consult the cardiology service. For every problem, consider the following issues.

### Is the patient acutely compromised?

If so, then urgent treatment is needed to minimize cerebral injury. For shock, lay the patient down and elevate the legs. Use IV fluids. Try to increase the heart rate using atropine (0.5 mg IV, repeated up to a total dose of 3 mg) and temporary pacing (external pads are quick and often well tolerated; if the situation persists, insert a temporary pacing wire).

Tailor your treatment to each individual. If the cause of the bradycardia is a catastrophic intracerebral event, putting the patient through a temporary wire is not sensible.

Try external paddles to increase the heart rate and see if this has a positive impact on consciousness level while a CT scan is organized. Conversely, an acute inferior MI may cause significant short-term problems with bradycardia yet little longer-term cardiac damage.

### Are there any symptoms?

If so, are they attributable to the bradycardia?

Is the condition likely to resolve? If it occurs after an acute MI (usually in RCA or RV infarcts), support the patient during the acute episode as needed (noninvasively, if feasible) with the likelihood that the bradycardia will resolve with reperfusion.

### How frequent are the symptoms?

- *Continuous:* A temporary wire may be needed before permanent pacing.
- *Exertional:* Consider bed rest pending permanent pacing instead of a temporary wire (this reduces risk of infection and makes insertion of permanent wire easier).
- *Infrequent:* An elective permanent pacemaker can be organized.
- *No symptoms:* No action is required unless there is a high risk of future asystole. This is the case with second-degree heart block type II, where there is also bundle branch block. It is also true of complete heart block. A pacemaker is required for these conditions (see Box 10.4).

### Are there any reversible factors?

- Check medication. Digoxin (especially with toxicity), amiodarone, beta-blockers, and calcium channel blockers can all cause or exacerbate bradycardia.
- Check thyroid function.
- Acutely, hypothermia can also cause bradycardia.

## Box 10.4 Permanent pacemakers

*Indications*
- Over 85% are used for patients over 64 years old.
- 50% are for sick sinus syndrome and AV block.
- Increasingly used for vasodepressor carotid sinus hypersensitivity (p. 100)
- Occasionally used for recurrent syncope where no cause is found
- Used with AV node ablation with refractory atrial fibrillation
- Cardiac resynchronization therapy for symptomatic heart failure
- May be combined with ICD

*Pacemakers*
- Dual-chamber pacemakers are more expensive but tend to produce a better cardiac output and less AF than single-chamber ones.
- In AV node ablation, single-ventricular pacers are used and chronic anticoagulation must be maintained.
- Permanent pacing should be programmed to minimize paced beats, allowing the intrinsic rhythm to get through as much as possible.
- With LV dysfunction, pacing may need to include multisite pacing as RV pacing can worsen dysynchrony and exacerbate LV failure.
- Cardiac resynchronization therapy (biventricular pacing) may reduce heart failure symptoms in patients with reduced LV function and wide QRS.

*Insertion*
- This is a relatively simple procedure, done while the patient is awake. It is usually well tolerated by even very frail patients, with often dramatic improvements in quality of life. Consider it in most patients where indicated.
- Technical problems can occur with insertion if the patient cannot lie flat.
- Although the procedure is usually straightforward, rare complications during insertion include arrhythmias (commonly AF) and, rarely, perforation of the right ventricle.
- An overnight hospital stay is required for IV antibiotics at the time of implantation.
- Later problems include sepsis and failure of pacemaker output.

Regular follow-up is required to check the pacemaker function and battery reserve.

# Common arrhythmias and conduction abnormalities

See Table 10.7.

**Table 10.7** Common arrhythmias and conduction abnormalities

| Condition | Clinical features | Treatment |
|---|---|---|
| Sinus bradycardia Intrinsic SA nodal disease<br>• Pulse rate <60<br>• Common incidental finding<br>• Drugs are common cause<br>• Acute onset associated with inferior MI and raised intracranial pressure<br>• Consider hypothyroidism Treat only if symptomatic (rarely causes problem)<br>• Check thyroid function Supraventricular ectopics Narrow complex QRS without a p wave, followed by a compensatory pause<br>• Patient may be aware of this, and describe an "early beat" with a gap afterwards Benign<br>• Reassure the patient<br>• No action required Sinoatrial block Intermittent inability of SA node to depolarize atrium<br>• ECG shows pauses that are multiples of the PR interval Usually asymptomatic<br>• Treat only if symptoms Slow AF Combination of AF and SA nodal disease very common<br>• Symptomatic pauses frequent Anticoagulation for stroke prevention<br>• High index of suspicion for pauses if suggestive symptoms—check with Holter monitor and treat with pacemaker Sick sinus syndrome | • SA node dysfunction (degenerative or due to ischemic heart disease) causing a bradycardia—includes sinus bradycardia and slow AF. Often associated with other conduction problems | • Treat symptoms<br>• Anticoagulate if AF |

**Table 10.7** Common arrhythmias and conduction abnormalities (*continued*)

| Condition | Clinical features | Treatment |
|---|---|---|
| Tachy–bradysyndrome | • Combination of slow underlying rate (sinus bradycardia of slow AF) with tendency toward runs of SVT that often terminate with a long pause <br><br>• Symptoms due to both slow and fast pulse | • Usually requires pacemaker for bradycardia and rate-limiting drugs to control tachyarrhythmias. <br><br>• Still need chronic anticoagulation |
| First-degree heart block | • PR >0.21 seconds | • Benign if isolated, but always check for coexisting second- or third-degree block <br><br>• No action required if isolated |
| Second-degree heart block, Mobitz type I (Wenckebach) | • PR interval increases progressively until a QRS is dropped | • Often occurs transiently post-MI <br><br>• Usually appropriate to monitor until resolves |
| Second-degree heart block, Mobitz type II | • Fixed PR interval, but conduction to ventricles does not occur on every beat. Usually in a fixed pattern (conducting every second, third, or fourth beat) <br><br>• Often associated with bundle branch block | • Often symptomatic <br><br>• High risk of progression to complete heart block <br><br>• Usually requires elective pacing |

(*continued*)

**Table 10.7** Common arrhythmias and conduction abnormalities (*continued*)

| Condition | Clinical features | Treatment |
| --- | --- | --- |
| Complete heart block (third degree) | • Complete dissociation of atrial and ventricular activity. P waves visible, but not conducted. QRS originates at ventricular pacemaker (escape rhythm). If this is in the AV node, the rate is around 60 and the QRS morphology narrow. If it is more distal, the rate tends to be around 40 with wide QRS complexes. | • Usually symptomatic, although if rate 50 may only be on exertion<br><br>• If chronic, limit activity until permanent pacing arranged<br><br>• If acute (e.g., post-MI) likely to resolve<br><br>• When associated with hypotension, angina or cardiac failure at rest, may need temporary pacing wire |
| Bundle branch block | • Widened QRS due to delayed conduction<br><br>• Not related to rate, so asymptomatic<br><br>• Right bundle branch block (RBBB) is a common finding in healthy older adults and is usually benign, but if acute, consider acute pulmonary embolism.<br><br>• Left bundle branch block (LBBB) is associated with hypertension and ischemic heart disease. | • Acutely, LBBB may indicate acute infarct<br><br>• If found incidentally, tell the patient (aids future emergency treatment) and consider giving a copy of the ECG to the patient. |

# Heart failure: assessment

Heart failure (HF) is very common, occurring in 1 in 10 of those over 65 and accounting for 5% of admissions to medical wards and 1%–2% of all health-care costs. Overall prevalence is 3–20 cases per 1000 population, but this doubles with each decade over 45 years.

HF is becoming more common as the population ages and survival from coronary events improves. In the older population, the incidence of HF with preserved systolic function (diastolic HF) is more common than systolic HF.

## Systolic heart failure

### Pathology

- Poor LV function decreases cardiac output, resulting in increased pulmonary pressures and edema.
- The sympathetic nervous system is activated (increased pulse, myocardial contractility, peripheral vasoconstriction, and catecholamines).
- The renin–angiotensin system is activated (which increases salt and water retention).
- Vasopressin and natriuretic peptides increase.

### Causes

HF is usually due to coronary artery disease (especially in Caucasians) and hypertension (especially in Blacks). Other causes include valve disease, tachyarrhythmias, pericardial disease, pulmonary hypertension (e.g., with COPD or multiple pulmonary embolisms), high-output states (look especially for anemia, thyroid disease, and Paget's disease), and cardiomyopathy (idiopathic, amyloid, alcohol).

### Diagnosis

Heart failure is a complex clinical diagnosis, with no universally agreed-upon diagnostic criteria. It is often difficult to diagnose accurately, particularly in older patients with increased comorbidity and symptoms.

Many older people are put on a diuretic for presumed heart failure, but diuretic use as a marker of HF is 73% sensitive but only 41% specific. This predisposes to postural symptoms and adds to polypharmacy.

### Symptoms

Ask yourself if these symptoms are cardiac and what the underlying disease is that is causing them. Exertional dyspnea is 100% sensitive for HF (i.e., every HF case has it), but only 17% specific (i.e., many other causes of exertional dyspnea exist, the main one being respiratory).

Fatigue and ankle swelling are also very common in HF but occur in many other diseases as well. Orthopnea and paroxysmal nocturnal dyspnea are much more specific, but occurring late in the disease are not sensitive.

### Signs

Again, early signs are sensitive, but not specific (e.g., tachycardia, pulmonary rales, peripheral edema). Later signs are more specific, but not sensitive (e.g., elevated JVP: 98% specific, 17% sensitive; gallop rhythm: 99% specific, 24% sensitive).

Overall, clinical features tend to be sensitive *or* specific, but not both. The multiple comorbidities, underlying aging changes, and multiple etiologies of HF in older patients pose a particular challenge in diagnosis. Clinical suspicion should thus be supported by investigation before embarking on a trial of treatment.

## How to investigate a patient with suspected systolic heart failure

Use investigations to support a clinical diagnosis and establish cause.
- *ECG* is abnormal in over 90% of cases (Q waves, T wave /ST segment changes, left ventricular hypertrophy [LVH], bundle branch block, AF). Consider Holter monitoring if there are paroxysmal symptoms.
- *Chest X-ray:* Look for cardiac enlargement (although this is absent with acute onset, e.g., post-MI or PE), upper-lobe blood diversion, fluid in the horizontal fissure, Kerley B lines, bat wing pulmonary edema, pleural effusions (usually bilateral; R > L if unilateral), or any other cause for breathlessness. The combination of a normal CXR and ECG makes HF very unlikely.
- *Blood tests:* CBC (? anemic), biochemistry (? renal function, sodium low in severe CF), glucose and lipids (CHD risk factors), liver function (? congestion, malnutrition, cirrhosis), thyroid function. Obtain urinalysis for proteinuria, B-natriuretic peptide (BNP) if available. See Box 10.6 B-Type Natriuretic Peptide (BNP), p. 311.
- *Echocardiography:* A 2D Doppler echocardigram should be done for all patients with suspected HF to confirm the diagnosis, establish cause, and grade disease severity. Use this to look for LV function (systolic and diastolic, see p. 310), estimate ejection fraction, and look for evidence of valve disease, cardiomyopathy, regional wall abnormalities from ischemic heart disease, pericardial disease, intracardiac shunts, LV aneurysms, or cardiac thrombus. Overall, only 25% of those referred for echocardiography have LV systolic dysfunction.
- *Pulmonary function tests* may help distinguish cardiac from respiratory breathlessness (PEFR and $FEV_1$ are reduced in HF, but less than in COPD). Remember, many patients have both.

# Acute heart failure

## Treatment
- Immediate treatment with oxygen, intravenous loop diuretic, and nitrates (if adequate blood pressure)
- Address the cause (e.g., acute myocardial infarction, arrhythmia).
- Consider ventilatory support (begin with noninvasive positive-pressure ventilation, which can be done in a non-ICU setting and does not present problems of weaning).
- After improvement is seen, begin ongoing treatment with a regular loop diuretic and slowly titrate an ACE inhibitor while initiating a beta-blocker as pressure tolerates this.

## Prognosis
Patients with acute heart failure look extremely unwell, yet can often make apparently "miraculous" recoveries as the precipitant is dealt with. Remember that it is the premorbid state and the nature of the acute injury—never age alone—that should determine how aggressively to manage the acute condition.

## Rapid atrial fibrillation and heart failure
- This is a common combination in older patients.
- It is rarely clear which came first.
- Treat both simultaneously.
- Anticoagulate with heparin first, with conversion to chronic anticoagulation.
- If symptomatic, consider TEE/cardioversion (see p. 286) after initial heart failure treatment.
- Digoxin may slow AF in this situation without depressing myocardial function. Assess renal function before using it and dose accordingly.
- Always look for a precipitant—sepsis, MI, pulmonary embolism, pneumonia, alcohol, hyperthyroidism, etc.

## Further reading
Cardiovascular Medicine. In *Oxford American Handbook of Clinical Medicine*. John A. Flynn, Editor. New York: Oxford University Press.

# Chronic heart failure

Begin by reviewing the basis for diagnosis, as chronic heart failure portends a poor prognosis and a commitment to a large number of medications. A multidisciplinary approach is preferable, involving the patient in monitoring where possible (e.g., daily weighing). This is best done by heart failure specialists with facilities for ongoing follow-up by cardiac-failure specialist nurses and social workers.

## Lifestyle

Address cardiovascular risk factors, reduce alcohol intake, minimize salt and fluid intake, and increase aerobic exercise (ideally, as part of a rehabilitation program).

## Medication

There is a large evidence base for a number of drugs (see Box 10.5). It may be tempting to limit the number of drugs in older patients, justified by concerns about side effects, but if the diagnosis is secure, all classes should be at least attempted. It is probably better to prescribe a low dose of an ACE inhibitor with a beta-blocker, rather than a maximum dose of ACE inhibitor, when the blood pressure may be insufficient to introduce the beta-blocker.

## Treating cause

- Atrial fibrillation should be slowed and anticoagulation started (cardioversion is unlikely to succeed if LV dysfunction is primary rather than secondary).
- Hypertension should be treated until disease progression drops cardiac output and, hence, blood pressure.
- Valvular disease should be assessed for surgical correction where appropriate (especially aortic valve disease—discuss this with the patient early after onset of HF).
- Treat anemia and thyroid disease.

## Vaccination

Offer influenza vaccination annually and pneumococcal vaccination.

## Monitoring

Monitoring should include the following:
- Clinical assessment of symptoms and functional capacity (e.g., how far can the patient walk without stopping)
- Blood pressure, including postural measurements
- Fluid status (weigh patient regularly). Estimate dry weight, record it, and use this to guide future management. Examine for elevated JVP, edema, and lung crackles.
- Cardiac rhythm (clinical and by ECG)
- Cognitive state (a common problem with HF due to vascular disease and low blood pressure). Evaluate cognition using the Mini-Cog or other instrument—see Appendix.

- Nutritional state (malnutrition is common in HF). Salt and fluid restriction must be balanced, but allow adequate protein and caloric intake. Ask patient about their appetite, and get a dietician's input.
- Medication review (is the patient on all appropriate drugs at maximum tolerated doses?)
- Side effects (especially ask about postural symptoms; check BUN, creatinine, and electrolytes)
- Psychological and social review (how are they and caregivers coping with problems of chronic disease? Do they need any social support?)

---

### Box 10.5 Medication for chronic cardiac failure

- *Loop diuretics:* (e.g., furosemide) Use to control symptoms. Begin with 20 mg (10 mg in the very elderly) and titrate upward (guided by symptoms and examination findings). Monitor renal function and electrolytes (hyponatriemia more common in elderly)
- *ACE inhibitors* should be started early in all patients with a diagnosis of systolic HF unless there is a valvular cause or renal artery stenosis is suspected. Again, begin low (e.g., ramipril 2.5 mg) and titrate upward, monitoring renal function and postural symptoms.
- *Beta-blockers* should be started in all stable patients with LV systolic dysfunction after diuretics and ACE inhibitors regardless of whether there are continuing symptoms (improves prognosis). Use a beta-blocker licensed for cardiac failure, e.g., carvedilol 3.125 mg, or metoprolol 25 mg twice a day, and titrate upward.
- *Spironolactone:* Use for continuing symptoms despite loop and ACE. Dose is 25 mg. Watch potassium levels, as ACE and spironolactone will raise this.
- *Digoxin:* Use in AF and when there are continuing symptoms despite maximal other therapy in sinus rhythm.
- *Thiazide diuretics* can be added to loop diuretics in end-stage HF, e.g., hydrochlorothiazide 25 mg, or metolazone 5 mg (monitor electrolytes closely; may be used on alternate days if it causes excess diuresis).
- *Warfarin:* Use in AF, or when echocardiogram has shown intracardiac thrombus, or if ejection fraction <20 %.
- *Angiotensin receptor blockers (ARBs)* (e.g., losartan) are useful when the patient is ACE intolerant. This class is rapidly gaining evidence of its efficacy in treating cardiac failure. There *may* be role for ARBs in addition to ACE inhibitors.
- *Aspirin/statins:* Use for risk factor modification if the cause is ischemic heart disease.

Additionally, discussion with older adults about implantation of an ICD for prevention of sudden cardiac death should be approached carefully (see When to consider an ICD, p. 281).

# Dilemmas in heart failure

### The cardiac failure seesaw

One of the most common dilemmas is balancing drugs in a patient who has both cardiac failure and chronic renal failure.

Aggressive diuretic use will improve the cardiac failure but lead to thirst, malaise, hyponatremia, uremia, postural hypotension, and, ultimately, anuria. Volume repletion to improve renal function will lead to worsening pulmonary edema.

Each patient will need a carefully planned balance, accepting moderate elevations in urea and/or a bit of edema, that enables the patient to exist in the greatest comfort. This balance will take time and skill to achieve.

The following considerations will help:
- Make all changes slowly and wait for the impact—large-dose changes increase oscillation between wet and dry states.
- If a patient is still losing weight on a therapy regime, he or she is likely to continue to do so. Do not discharge after an acute event until steady state is reached; otherwise the patient will come back into the hospital with volume depletion and renal failure.
- Get to know the patient's ideal weight and use this to guide therapy.
- Involve patients and caregivers wherever possible.
- Admit and stabilize the patient in the hospital, with nursing and medical house calls following.
- Get to know the patient—continuity of care is very helpful, and HF case management nurses may play a key role in this.

### Terminal care

- Chronic heart failure is a grim diagnosis with a poor outlook (only 25% will survive 3 years, which is worse than many cancers).
- Consider hospice care.
- Consider broaching this with all patients in clinic (ideally, in a stable phase of the illness) to allow future plans to be made and resuscitation issues discussed.
- As the disease progresses, ensure that appropriate palliative care measures are taken, with careful review of symptoms and of patient and family anxieties.
- Opiates (morphine) can be given to help relieve the distress of dyspnea and allow rest.
- Continuous oxygen therapy may ease discomfort.
- Intermittent IV boluses of furosemide in an ambulatory setting can keep people out of hospital.

### Further reading

Stewart S, McMurray JJV (2002). Palliative care for heart failure. *BMJ* **325**:915–916.

# Diastolic heart failure

- This is a clinical syndrome of cardiac failure with preserved LV ejection fraction seen on echocardiography (>50%), where there is no major valvular disease.
- It accounts for about a third of clinically diagnosed heart failure and is more common in older patients, especially females, hypertensive patients, and those with left ventricular hypertrophy (LVH).
- Diastolic heart failure is not a benign condition; ambulatory patients do better than those with systolic heart failure, but the mortality is equivalent in older patients or those hospitalized. There is a 4-fold increase in mortality compared with controls without heart failure.

This condition is important to recognize and treat. Do not discontinue treatment for heart failure on the basis of normal LV function.

## Pathology

The left ventricle has a thick wall with a small cavity and is slow to relax and allow filling in diastole. This causes increased diastolic pressures (hence pulmonary pressures and dyspnea) and a low cardiac output (hence fatigue). Much of the pathophysiology is unknown. Patients are very sensitive to volume.

## Diagnosis

- **Clinical suspicion** (history as for all systolic heart failure [SHF]) and examination findings (elevated JVP, pulmonary edema, hypertension, murmur in the aortic area, fourth heart sound) are key.
- **Chest X-ray** will show pulmonary congestion, and the **ECG** will show evidence of hypertension.
- **Echocardiography** shows preserved LV function and evidence of abnormal diastolic relaxation (Doppler studies show a reduced ratio of early (E) to late or atrial (A) ventricular filling velocities—E:A <0.5 is suggestive of diastolic dysfunction). Tissue Doppler examination helps further, as it is a load-independent measure of LV filling. Because these changes are common in older ventricles, treatment is based on symptoms, not echocardiographic results.
- **BNP** (see Box 10.6) may be useful in cases where there are multiple possible etiologies of dyspnea, as a negative result makes heart failure unlikely, helping to limit polypharmacy.

## Management

- **Prevention** is by blood pressure control at population level.
- **Relieve precipitants**: Treat tachyarrhythmias, anemia, thyroid disease, ischemia, and malnutrition. The patient needs to track daily weight and follow salt and volume restrictions.
- **Acute symptoms**: Control blood pressure with oral agents as priority. Use diuretics cautiously as they can drop cardiac output still further by decreasing preload.
- **Chronic disease management**: There is less evidence for DHF than for SHF. Control of blood pressure is key. Diastolic-relaxation agents (e.g., beta-blockade) are not proven, but rate control with these or CCBs, especially when there is dual indication, e.g., AF or ischemic

heart disease, may help. ACEs and ARBs are likely to help (there is some trial evidence that ARBs reduce readmission rates modestly). The patient should improve exercise tolerance with physical activity.

### Box 10.6  B-type natriuretic peptide (BNP)

Three types of natriuretic peptide are known, with effects on heart, kidneys, and the nervous system. B-type is found mainly in the heart in humans and increases with pressure overload of the heart, acting as a biochemical marker for cardiac failure. BNP concentration correlates with the severity of heart disease and is 97% sensitive and 84% specific for the diagnosis in symptomatic primary care patients.

### Problems

- What is a high level? Different assays produce different numbers, and there is a continuum of results making a diagnostic cutoff necessary.
- What is the gold standard for diagnosis in order to evaluate the test? (Echocardiography has limitations.)
- Cost-effectiveness is unknown.
- There is limited clinical trial evidence.
- Significance of a high level in an asymptomatic patient is unclear.

Overall, a "negative" (i.e., very low) result in a breathless patient makes cardiac failure very unlikely, and other causes should be sought. It may be useful to help pre-select patients for echocardiography.

# Valvular heart disease

Most valvular heart lesions are degenerative (e.g., calcification is the main cause of aortic stenosis), so valve defects are very common in older patients. The following points must be remembered:

- Listen to the heart for murmurs in all older patients, as many valve lesions are detected incidentally.
- Think of valvular disease when a patient presents with dyspnea, heart failure, angina, palpitations, syncope, or dizziness. Examine them carefully (see Table 10.8).
- When a murmur is heard, echocardiography should be requested to document the valve lesion and formulate a management plan.
- Remember to consider endocarditis, which is more common in older adults because of turbulence around valves, dental issues, and undergoing more procedures. Fever is not necessarily present in an older patient with endocarditis, who may present with malaise, fatigue, and the "dwindles." Blood cultures, ↑ ESR, and echocardiography help with the diagnosis.
- Once the valve lesion is known, decide whether valve replacement is indicated (see Table 10.8). In many lesions (e.g., mitral valve disease and aortic regurgitation) the progression of symptoms alerts to the need for pre-emptive surgery. In aortic stenosis, however, a prompt response to the development of early symptoms is required, and so the approach is different.
- After deciding whether intervention is required, consider whether or not the patient is a surgical candidate. Some lesions may be amenable to percutaneous interventions (feasible in much frailer patients). Always ask the patient what he or she thinks—often there will be strong views that come as a surprise to the physician. Make it clear that obtaining a surgical opinion is not committing the patient to surgery. Indeed, the surgeon may feel that the risks outweigh the benefits, but talking with the surgeon is an important first step.
- If surgery is not yet indicated, ensure that there is some sort of follow-up or surveillance system in place, whether repeat echocardiography, or clinic review, or simply confirm that the patient knows what symptoms should trigger medical review.
- The risk of valve surgery increases if concomitant CABG is performed.
- If it is decided that surgery is not an option, ensure that full palliative care measures are in place.
- See guideline for prevention of bacterial endocarditis (p. 741).

## Talking to patients about potential surgery

Many older people are terrified at the prospect of surgery, and the gut reaction may be to avoid it at all costs. Others will not want to take responsibility for the decision—"Whatever you think, doctor," is a common response. Having a frank and useful discussion about risks and benefits is often difficult, but should always be attempted before referral is made.

Bioprosthetic valves can be used in older patients, which have a shorter life span than metal valves, but obviate the need for warfarin.

Be sure you have enough time for this discussion and give plenty of opportunity for questions. The patient may wish to go away and think about it, perhaps returning with a spouse or child—encourage this and do not force a decision.

Table 10.8 Common valve lesions

| Valve lesion | Symptoms | Complications | Treatment | Who to consider for surgery? |
|---|---|---|---|---|
| Mitral stenosis | Dyspnea<br>Fatigue<br>Palpitations<br>Chest pain<br>Hemoptysis | Atrial fibrillation<br>Systemic emboli<br>Pulmonary hypertension<br>Pulmonary edema<br>Pressure effects from large LA<br>Endocarditis | Rate control of AF (digoxin and/or beta-blocker)<br>Anticoagulation if AF<br>Diuretics if CF<br>Antibiotic prophylaxis for invasive procedures | Symptoms despite medical management.<br>If pliable valve, may be candidate for balloon valvuloplasty (difficult in older patients due to calcification) |
| Mitral regurgitation | Dyspnea<br>Fatigue<br>Palpitations | Pulmonary edema<br>Atrial fibrillation (AF)<br>Endocarditis | Rate control of AF<br>Anticoagulation if AF<br>Diuretics if CF<br>Antibiotic prophylaxis for invasive procedures | Deteriorating symptoms—aim to replace valve before extensive LV damage<br>Condition progresses slowly. Repair may be possible and not delayed. New-onset AF or increased pulmonary hypertension should be considered for surgery. |
| Aortic stenosis | Angina<br>Dyspnea<br>Cardiac failure (CF)<br>Dizziness<br>Syncope<br>Sudden death | Angina<br>Pulmonary edema<br>Syncope<br>Sudden death<br>Endocarditis | Consider surgical referral<br>If not suitable, then treat angina and HF symptomatically<br>Avoid ACE inhibitors<br>Antibiotic prophylaxis for invasive procedures<br>Statins may slow progression | Once symptomatic, prognosis is poor (2–3 years), so refer for valve replacement early after symptom onset<br>Asymptomatic patient with deteriorating ECG should also be referred<br>Valvuloplasty may be an option for frail patients |

| | | | | |
|---|---|---|---|---|
| Aortic sclerosis | None | None | Statins may slow progression of aortic stenosis<br>Follow patients for progression with echo; some will progress, some remain stable | Not applicable |
| Aortic regurgitation | Dyspnea<br>Palpitations<br>Cardiac failure | Pulmonary edema<br>Endocarditis | Diuretics if CF<br>Antibiotic prophylaxis for invasive procedures | Worsening symptoms, worsening cardiomegaly,<br>ECG deterioration<br>Aim to replace valve before extensive LV damage |

# Peripheral edema

Swollen ankles are extremely common in older patients. Starting a diuretic must not be an immediate reaction, as this treats only one of several causes and may cause harm. As with all geriatric medicine, a careful assessment, diagnosis, and appropriate treatment should be carried out.

Swollen ankles do not always indicate cardiac failure.

## Causes

- Often, mild ankle swelling occurs in an otherwise fit person: this tends to be worse on prolonged standing and in the heat (sometimes referred to as "dependant edema"). It is likely that there is some minor venous disease causing the edema, but it is essentially benign.
- Peripheral venous disease is chronic edema due to damage to deep veins causing venous hypertension, increased capillary pressure, and fibrinogen leakage. It is usually bilateral, but one side is often worse than the other (see p. 626).
- Cardiac failure is usually bilateral; look for associated signs, e.g., raised JVP, cardiac enlargement, S3, atrial fibrillation, pulmonary crackles, and hepatojugular reflux.
- Acute edema may be due to superficial thrombophlebitis (red, hot, very tender venous cord with surrounding edema) or a new deep vein thrombosis (DVT) (painful swollen calf with pitting edema of ankle. Review thrombotic risk factors).

Always consider DVT with new-onset unilateral swelling.

- Drug side effect: commonly calcium channel blockers (especially amlodipine) and NSAIDs, some SSRIs
- Low-serum albumin from nephrotic syndrome, gastrointestinal loss, malnutrition, chronic disease, acute sepsis, chronic liver disease, etc.
- Lymphatic obstruction: consider obstructing pelvic tumors. If edema is severe, perform rectal and groin examination.
- Traumatic: after forcefully dorsiflexing the foot (usually when walking), leading to rupture of the plantar tendon or injury to gastrocnemius. This edema tends to be unilateral, tender, above the ankle, and with associated bruising to the calf. Treat with rest and NSAIDs.
- Other causes include hypothyroidism, osteoarthritis of the knee, ruptured Baker's cyst, gout, and post-stroke paralysis.

## Assessment

- *History:* How acute was the onset? Is it unilateral or bilateral? Is it painful, red, and hot? What are the associated physical symptoms—importantly, dyspnea (may indicate PE or heart failure)?
- *Examination:* Look for physical signs as above. Always listen to the heart and lungs and look for sacral edema when ankle swelling is found. Consider rectal or groin examination.
- *Investigations* should be guided by your clinical suspicion. Consider ECG (unlikely to be normal in heart failure), BUN and electrolytes, albumin, full blood count, liver function tests, and thyroid function tests.

D-dimer in elderly patients with swollen ankles is rarely helpful. While a negative result effectively rules out DVT, many older patients will have an elevated D-dimer. Only use the test if you would proceed to ultrasound scanning in the event of a positive result.

## Treatment

All patients with ankle swelling should have a careful assessment for disease as above, with treatment dependant on cause:

- Stop drugs if they are responsible (replace with alternatives).
- If there is heart failure, then full assessment and treatment is required.
- For chronic venous disease use leg elevation and compression stockings (p. 626).
- With severe lymphedema, massage and pneumatic boots can be useful.
- If there is low albumin treat the cause. Most causes do not respond to increased dietary protein intake.

If no disease is found management is pragmatic. Patients may find the ankle swelling unsightly, have difficulty fitting on their shoes, or even complain of an aching pain. Support hose may help.

It may then be appropriate to start a low dose of thiazide diuretic (e.g., hydrochlorothiazide 25 mg), but this will necessitate occasional monitoring of electrolytes and clinical review to ensure that the benefits of treatment still outweigh the risks. Many patients may be happy to tolerate the minor inconvenience once they have been assured that there is no serious pathology.

### Ankle swelling and nocturnal polyuria

During the day, a large amount of fluid can collect in the interstitial space in the ankles. At night, when the legs are elevated, this fluid is partly returned to the circulating volume and can cause a diuresis, hence nocturnal polyuria.

Paradoxically, treating such a patient with diuretics to limit the swelling will ultimately help with the polyuria.

# Peripheral vascular disease

Peripheral vascular disease (PVD) is common in older patients, causing symptoms in 10% of those over 70 years. Only a third of older patients will have the classic symptoms of intermittent claudication, and often decreasing activity levels will mask developing disease. It may be difficult to distinguish pain from osteoarthritis, or the patient may assume their pain is due to arthritis and not mention it.

Claudication pain may progress to ischemic rest pain (night-time pain, often relieved by hanging the foot over the bed), then to ulceration, due to trauma with poor healing (small, punctate, painful ulcers at pressure points, e.g., toes, lateral malleolus, metatarsal heads), and possibly gangrene. Diabetics are especially at risk for this.

Around 80% of patients with claudication remain stable or improve; only 20% deteriorate, and 6% require amputation (longtime smokers and diabetics are most at risk).

Examination reveals a loss of pulses (best discriminator is an abnormality of the posterior tibial pulse), possibly bruits, coolness to touch, slow capillary refill (over 2 seconds), shiny hairless skin with atrophic nails, and poor wound healing.

## PVD as a marker of other vascular disease
- 5-year mortality in PVD is 30%, mostly due to cardiovascular disease.
- It is easy to detect PVD noninvasively by measuring ABPI (see How to measure an ankle–brachial pressure index, p. 319).
- The impact of broad vascular-risk management on subsequent vascular disease burden has yet to be quantified but is likely to be substantial.

If a patient complains of leg pains, screen for PVD and if detected, initiate full vascular secondary prevention.

## PVD as a cause of significant morbidity
Although PVD is very common, many older people will modify their lifestyle to reduce symptoms. It is important to actively ask about symptoms. Adopt the following treatment approach:
- Modify risk factors.
- Advise increasing exercise (NOT decreasing).
- Commence antiplatelet agent, commonly aspirin.
- Consider other drugs—phosphodiesterase inhibitors (e.g., cilostazol) have antiplatelet activity and act as vasodilators. Clopidogrel may also lessen symptoms.
- Do not necessarily stop beta-blockers, even though traditionally they were thought to worsen claudication. The evidence for this is weak and beta-blockers have a major role in modifying cardiac risk.
- Refer for revascularization when appropriate. Percutaneous revascularization is a relatively low-risk procedure and should be considered for lifestyle-limiting claudication that does not respond to medical therapy, when there is a focal stenosis, or when there is limb-threatening ischemia in a patient who is not fit for surgery. Elective surgery is usually reserved for low-risk patients (under 70 years with no diabetes and no distal disease) who are fit enough to tolerate

the procedure. Age has a significant impact on surgical risk—relative risk of mortality increases by 1.62 with each decade.

## How to measure an ankle brachial pressure index (ABPI)

### When?
- To confirm PVD as a cause of claudication
- To diagnose vascular disease before implementing secondary prevention
- To diagnose the etiology of (venous) ulcers
- To ensure compression bandaging is safe

### Equipment
- Blood pressure cuff with sphygmomanometer
- Hand-held Doppler probe

### Method
- Inflate the cuff around the upper arm as usual and use the Doppler probe over the brachial artery to measure systolic blood pressure.
- Repeat in the other arm.
- Next, inflate the cuff around the ankle and use the probe to measure the systolic pressure in the dorsalis pedis and posterior tibial arteries.
- Take the highest of the four ankle readings and divide by the higher of the two arm readings to give the ABPI.

### Interpretation
- >1.4    Noncompressible calcified vessels—reading has limited value and suggests vascular stiffness
- 1.0–1.4  Normal range
- <0.9    Angiographic peripheral vascular disease is very likely
- 0.4–0.9  Likely to be associated with claudication
- <0.4    Advanced ischemia

# Gangrene in peripheral vascular disease

The onset of gangrene is relatively common in people with severe PVD and causes considerable distress. It often poses management difficulties, as many frail elderly are judged inappropriate for surgery.

## Slowly progressive disease with dry gangrene

- Cyanotic anesthetic tissue with necrosis
- Distal, with clear demarcation
- Often a low-grade inflammatory response (elevated WBC and CRP). The patient may feel unwell and anorexic.
- Non-urgent surgical review is appropriate, but the approach is often to allow autoamputation, a lengthy and sometimes distressing process for patient and family.

Surgical amputation may be considered, but as there is often inadequate local circulation to allow healing. This may need to be extensive or combined with bypass (the latter carrying a significant operative risk). Sometimes amputation vastly improves the quality of life for a bed-bound patient with gangrene.

Discussion about possible amputation should be approached with tact and sensitivity—patients are often very opposed to losing a limb, even when they have not walked for years. Ensure that the patient and family are aware of the rationale for treatment, and that there is regular review of analgesia requirements.

## Wet gangrene

This is a life-threatening condition, and urgent surgical review is required in all but the most terminal of patients.

- Moist, swollen, and blistered skin develops, usually in diabetics.
- The usual approach to management is for debridement and amputation.

## Acute ischemia

This is a limb-threatening condition and demands urgent action.

- It is usually due to embolization.
- **Distal emboli** cause so-called blue toe syndrome. The main object of treatment is to prevent recurrence as little can be done to salvage occluded small vessels. This may include angiography to establish the source and/or anticoagulation depending on the fitness of the patient.
- **Proximal emboli** cause diffuse acute ischemia. Revascularization of the limb is nearly always attempted (unless there is already irreversible ischemic changes) and the approach can be tailored to the frailty of the patient, ranging from thrombolysis, percutaneous thromboembolectomy (possible under local anesthetic), to emergency bypass procedures.

# Vascular secondary prevention

Atheromatous vascular disease (cardiac, peripheral vascular, and cerebral) accounts for a huge amount of morbidity, mortality, and expenditure. Secondary prevention measures (see Table 10.9) evolve continually as individual clinical trials reach completion.

Although some interventions are primarily applied to a specific pathology (e.g., statins in cardiovascular disease), most affect all vascular systems. The cumulative effect of therapies is not known, but the consensus is that they substantially reduce the burden of future vascular events.

Traditionally, older patients have been under-provided with secondary prevention measures, for a number of reasons:

- There is often polypharmacy, and patients and health-care professionals are reluctant to add to this.
- It was thought that secondary prevention benefits were seen only with long-term (perhaps 5–10 years) treatment. Unless life expectancy was greater than this, therapy was not begun.
- It may be "shutting the door after the horse has left the barn"—the damage has already been done.

But consider several contrary points:

- Recent evidence suggests that some therapies (statins and ACE inhibitors) act quickly, possibly due to endovascular stabilization.
- Although older patients are underrepresented in clinical trials, when they have been included (e.g., the Heart Protection Study) the benefits have been equal if not greater than those in younger patients.
- Do not assume that a disabled person will not benefit from prevention of further events. In a bed-bound stroke patient who has to be spoon-fed, a further stroke that removes swallowing ability altogether may deprive that person of their only pleasure in life.
- As with much of geriatric medicine, frank discussion with the patient is advised.
- Drug doses are determined by clinical trial evidence—often a high dose in generally robust patients. Adopt a pragmatic approach for frail patients, with lower doses, as these may be effective.
- Always calculate creatinine clearance when dosing renally cleared medications.

We do not advocate blind prescription of all secondary prevention to all older patients. Such an approach would be clinically inappropriate for some and unlikely to be cost-effective. What we do suggest is that each case be considered on an individual basis and, when possible, prevention discussed with the patient to reach an individually tailored action plan.

## Further reading

A randomised, blinded, trial of clopidogrel versus aspirin in patients at risk of ischaemic events (CAPRIE) (1996). *Lancet* **348**:1329–1339.

Heart Protection Study Collaborative Group (2002). MRC/BHF Heart Protection Study of cholesterol lowering with simvastatin in 20,536 high-risk individuals: a randomised placebo-controlled trial. *Lancet* **360** (9326):7–22.

Yusef S, Sleight P, Pogue J, et al. (2000). Effects of an angiotensin-converting-enzyme inhibitor, ramipril, on cardiovascular events in high-risk patients. The Heart Outcomes Prevention Evaluation Study Investigators. *N Engl J Med* **342**:145–153.

Table 10.9 Main secondary prevention agents

| Agent | Dose | Action | Outcome | Special points for older patients |
|---|---|---|---|---|
| Aspirin | 75–300 mg daily | Antiplatelet activity | Prevention of all vascular events | Use lower doses<br>Beware of gastric irritation<br>Consider co-prescription of proton pump inhibitor<br>Enteric-coated formulations unlikely to be very useful |
| Clopidogrel | 75 mg daily | Antiplatelet activity | Mainly as an alternative to aspirin when not tolerated, or as an addition in cardiac disease | Reportedly, lower gastric side effects than with aspirin<br>Slightly higher efficacy than that of aspirin as monotherapy |
| Antihypertensives | Various agents | Blood pressure reduction | Prevention of all vascular events | The lower the blood pressure, the greater the benefit, but take care to avoid hypotensive side effects. |
| ACE inhibitors | e.g., Ramipril 10 mg daily | Blood pressure reduction and possible endovascular effect | Prevention of all vascular events | Dose stated is often not tolerated in older patients—aim as high as tolerated, but start with 1.25 mg |
| Statins | e.g., simvastatin 40 mg daily | Cholesterol lowering and possible endovascular effect | Prevention of all vascular events | Should be prescribed for vast majority<br>Lower doses (e.g., 10 mg) may be better tolerated<br>Higher doses associated with ↑ LFTs,<br>Watch for myalgias, |

Note: consider also smoking cessation, increasing physical activity, and, for stroke, endarterectomy and AF prophylaxis.

# Pulmonary medicine

**Robert Wise**

# The aging lung

Most of the functional impairment of the lungs seen in older people is due to disease, often smoking related. Intrinsic aging leads only to mild functional deterioration. The respiratory system has a capacity well in excess of that required for normal activity. Therefore, intrinsic aging
- Does not lead to symptoms in the nonsmoker without respiratory disease.
- In those with respiratory disease (e.g., emphysema) will cause progressively worsening symptoms with age, even if the disease itself remains stable.
- In acute disease, e.g., pneumonia, may cause earlier decompensation or a more severe presentation.

The specific changes seen in healthy older people are similar to those seen in mild chronic obstructive pulmonary disease (COPD):
- Decreased elastic recoil, causing airflow limitation and air trapping (elevated residual volume)
- Increased chest wall stiffness, due to
  - Degenerative change in intercostal, intervertebral, and costovertebral joints
  - Osteoporosis and kyphoscoliosis
- Weaker respiratory muscles that may have lower endurance
- Increased ventilation–perfusion mismatch, causing lower levels of arterial oxygen ($PaO_2$)
- Impaired chemoreceptor function, leading to lessened ventilatory response to decreased $PaO_2$ or increased $PaCO_2$.
- Impairment of microbial defense mechanisms. There is less effective mucociliary clearance and a less sensitive cough reflex.

Generally observed consequences of these changes include the following:
- Increased susceptibility to infection (decreased cough and gag reflexes and difficulty clearing mucus from dependent lung zones)
- An approximately linear fall in $PaO_2$ with age (0.25 mmHg/year). Since alveolar oxygen tension remains stable, the alveolar–arterial (A-a) oxygen gradient increases.
- Reduced exercise capacity. However, maximum oxygen consumption and cardiac output decline in proportion to lung function, so the lungs are rarely the limiting factor in exercise performance with normal aging, except in highly trained senior athletes.

Breathlessness in older people is often multifactorial:
- Chronic breathlessness in an individual may be the result of, e.g., decreased fitness, obesity, an inefficient gait (osteoarthritis or stroke), kyphosis, previous lung damage (e.g., apical fibrosis due to tuberculosis [TB]), and intrinsic aging. In this example, note that only one of the factors is specific to the lung.
- In the acutely breathless patient, several pathologies commonly coexist, e.g., infectious, cardiac, and respiratory disease. Empiric treatment of more than one condition is often, therefore, justified.

# Respiratory infections

Cough with or without sputum, shortness of breath, fever or chest pain is a very common presentation in older patients. It is very important to try to distinguish which part of the airway is primarily affected because this implies different pathogens, prognoses, and treatment strategies. Treatment, therefore, should be individualized on the basis of etiologic agent, presence of comorbidities, and acuity of the presentation.

## Upper respiratory infection (URI)

These are caused by viruses, most commonly, rhinovirus, parainfluenza virus, coronavirus, adenovirus, respiratory syncytial virus, coxsackievirus, and influenza virus. Symptoms include nasal discharge and congestion, fever, and sore throat. These may extend to the lower tract and then include cough, wheeze, sputum production, or worsening of existing cardiopulmonary disease.

With increasing age:
- URIs becomes less frequent, but more severe.
- The risk of complications increases. These include the following:
  - Lower respiratory tract infection, such as bronchitis or pneumonia, which may be bacterial or viral
  - Bronchospasm
- Post-infection weakness, fatigue, and anorexia are more severe and prolonged, sometimes lasting several weeks.
- Frequency of hospital admission and mortality increase substantially.

# Influenza

This is the most serious viral respiratory tract infection and is often a severe, systemic illness with pulmonary bacterial superinfection (*Staphylococcus aureus, Hemophilus influenzae, Streptococcus pneumoniae*). It occurs most commonly in December–February. Antigenic shifts result in periodic pandemics (large-scale epidemics).

## Presentation

Presentation is similar in young and old, i.e., rapid onset of fever (rigors, chills), myalgia, headache, and fatigue with variable degrees of prostration. Influenza can be distinguished from a URI by the sudden onset of symptoms: prostration, fever, headache, and myalgias.

Typical URIs, in contrast, usually have a 1- to 2-day prodrome and milder constitutional symptoms.

## Diagnosis

Diagnosis is usually based on combining clinical assessment with epidemiological data, particularly current influenza incidence. Some other viruses can cause an identical clinical syndrome, and serological test results are not immediately available. Thus an initial assessment cannot produce an absolutely confident microbiological diagnosis. The syndrome may therefore most precisely be labeled "influenza-like illness."

Positive virological diagnosis in the context of increased community incidence or a nursing home outbreak is helpful by prompting vigorous attempts to reduce transmission of infection (see below and p. 329).

## Reducing viral transmission

Mass outbreaks of respiratory viral infection are common in nursing homes and hospitals. They can occur at any time of year but are most common from autumn to spring. Viruses are spread by aerosol or hand-to-hand contact (sometimes indirect, via fomites).

During an outbreak:
- Reduce transfers of healthy patients into, or symptomatic patients out of, the affected area.
- Reduce staff movement across work areas (especially applicable to short-term staff who may work in many clinical areas in a short time).
- Care for symptomatic patients in single rooms, with appropriate aerosol droplet precautions, i.e., the use of a facemask within 3 feet of an infected patient.
- Exclude visitors who have respiratory or other symptoms of viral illness from the ward.
- Ensure that staff caring for patients have been immunized against influenza.
- Ensure that scrupulous hand-washing procedures are followed.
- Staff caring for symptomatic patients should wear face masks.
- Avoid crowding of patients (the zone of aerosol droplet deposition is 3–6 feet around the patient).

## How to treat influenza-like illness in older people

The following guidance is generic and should be tailored to the patient, their illness, and their care environment. If the highest quality care cannot be provided, then a prompt step-up of care should be arranged. This may include hospital admission.

- Do not underestimate the disease. Mortality and morbidity increase exponentially with age and frailty.
- Give supportive and symptomatic care.
  - *Fluids:* Reduced intake and increased losses lead to volume depletion and end-organ dysfunction. Encourage frequent oral fluid. Consider early initiation of intravenous fluids if dehydration and poor intake seems likely.
  - *Nutrition:* Encourage adequate nutrition. Nutritional supplements may be needed.
  - *Acetaminophen:* If there is fever, discomfort or pain occur.
  - *Maintain mobility.* Physical therapy can prevent orthopedic complications and hasten recovery and self-care.
- Identify and treat complications promptly.
  - Caregivers may need information about important warning signs and the need to seek prompt medical advice.
  - Perform regular observations of blood pressure, pulse, temperature, and oxygen saturation.
  - Common serious complications include delirium, secondary bacterial infection, bronchospasm, pressure sores, and circulatory collapse.
- Antiviral agents (the neuraminidase inhibitors zanamivir and oseltamivir) can reduce both the severity and duration of influenza.
  - Recently introduced, they are not yet widely used.
  - They are indicated in patients over 65 years who have an influenza-like illness during a period of high community incidence providing they present early (<48 hours).
  - They are well tolerated and reduce symptom severity and duration of the illness.
  - Zanamivir is inhaled (10 mg bid for 5 days; two blisters of 5 mg each via dry-powder inhaler). Oseltamivir is taken orally (available as capsules or suspension; 75 mg bid for 5 days)

# Lower respiratory tract infection

This includes bronchitis and pneumonia.

### Acute bronchitis

This illness, characterized by cough and phlegm, has fewer systemic symptoms and a better prognosis than pneumonia. Acute bronchitis can be differentiated from pneumonia by the absence of fever, chills, pleurisy, chest crackles, and oxygen desaturation. If bronchospasm is a component, then wheezing and dyspnea may result.

In a typical, uncomplicated case, a chest radiograph is not necessary unless there are findings suggesting pneumonia or if the cough persists for more than 2 weeks.

Acute bronchitis can be managed less aggressively, with more reliance on bronchodilators than antibiotics. Often viral in origin, bacterial infections can occur as a superinfection. Antibiotics should be reserved for those with purulent sputum and an underlying chest condition such as COPD or bronchiectasis. In such cases, a macrolide antibiotic such as clarithromycin or azithromycin should be prescribed.

If a nonproductive cough with severe paroxysms persists for several weeks, consideration of pertussis infection should be considered in the elderly population who exhibit diminished protection from childhood immunizations.

Chest imaging for evolution into pneumonia should be considered if an elderly patient exhibits declining mental status, fever, or oxygen desaturation.

### Pneumonia

This is a syndrome of acute respiratory infection with infiltrates on the chest radiograph. Symptoms may be mild and may be nonspecific, such as declining mental status, poor oral intake, arrhythmia, cardiac ischemia, or dehydration with renal failure.

Frail older patients can sometimes present with septic shock, coma, and adult respiratory distress syndrome (ARDS).

Pleuritic chest pain, dyspnea, and high fever are less common than in younger people. Signs may be minimal:
- The patient may appear well or sick. Assess severity using the CURB criteria (**C**onfusion, **U**remia, **R**espiratory rate, and **B**lood pressure) (p. 334).
- Fever may be absent, but vasodilatation is common.
- Tachypnea is a sensitive sign, as is hypoxemia (<92% $SpO_2$ on room air).

Tests often guide management.
- Chest radiograph often reveals small infiltrates. Comorbid conditions can include malignancy, pleural effusion, or heart failure.
- Blood cultures should be sent, but sputum culture is not useful unless TB is suspected.
- White cell count (WBC) may be elevated, normal, or decreased. Early WBC precursors are usually increased.

- Urea, creatinine, and electrolytes guide fluid management. Renal impairment is a poor prognostic sign.
- Arterial blood gas (ABG) sampling is not usually necessary, unless oxygen saturations are <90%. Pulse oximetry is much better tolerated and usually sufficient to guide oxygen therapy.

*Organisms* (see Table 11.1)

- Often no causative organism is identified.
- Pneumococcus is a common pathogen in all settings.
- Viral pneumonia, especially influenza, is often missed outside of a known epidemic.

Legionella pneumonia varies in prevalence depending on local conditions. Hospital and nursing home water sources may be the source of epidemics. Mycoplasma pneumonia is uncommon in older adults except during epidemics.

Unusual organisms are more common in frail patients, in health-care settings, and in those who have recently received courses of antibiotics. These organisms include Gram negatives (which colonize the oropharynx) and anaerobes (a result of aspiration of gut contents).

Community-acquired methicillin-resistant *Staphylococcus aureus* (MRSA) is an increasingly common and serious cause of systemic infections including pneumonia, often occurring in previously healthy individuals. The prevalence and severity of this infection vary geographically for unknown reasons.

**Table 11.1** Pneumonia pathogens in various care settings, in approximate order of frequency

| Community acquired | Chronic care facility | Hospital |
|---|---|---|
| Streptoccus pneumoniae (>30% of cases) | Streptoccus pneumoniae (>30% of cases) | Gram-negative aerobic bacilli, e.g., Klebsiella, Pseudomonas aeruginosa |
| Viral, e.g., influenza, parainfluenza, respiratory syncytial virus (RSV) | Viral, e.g., influenza, parainfluenza, respiratory syncytial virus | Anaerobes, e.g., Bacteroides, Clostridium. Especially in those at risk of aspiration, e.g., immobility, swallowing difficulty, prolonged recumbency, or impaired conscious level |
| Hemophilus influenzae | Gram-negative aerobic bacilli, e.g., Klebsiella, Pseudomonas aeruginosa | Staphylococcus aureus |
| Gram negative bacilli, e.g., Klebsiella, Pseudomonas aeruginosa | Hemophilus influenzae | Streptococcus pneumoniae and Hemophilus influenzae. These may be the most common pathogens<br><br>• In non-acute settings, e.g., rehabilitation wards<br><br>• In the well, less frail patient |
| Legionella pneumophila. Mycoplasma pneumoniae if epidemic | Anaerobes, e.g., Bacteroides, Clostridium. Especially in those at risk of aspiration, e.g., immobility, swallowing difficulty, prolonged recumbency or impaired conscious level | Viral, e.g., influenza, parainfluenza, respiratory syncitial virus |
| Other, e.g., TB | Other, e.g., TB | |
| Following influenza, think of secondary bacterial infection, especially with Streptococcus pneumoniae (most common), Haemophilus influenzae, or Staphylococcus aureus | Following influenza, think of secondary bacterial infection, especially with Streptococcus pneumoniae (most common), Haemophilus influenzae, or Staphylococcus aureus | |

# Pneumonia: treatment

Treatment involves more than antibiotics alone.

- Assess and optimize fluid volume status; give oral or IV fluid as appropriate. Concurrent heart failure is common, but volume depletion even more so.
- Assess and optimize oxygenation. If there is dyspnea or hypoxemia, supplemental oxygen should be titrated to achieve arterial oxygen saturations >90%.
- Exercise caution in COPD: observe the patient closely, both clinically and with serial arterial blood gas sampling.
- Encourage mobility. If the patient is immobile, sit upright in bed in a chair as tolerated.
- Maintain head of bed at 30-degree elevation to reduce risk of aspiration.
- If dyspnea, anxiety or pain is distressing, consider small doses of opiates and titrate to effect.
- Administer nebulized bronchodilators if there is associated broncho-constriction.
- Respiratory therapy with suctioning and coughing help with secretions.
- Minimize risk of thromboembolism through early mobilization, compression stockings, and prophylactic heparin.
- Assess pressure sore risk and institute preventive measures (p. 522).
- Anticipate possible deterioration and decide in advance on the appropriate levels of intervention. Would renal dialysis, mechanical ventilation, and/or cardiopulmonary resuscitation be consistent with the patient's advance directives?
- Keep the family informed. When possible, enlist their help, e.g., in encouraging eating and drinking.

---

**Box 11.1 Characteristics of severe pneumonia: the CURB-65 score**

Five key criteria (acronym *CURB-65*) determine prognosis; 1 pt each:
1. Confusion
2. Urea (serum urea >20 mg/dL)
3. Respiratory rate (≥30/min)
4. Blood pressure (<90 systolic or ≤60 mmHg diastolic)
5. 65 years of age or more

The score has a 6-point scale (0–5 adverse prognostic features):
- Score 0 or 1. Low risk of death (0–3%). Possibility of home treatment (but consider other factors, e.g., functional status, hypoxemia)
- Score 2. Intermediate risk of death (13%). Hospital treatment is indicated.
- Score 3, 4, or 5. Severe pneumonia, with high risk of death (score 3: mortality 17%, 4: 41%, 5: 57%). Consider intensive care admission.

A 5-point scale (CRB-65; urea excluded) can be applied outside the hospital and also discriminates effectively between good and poor prognoses (e.g., mortality with score 1: 5%, score 3: 33%).

## Antimicrobials

The choice of antibiotic depends on local pathogen sensitivities and drug costs. In the initial 24 hours of treatment of acutely ill patients with community-acquired pneumonia, adequate coverage should include the rapidly fatal forms of pneumonia: pneumococcus, streptococcus, and Legionella. Thereafter, the antibiotic choice depends on the identification of the organism and specific sensitivities, if known.

### Community or nursing home settings

- Doxycycline 100 mg bid for 7–10 days or azithromycin 500 mg once daily for 3 days is adequate empiric treatment for patients who can take oral medications and who have mild–moderate symptoms.
- For patients with comorbidities (e.g., diabetes, COPD, congestive heaert failure [CHF]) or recent hospital exposure, empiric treatment with a fluoroquinolone can be initiated (e.g., levofloxacin 750 mg/day PO x 5 days or moxifloxacin 400 mg/day PO x 7 days).
- Intravenous antibiotics are necessary if the patient is very ill or unable to swallow. Give intravenous (IV) fluoroquinolones (e.g., levofloxacin 750 mg/day IV x 7–10 days, or moxifloxacin 400 mg/day IV x 7–10 days), or a combination of an advanced-generation cephalosporin (e.g., ceftriaxone 1 g IV daily or cefotaxime 1 g IV q8h) with a macrolide such as azithromycin or clarithromycin as above.
- If aspiration pneumonia is a consideration, then clindamycin 600 mg IV q8h with a fluoroquinolone is given. Alternatively, a combination penicillin such as amoxicillin-clavulanate (Augmentin®), Ticarcillin-clavulanate (Timentin®), or piperacillin-tazobactam (Zosyn®) can be employed pending culture and sensitivities.
- Hospital-acquired infections are often caused by antibiotic-resistant organisms including *Staphylococcus aureus* and gram-negative bacilli. In these cases, empiric treatment with broad-spectrum agents such as those described under intravenous antibiotics (above) can be initiated and the antibiotic choice tailored to the cultures and sensitivities of the patient's blood and respiratory secretions.

## How to manage the patient with pneumonia who fails to respond to treatment

*Is the diagnosis correct?*
- Consider other chest pathology such as heart failure, pulmonary embolism, pleural effusion, empyema, cancer, cryptogenic organizing pneumonia, aspirated foreign body, or bronchial obstruction.
- Consider further tests such as chest CT, echocardiogram, and bronchoscopy.

*Is there a complication?*
- For example, effusion, empyema, heart failure, silent myocardial infarction, or pulmonary embolism

*Is the antibiotic being taken regularly and in adequate dosage?*
- Is drug adherence a problem? Could a friend or relative supervise medication-taking, or would a pill-counting box help?
- If there are pill-swallowing difficulties, drugs can be crushed or given with applesauce. Liquid formulations are available for some antibiotics. Consider whether intravenous therapy may be necessary.

*Is the organism resistant?*
- Take more blood cultures.
- Consider a change in antimicrobial, taking into account likely pathogens and their known sensitivities.
- Consider atypical infection: send urine for Legionella antigen test, especially if the patient is immunocompromised or if a patient with a community-acquired pneumonia appears disproportionately unwell.

*Could other elements of care be more effective?*
- For example, fluid balance, oxygenation, nutrition, posture, and chest physiotherapy

*Is this an end-of-life situation?*
Not all pneumonias require aggressive treatment. Pneumonia is often the final complication of other serious illness such as advanced dementia, heart failure, cancer, chronic liver failure, or renal failure. Consider the patient's advance directives for patients with severe comorbidities as a guide to how aggressively to treat this condition. Involve the family and surrogate decision-makers in end-of-life decisions. If palliative care is the goal of therapy, relief of dyspnea and pain should be the primary goals of treatment. Supplemental oxygen, narcotics, and nursing care are helpful in relief of these symptoms.

# Vaccinating against pneumonia and influenza

## Vaccine delivery

Influenza vaccine should be offered in October or early November to all individuals over 50 years of age and to caregivers of older adults. Because protective antibody levels can be achieved within 2 weeks, it is recommended that persons who miss their autumnal immunization should receive it up until the end of influenza season.

Pneumococcal polyvalent immunization should be given at least once to individuals over the age of 65. Antibody levels decline over 5–10 years; however, it is not clear whether revaccination for those who were vaccinated after the age of 65 is of benefit. Nevertheless, some experts recommend a single revaccination if >5 years since first vaccination. The incidence of bacteremic pneumococcal infections is decreased, but it is not known whether the incidence of pneumonia is diminished.

## Post-exposure antiviral prophylaxis

Immunized or unimmunized residents of nursing homes where there are new cases of influenza-like illness should be offered prophylaxis regardless of immunization status. The neuraminidase inhibitor oseltamivir (see p. 329) is recommended (available as capsules or suspension; 75 mg daily for at least 7 days; consider for up to 6 weeks during an epidemic).

# Pulmonary fibrosis

This uncommon disease is often overlooked in the elderly and may be mistaken for CHF or COPD. The presenting symptoms are dyspnea associated with "Velcro"-like crackles in the chest and interstitial infiltrates on chest radiograph or CT.

## Causes

- Idiopathic: the most common type in older people, known as usual interstitial pneumonia (UIP)
- Connective tissue disease, e.g., rheumatoid arthritis (most common) or scleroderma
- Drugs (e.g., amiodarone, nitrofurantoin rarely)
- Occupational exposure, e.g., asbestos, silica
- Hypersensitivity pneumonitis (e.g., farmer's lung or pigeon-breeder's lung)

## Tests

The diagnosis is usually confirmed by high-resolution CT scanning, which can also help distinguish subgroups likely to respond to immunosuppressive treatment. Subpleural cystic changes at the base of the lung usually signify a diagnosis of UIP, whereas ground-glass densities are more often found in nonspecific interstitial pneumonitis (NSIP) or desquamative interstitial pneumonitis (DIP), which is more responsive to steroids.

Respiratory function tests show a restrictive ventilatory defect with decreased diffusing capacity.

Although pulmonary fibrosis is often rapidly progressive in younger and middle-aged adults, the disease may show slow progression in the elderly. The need for lung biopsy depends on the likelihood of the diagnosis based on imaging, history, and laboratory tests. Specialist consultation should be requested if a lung biopsy might be necessary for diagnosis or immunosuppressive treatment instituted.

## Treatment

- Treat or remove any underlying cause, e.g., drugs.
- A minority respond slowly to immunosuppression, usually with steroids (e.g., 30–60 mg daily prednisone and azathioprine). Monitor closely for side effects (see p. 130). In the elderly, long-term steroids usually cause more adverse effects than benefits. In nonresponders, the treatment should be tapered and stopped. Patients requiring long-term steroids should have an adequate bone-protection program with vitamin D, calcium, and bisphosphonates. Prophylaxis against pneumocystis should be considered when the dose of prednisone is >20 mg/day.
- Home oxygen therapy is often useful.
- Give opiates for distressing dyspnea and cough.
- In those in whom dyspnea progresses, consider end-of-life issues including treatment limitation, and a change of focus from life-extending measures to a purely palliative approach.
- Lung transplantation is usually not an option for individuals over the age of 60 years.

# Rib fractures

These are common in older people.

- They are often a result of falls or even minimal stresses such as coughing or rolling over in bed for a person with osteoporosis.
- Consider the possible contribution of alcohol, which causes both falls and osteoporosis.
- Fractures should be diagnosed clinically—point tenderness and crepitus are found. If anterior–posterior compression of the chest causes pain in a lateral rib, a fracture over that site is likely (positive "bow" sign). Even with multiple projections the chest radiograph is insensitive to fracture but is useful in excluding early complications such as pneumo- or hemothorax.
- Technetium bone scans are very sensitive to fractures, but usually do not change the treatment.
- Rib fractures heal without specific treatment. The major problem is pain, which commonly leads to voluntary splinting of the injured area. There is hypoventilation and a failure to clear secretions, and secondary pulmonary infection can occur. The patient should be encouraged to breathe deeply and to cough.
- Supporting the injured area when coughing, using a small pillow, minimizes pain.
- Regular analgesia should include acetaminophen, plus a weak opiate in most cases. A short course of NSAIDs may be helpful.
- In cases of severe pain (e.g., multiple fractures), consider strong opiates or intercostal/paravertebral blocks. A fentanyl patch or long-acting oral narcotics can often prevent the need for hospitalization. Elderly narcotic users should be monitored closely for signs of delirium.

# Pleural effusions

This is a frequent (clinical or radiological) finding, sometimes incidental. Common causes are heart failure, parapneumonic effusions, and malignancy, especially adenocarcinoma, primary to the lung or metastatic from breast, colon, stomach, or ovary.

The differential diagnosis is wide, but narrowed when the results of the chest radiograph and pleural fluid aspiration are known (see Table 11.2).

**Table 11.2** Differentiating cause, by protein level

| Transudate (protein <25 g/L) | Exudate (protein >35 g/L) |
| --- | --- |
| Heart failure | Malignancy |
| Hepatic cirrhosis | Infection, including TB |
| Hypothyroidism | GI causes e.g., pancreatitis |
| Nephrotic syndrome | Collagen diseases e.g., rheumatoid arthritis or systemic lupus erythematosus (SLE) |
| (Exudative causes if low-serum protein) | (Heart failure after diuresis) |

- Empyemas, malignancy, and TB produce exudates with low pH (<7.2), low glucose (<40 mg/dL), but high lactate dehydrogenase (LDH).
- Transudates are usually not due to focal lung pathology and so usually affect both lungs. Unilateral effusions due to transudates occasionally do occur, more commonly on the right side, particularly with CHF.
- Effusions due to heart failure are typically small and bilateral, with cardiomegaly; they can be unilateral, but usually a tiny contralateral effusion is seen, manifesting as blunting of the costophrenic angle. If the angle remains sharp, other causes are more likely.
- A massive unilateral effusion is usually due to malignancy.
- A uniformly hemorrhagic effusion is usually due to infection, embolism, malignancy, or trauma.
- Chronic exudative effusions may occur following coronary artery bypass surgery. The etiology is unknown, but may be an autoimmune process.

## Chronic effusions

- If there are bilateral transudates, the patient should be treated as for heart failure.
- If the diagnosis is not clear after chest imaging and aspiration, consider pulmonary specialist referral and tests including CT, pleural biopsy (CT-guided rather than blind), thoracoscopy, and echocardiogram.
- For large, recurrent effusions, consider pulmonary specialist referral for continuous outpatient external fluid drainage via a semi-permanent intrapleural catheter.

- Large recurrent effusions that are symptomatic may require a video-assisted thoracoscopy (VATS) for biopsy and pleurodesis.

Frail patients may not tolerate, or desire, the more invasive tests. In this case, consider the following:
- Repeated aspiration, combining diagnostic with therapeutic taps and sending larger volumes of fluid for cytology and acid-fast bacilli (AFB) culture.
- "Watching and waiting," with regular clinical review
- A trial of diuretics, especially if the effusion is a transudate

# Pulmonary embolism

Pulmonary embolism (PE) is common, but the diagnosis can be difficult and is often overlooked. It commonly coexists and is confused with other lung disease, e.g., pneumonia, heart failure, and COPD, and is a cause of clinical deterioration in such patients.

## Presentation

The classic symptom triad of pain, dyspnea, and hemoptysis is seen less commonly in older people.

Common presentations include the following:
- Brief paroxysm(s) of breathlessness or tachypnea
- Collapse, cardiac arrest, syncope, presyncope, or hypotension
- Pulmonary hypertension and right heart failure, presenting as chronic, unexplained breathlessness
- Pulmonary emboli may present with nonspecific clinical signs such as fever, wheeze, pulmonary edema, arrhythmia, confusion, or functional decline.

## Diagnostic testing

Determining the likelihood of PE rests on combining clinical judgment (the product of history, examination, and immediately available tests such as the chest radiograph) with appropriate imaging such as ventilation–perfusion (V/Q) lung scan or CT angiogram. The common clinical features of PE—tachypnea, tachycardia, and modest degrees of hypoxemia—are common in older patients for many reasons, so clinical judgment alone is rarely enough.

Moreover, a confident diagnosis is essential because of the following:
- The risk of anticoagulation is higher in older adults.
- The risk of a missed diagnosis is higher in older people because they have less cardiorespiratory reserve capacity.

Possible PE in older people should be investigated in the usual way, with the choice of tests guided by local facilities and expertise. The following issues are especially relevant:
- In a patient without known lung disease, the combination of breathlessness and a chest radiograph showing clear lung fields raises the possibility of PE. Further tests, usually a V/Q lung scan or CT angiogram, are indicated.
- In patients who cannot have such studies, Doppler venograms are useful. A normal Doppler venogram is reassuring that a large, subsequent PE is not likely. However, a negative venogram does not absolutely rule out PE. A positive Doppler venogram provides an indication for anticoagulation, regardless of whether a PE has occurred.
- Chest radiographic abnormalities may be minor (atelectasis or small effusions) or major (usually reflecting comorbid conditions rather than PE itself). Classical pleural-based wedge-shaped densities or unilateral oligemia are rare. The most common abnormality is unilateral elevation of the diaphragm.

- Arterial blood gases have some value in diagnosis, but the common abnormalities (low $PaO_2$, low $PaCO_2$, and increased A–a oxygen gradient) are neither sensitive nor specific.
  - In healthy older people, an increased A–a gradient is common.
- Echocardiogram may be normal following PE. However, in a patient with a high clinical probability, typical features of PE on echocardiogram usually provide sufficient diagnostic confidence to permit anticoagulation without further imaging.
- In the patient with unexplained right heart failure, consider PE: obtain an ECG and echocardiogram (ask for pulmonary artery [PA] pressures) and request imaging that details the lung parenchyma (high-resolution CT: pulmonary fibrosis?) and the vasculature (CT pulmonary angiogram [CTPA]: pulmonary embolism?).
- In the patient who does not respond to treatment for chest infection, heart failure, or acute exacerbation of COPD, consider whether PE may be responsible.

## Treatment

### Anticoagulation

Standard treatment is anticoagulation with either unfractionated or low-molecular-weight heparin (LMWH) (e.g., enoxaparin) followed by warfarin. Once the possibility of PE is raised, it is essential to treat with heparin pending diagnostic study results, unless there are particular treatment risks.

To minimize bleeding risk with warfarin, start with maintenance therapy (usually 5 mg /day) for the first 3 days. Subsequent doses should be guided by the prothrombin time with a goal INR of 2.0–3.0. The duration of treatment following a PE should be 6–12 months.

In the very frail, sick, unstable patient in whom anticoagulation with warfarin would present significant risk, consider a period of anticoagulation with unfractionated heparin or LMWH. Start warfarin when clinical stability returns.

### Thrombolysis

Consider thrombolysis when there is a massive PE, manifesting as acute right heart strain and systemic hypotension.

### Inferior vena cava (IVC) filter

Consider an IVC filter. These are inserted by interventional radiology, and some models can be removed after placement. Indications include the following:

- Strong contraindication to anticoagulation, e.g.:
  - Active bleeding
  - A high risk of bleeding, e.g., recent hemorrhagic stroke
- Massive thromboembolism with contraindication to thrombolysis
- Ongoing thromboembolism despite anticoagulation
- Chronic thromboembolic pulmonary hypertension

# Pulmonary aspiration

The involuntary aspiration of extrinsic material into the pulmonary airways is a common problem, ranging from subclinical microaspiration of oropharyngeal mucus to major inhalation of gastric contents.

If a bolus of food is aspirated into the upper airway it can simulate sudden death ("café coronary"). Older adults are prone to such aspiration if they have poor dentition and are unable to masticate their food.

## Causes
- Swallowing problems
- Gastroesophageal reflux
- Impaired conscious level, including seizures
- Sedative drugs and alcoholic delirium
- Previous aspiration or non-aspiration pneumonia
- Artificial feeding—either nasogastric or gastrostomy

## Diagnosis
The occurrence of pneumonia in a patient with risk factor(s) suggests the diagnosis.

If the patient aspirates in the recumbent position, the lower lobes are most likely to be affected. If the patient aspirates while sitting upright, the right middle lobe is the most likely site. However, aspiration pneumonia can affect any area of the lung.

## Treatment
The role of antibiotics is controversial. Much of the radiographic response may be a chemical pneumonitis, i.e., an inflammatory reaction to the acidic gastric contents, rather than infective pneumonia. In chronically ill patients, however, the upper airway becomes colonized with gram-negative bacteria, making them more prone to develop secondary bacterial infections. Aspiration of upper-airway contents is the likely etiology of much hospital-acquired pneumonia.

The choice of antibiotics is also contentious. Mild cases respond well to amoxicillin or amoxicillin-clavulanate, but consider broad-spectrum intravenous antibiotics to cover Gram negatives and anaerobes in very frail or chronically ill patients, or those who reside in a long-term care facility.

If possible, treat the underlying cause. If risk factors persist (e.g., impaired swallow or continual seizures), consider an NPO order until they are addressed.

Where the swallow may be impaired, perform a formal swallowing assessment (see p. 180) and manage according to the results.

In advanced dementia, it is often appropriate to accept the risk of aspiration. Insertion of a gastrostomy feeding tube (commonly a percutaneous endoscopic gastrostomy [PEG]) is effective if swallowing prevents adequate nutrition, but does not significantly reduce the risk of aspiration.

The risk of feeding patients prone to aspiration must be balanced with the benefits of oral nutrition. The administration of honey-thickened liquids and pureed food, avoidance of drinking straws, and elevation of the head of the bed all diminish the risk of aspiration. Some patients may require supervised feeding with ready availability of a suction apparatus.

# Chronic cough

This is a common problem, with causes ranging from the trivial to serious. Even when the underlying cause is benign, chronic cough can be both distressing and disabling.

## Causes

- Asthma. Cough is a common presenting symptom in older people.
- Silent pulmonary aspiration or an aspirated foreign body (e.g., a tooth).
- Gastroesophageal reflux disease (GERD)
- Postnasal drip, due to the following:
  - Sinusitis
  - Chronic rhinitis. Frequently allergic in origin, but in older people, symptoms are often perennial
- Drugs e.g., ACE-inhibitors
- Persistent benign cough following URI. May persist for 3–6 months
- Chronic pulmonary pathology, e.g., COPD, TB, bronchiectasis or pulmonary fibrosis
- Thoracic malignancy, either primary or secondary

## Diagnostic tests

Consider both tests and trials of treatment. Their pace and extent depend on the differential diagnosis following careful history and examination. Consider the following tests:

- Chest radiograph or CT for coughs that persist longer than 2 weeks without improvement
- Sinus X-rays or CT
- Spirometry, with assessment of response to bronchodilators
  Next, consider a trial of treatment for the most likely cause, e.g.:
- Bronchodilators (and inhaled steroids) for possible asthma
- A proton pump inhibitor for possible GERD
- Assess the effect of treatment of possible chronic rhinitis with nasal corticosteroids, e.g., beclomethasone, budesonide, or fluticasone.

In all cases, trials of treatment need to be prolonged (≥8 weeks).

## Treatment

Treatment is of the underlying cause. When this cannot be treated effectively (e.g., advanced malignancy), specific treatments aimed at reducing cough may be of benefit. These include opiates such as codeine (15–60 mg 4-hourly) or morphine (starting dose 5 mg q4h). Simple cough syrups such as guaifenesin, 100–300 mg qid, may be useful for irritating dry cough following URI.

# Lung cancers

Lung cancer is the most common cause of cancer death, and largely a disease of older people.

Symptoms may be nonspecific (e.g., fatigue, weight loss) or pulmonary in origin but attributed to existing nonmalignant pathology (e.g., dyspnea in a patient with COPD). Brain metastases may present as seizures or a stroke. Paraneoplastic syndromes may cause electrolyte disturbance or muscle weakness. Vocal cord paralysis due to recurrent laryngeal nerve involvement may present as hoarseness.

Have a high index of suspicion and a low threshold for further diagnostic testing, particularly in current or former smokers, who account for about 90% of lung cancer cases.

In those presenting with pneumonia, features suggestive of lung cancer include the following:
- Hemoptysis, especially if significant, e.g., with persistent blood clots
- Regional or generalized symptoms of cancer (e.g., hoarse voice, weight loss)
- Cough and consolidation without obvious infectious symptoms (e.g., fever)
- Symptoms that continue to be troublesome despite antibiotics
- Failure of a pneumonia to resolve within 8 weeks

If these features are present, a chest CT with and without IV contrast is useful. Bronchoscopy or lung biopsy is needed for definitive diagnosis. Positron emission tomography (PET) scans can help determine the presence of metastatic disease. Treatment is rapidly changing, so treatment should be directed by a specialist in thoracic oncology.

Older people with probable lung cancer tend to be undiagnosed and untreated.
- Tests such as bronchoscopy and a histopathological diagnosis are less commonly obtained. This makes palliative treatment and prognostication difficult.
- Treatment such as surgery or chemotherapy is less commonly considered or administered. To an extent, this reflects appropriate decision-making based on functional status.

Treatment decisions should be made by expert teams who consider the patient's functional status, comorbidities, and cancer characteristics.

### Non–small cell carcinoma (squamous cell, adenocarinoma, and large cell carcinoma)
Surgery may lead to cure if
- There is adequate pulmonary function (i.e., the postoperative $FEV_1$ exceeds 0.8 L).
- There is no distant spread (but 70% of cancers have spread at presentation).
- The patient is relatively well with good functional status and no serious comorbidity.

Surgical procedures are high risk (e.g., at 70 years, lobectomy has 5% perioperative fatality, and pneumonectomy 10%). However, the condition is always fatal without treatment, so the patient's view is critical.

When surgery is not feasible, either because of the nature of disease, or the fitness of the patient, then radiotherapy may be used:

- For palliation, i.e., to control symptoms (see below)
- High-dose radiation therapy with stereotactic guidance can be curative in some cases of localized tumors, though the success rate is lower than with surgery.
- Combination radiation and chemotherapy may be used prior to surgery (neoadjuvant therapy) to reduce tumor cell burden. Such treatments show promise of improved survival compared to surgery alone.

## Small cell carcinoma

This is relatively more common in older people, with >20% of cases.

Most cases present with bulky mediastinal or hilar adenopathy and thus are advanced at presentation. For this reason, surgical resection is usually not attempted, and treatment is palliative.

Most tumors are chemoresponsive. Frail patients are unlikely to tolerate aggressive treatment and it risks reducing the quality of the brief life that remains. Therefore, chemotherapy regimes are tailored to the patient, determined by structured assessment of performance status. In general, frail patients undergo fewer but similar chemotherapy cycles compared to those who are more robust.

## Palliative interventions

- Radiotherapy for superior vena cava obstruction, bronchial obstruction, chest pain, hemoptysis, or painful bony metastases. This is generally well tolerated, although 5% develop radiation pneumonitis weeks after treatment, which can be more severe in the elderly because of diminished physiologic reserve capacity.
- Opiates for cough
- Oxygen to relieve breathlessness
- Aspiration of pleural effusion for breathlessness
- Endobronchial therapy (e.g., stenting, laser resection, brachytherapy)

# Tuberculosis: presentation

In older people, tuberculosis (TB) has the following traits and history:

- Incidence is higher, especially in the very old, because of the higher rates of previous primary infection and the diminished immune memory.
- Mortality from TB is higher in the elderly, who are prone to having disseminated disease.
- It is most commonly due to reactivation of previous disease, the primary infection having been asymptomatic or unrecognized many years prior. In the early twentieth century, primary infection of young adults was common. By the mid- to late twentieth century, primary infection of younger people had diminished. Thus, it is likely that the prevalence of TB in the elderly will decline over time.
- Reactivation (post-primary disease) occurs because of decreased immunity (see p. 640), which itself is due to intrinsic aging, disease (e.g., diabetes mellitus, renal failure), malnutrition, or immunosuppressive drugs (e.g., steroids or anti-TNF treatments).
- A few patients develop new infection from unrecognized cases of active disease. Nursing home residents are most vulnerable.

## Presentation

### Pulmonary disease

- Usually similar to that in younger people, i.e., cough, sputum, fatigue, weight loss, and anorexia
- Night sweats, fevers, and pulmonary symptoms may be less common.
- May present as an upper lobe pneumonia that fails to resolve, or as an incidental finding, suggested on chest radiography

### Extrapulmonary disease

Most presentations are pulmonary, but extrapulmonary cases are relatively more common in older people.

#### Miliary

This is diffuse, overwhelming infection with fever, weight loss, and hepatosplenomegaly. Hematological abnormalities are common, causing the diagnosis to be confused with myelodysplastic syndromes.

#### Urogenital and renal

Disease may affect any part of the renal tract. Sterile pyuria and microscopic hematuria are typical presentations,

#### Meningeal

Consider this in the very frail, malnourished, or immunosuppressed patient with nonspecific cerebral signs (e.g., confusion, dementia-like syndrome, headache, or reduced consciousness level). Meningism (nuchal rigidity, photophobia, and headache) are usually absent, and the cerebrospinal fluid (CSF) has a mild *pleiocytosis and elevated protein*. On occasion, the CSF may be normal. Organisms are usually absent in the CSF and a positive polymerase chain reaction (PCR) for *M. tuberculosis* is diagnostic, but does not rule out the diagnosis.

*Skeletal*

Bone infection most commonly affects the spine (usually thoracic or lumbar), presenting as pain and tenderness. Deformity leading to kyphosis can be mistaken for osteoporotic compression fractures. Advanced disease may present as paraplegia requiring urgent laminectomy. TB arthritis usually affects large weight-bearing joints.

# Tuberculosis: diagnosis

### Chest radiograph

Changes in the elderly are more variable than in younger people, and may mimic other benign or malignant disease (e.g., pneumonia, cancer).

- Usually apical infiltrates with cavities, but also as miliary (diffuse nodular) infiltrates
- Healed old disease, e.g., calcified hilar nodes, a calcified nodules, pleural or pericardial thickening, bronchiectasis, or apical fibrosis
- Pleural effusions usually follow primary infection, and are less common in reactivated disease.
- Endobronchial disease may present with hemoptysis and a normal chest radiograph.

### Sputum for microscopy and culture

This is the standard method of confirming TB.

- Conventionally, three early-morning sputum specimens are obtained and stained by acid-fast staining (e.g., Ziehl–Neelsen or fluorochrome). A negative microscopic exam does not rule out TB until the culture is negative on multiple specimens.
- If a patient cannot expectorate, obtain "induced sputum," through physiotherapy, or nebulized normal saline. If clinical suspicion is high despite negative smear and culture, bronchoscopy with lavage can be diagnostic, particularly in disseminated miliary TB.

### Other tests

- Raised ESR and CRP are usual.
- The WBC is usually normal with a lymphocytosis. With disseminated disease, pancytopenia may be present.
- Obtain three early-morning urine specimens for mycobacterial culture to diagnose renal TB.
- Tissue sampling. Where possible, sample tissue, e.g., lymph node, pleura, bone marrow. Send samples to both microbiology (microscopy and culture) and to histology. Typical histological features of caseous necrosis with granuloma formation (with or without acid-fast bacilli) strongly support the diagnosis of TB.
- Tuberculin skin testing is mandatory if the patient is not known to have a positive test.

## How to perform and interpret a tuberculin skin test

In these diagnostic tests, tuberculin purified protein derivative (PPD) is injected in a standardized manner, and the reaction assessed quantitatively.

The PPD (Mantoux) test is performed where TB is suspected in an individual patient. PPD is injected intradermally and the size of the indurated area after 48 hours is measured.

- The standard dose is 5 tuberculin units (0.1 mL) administered as an intradermal skin wheal with a 27-gauge needle and tuberculin syringe.
- Edema may cause induration for the first 24 hours, which will thereafter abate.
- After 48 hours measure the diameter of induration, reflecting the extent of the cell-mediated immune response. A ballpoint pen can be used to draw the borders of the indurated area.
- A positive test indicates prior (often asymptomatic) primary infection, not necessarily an active infection or reactivation.
- The degree of induration correlates approximately with the likelihood of infection. However, the post-test probability of infection is a product of both the pre-test probability and the test result.
  - 10–15 mm indicates a significant reaction and increases the probability of active infection.
  - 5–10 mm may be significant if pre-test probability is high or if the patient is immunosuppressed.
  - <5 mm is negative, usually indicating a low probability of active infection. However, if the pre-test probability is very high, consider treatment.
- The test may be falsely negative (or equivocal) with steroid use, lymphoma, malnutrition, sarcoid, overwhelming TB infection, or when there is concurrent other infection.
- Aging itself impairs the immune response to TB, and may produce a false-negative or equivocal test in patients previously infected with TB. Giving a second (booster) tuberculin dose after the first often produces a positive test, defined as when induration >10 mm and augmentation of induration (test 1 – test 2) exceeds 6 mm.

# Tuberculosis: treatment

Given the complexities of treatment, specialist referral is necessary.
- All proven cases should be reported to the health department for surveillance of exposed household members or caregivers.
- If the suspicion of TB is high, empiric treatment is often initiated pending results of cultures.
- Respiratory isolation is mandatory in medical facilities. TB infection is spread by droplet nuclei that can persist in the air for days, depending on ventilation. Ultraviolet light can sterilize TB-contaminated air.
- Pulmonary disease: Usually 6 months of rifampin and isoniazid (INH), with pyrazinamide (and ethambutol) for the first 2 months only. Longer treatment periods may be needed for extrapulmonary disease.

*In older people*
- Drug resistance is rare in the elderly, as most infections are recurrences of primary disease, contracted decades ago. However, future generations of the elderly, particularly those from endemic regions, will be more likely to have drug resistance.
- Failures of treatment are usually due to poor adherence. Directly observed therapy is considered the best approach in patients who may not be compliant with treatment.
- Side effects are more common in older patients, including ocular toxicity from ethambutol (reduce dose in renal impairment) and hepatitis from isoniazid. Monitoring is important.

# Atypical mycobacteria

## Presentation

Atypical mycobacteria can mimic pulmonary tuberculosis and are more common in elderly individuals with underlying structural lung disease (e.g., bronchiectasis or pneumoconiosis) or those with poor nutritional status. The most common organisms are *Mycobacterium avium-intracellulare* (MAI) or *Mycobacterium kansasii*. The chest radiograph mimics tuberculosis or may present as micronodular infiltrates that coalesce.

## Treatment

Treatment of atypical mycobacteria depends on identification of the organism, which is facilitated by rapid culture methods and PCR.

- Often a combination of multiple antituberculous drugs and macrolide or fluoroquinolone antibiotics is needed for treatment, which may be prolonged.
- Atypical mycobacteria are not spread from person to person, so respiratory isolation and case-finding in exposed individuals is not necessary.

# Asthma and COPD: assessment

## Presentation

Asthma and chronic obstructive pulmonary disease (COPD) in older people
- Are both diseases characterized by airflow obstruction.
- Commonly coexist, e.g., in the childhood asthmatic who has smoked.
- May both be mimicked by other common diseases, e.g., pulmonary embolism, heart failure.
- May present late. Inactive older people can be less aware of hypoxemia, breathlessness, or bronchoconstriction.
- Are underdiagnosed and undertreated, especially in older people.

### Asthma
- May present in old age as "late-onset asthma." This often follows an influenza-like illness.
- Long-standing asthma causes remodeling of the airways with fixed airway obstruction that can be hard to distinguish from COPD.
- Older asthmatics tend to have less allergic component to their disease.
- In older people, cough may dominate, symptoms fluctuate less, triggers (e.g., cold, smoke, allergens) are less frequent, and the association with hay fever or eczema is less strong.
- Nocturnal cough or dyspnea, including paroxysmal nocturnal dyspnea, may be caused by asthma.
- NSAIDs and beta-blockers (oral or ocular) may worsen bronchoconstriction.

### COPD
- COPD is much more common in older age, the consequence of intrinsic aging and progressive disease.
- It is most often caused by cigarette smoking, in susceptible people. However, some nonsmokers can develop a variant of COPD called "senile emphysema" as a result of accelerated aging of the lung.
- Compared to asthma, symptoms are usually more chronic with less day-to-day variability.
- If bronchitis is significant, there is a productive cough. Fatigue and sleep disturbance are common.
- COPD is a systemic inflammatory disease that can be associated with osteoporosis, muscle atrophy, malnutrition, and depression.
- Anemia of chronic disease may coexist with COPD and exacerbate dyspnea.
- Beta-blockers, if indicated for coexistent cardiac disease or glaucoma, should not be avoided in treating COPD.

## Diagnostic tests
- Oximetry will determine the presence and degree of hypoxemia. If the room air oxygen saturation is <90%, oxygen supplementation is usually indicated.
- Chest radiograph, electrocardiogram, and complete blood count (CBC) will help to exclude other pathology, e.g., anemia, arrhythmia.

- Spirometry. An $FEV_1/FVC$ ratio of <70% suggests obstruction. The severity of obstruction depends on the degree of impairment of $FEV_1$ compared to reference values.

Older people often have difficulty performing pulmonary function tests, so good coaching, patience, and assessment of quality of the testing are essential.

Assessments for bronchodilator responsiveness do not distinguish reliably between asthma and COPD. However, airflow obstruction that completely reverses after bronchodilator strongly suggests asthma.

Failure to respond acutely to a bronchodilator should not preclude such therapy.

# Asthma and COPD: drug treatment

In general, treatment principles are similar to those for younger people. A step-wise approach is indicated depending on the severity of the disease. The major differences between treatment of asthma and COPD are as follows:

- Inhaled corticosteroids are the initial treatment of persistent asthma, whereas they are reserved for COPD patients who have recurrent exacerbations.
- Long-acting bronchodilator monotherapy is often used in COPD, but is discouraged in asthma.
- Long-acting anticholinergic bronchodilators are indicated for COPD, but their role in asthma in the elderly is not established.

### Bronchodilators

- High-dose beta-agonists, e.g., from nebulizers, may cause tremor, tachycardia, or rate-related angina.
- Nebulizers can often be replaced by a metered-dose inhaler (MDI) with a spacer or a dry-powder inhaler (DPI).
- Nebulizers are often attractive to older adults because the drug costs are covered by Medicare, but this should not be the reason to prescribe them.
- For patients who require frequent dosing of short-acting bronchodilators such as albuterol or ipratropium, consider long-acting bronchodilators. Long-acting beta-agonists include formoterol and salmeterol. A long-acting antimuscarinic is tiotropium.
- Anticholinergic bronchodilators may cause urinary retention in elderly patients with bladder neck obstruction. If the agents are sprayed directly into the eye they may cause acute narrow-angle glaucoma, but do not cause open-angle glaucoma, which is the common type in older people.
- Long-acting beta agonists can be overdosed in the elderly if they do not understand that they are for maintenance therapy rather than rapid relief of symptoms. For this reason, a rapid-relief, short-acting inhaler should usually be prescribed with a long-acting bronchodilator.

### Corticosteroids

- The benefits of long-term oral steroids usually do not outweigh the adverse effects.
- In those receiving repeated courses of oral steroids for acute exacerbations, give osteoporosis prophylactic treatment.
- Inhaled steroids in moderate doses probably do not cause osteoporosis, but screening and treatment are indicated in older patients as a component of general medical care.
- Combination inhaled steroids and long-acting bronchodilators have additive benefit in treating both asthma and COPD.

### Theophylline

- Toxicity is common in older people. Plasma levels are increased by febrile illness, heart failure, and drugs, e.g., erythromycin and ciprofloxacin. Anorexia, nausea, tremor, palpitations, and seizures may be signs of toxicity.

- Low-dose, long-acting theophylline (e.g., 200–400 mg/day) is usually well tolerated and does not require monitoring of drug levels without signs of toxicity.
- Theophylline is protein-bound, so drug levels may be misleading in older people with malnutrition.
- Although inhaled therapy is preferred, oral theophylline is an inexpensive adjunct in those elderly persons who cannot afford to purchase more expensive inhaled agents.

### Other

- Influenza and pneumococcal vaccine should be given (see p. 752).
- Exercise caution in the use of respiratory depressants such as sedatives or opiates for the following patients:
  - Acutely ill patients with $CO_2$ retention
  - Stable patients with advanced disease

In severe, end-stage COPD, consider titrating opiates to relieve cough and dyspnea while maintaining as much alertness as possible. Give small doses initially, but increase it as needed to relieve distress, even if respiratory function deteriorates. Explain the rationale to caregivers, as well as to relatives and the patient, if appropriate.

### How to improve drug delivery in asthma or COPD

- The traditional metered-dose inhaler (MDI) alone is rarely adequate, due to difficulties in coordinating device activation and the onset of inhalation.
- Adding a spacer device reduces the need to coordinate activation and inhalation, improving drug delivery and reducing side effects (e.g., oral thrush).
- Breath-activated devices and dry-powder inhalers provide an alternative to the MDI. Because of the varied designs, proper instruction and monitoring are important.
- Assess and advise on technique regularly, involving both hospital and community teams (doctor, nurse, and pharmacist) as well as the family and other caregivers.
- Nebulizers are rarely required. An MDI with a spacer device is usually just as effective. Patients in whom nebulized drugs are being considered should be referred for specialist assessment.
- Rarely, inhaled drugs are administered too frequently by cognitively impaired people. Long-acting beta-agonists with slow onset of action may be particularly dangerous if confused with a short-acting rescue inhaler.

# Asthma and COPD: non-drug treatment

- *Pulmonary rehabilitation* is effective in improving patients' quality of life and exercise capacity. It should be considered for those patients who may benefit, regardless of age. It is a complex intervention tailored to the individual, with exercise, behavioral, and educational components. Individual action plans can be followed by older people, facilitating self-management and early intervention.
- *Smoking cessation* should be strongly counseled in all cases, and pharmacological adjuncts such as nicotine replacement, bupropion, and varenicline should be offered.
- *Nutritional depletion* (low BMI) is common with advanced disease, as the work of breathing exceeds calorific intake, and nutritional supplements may be needed.
- *Comorbidities* including depression, osteoporosis, coronary artery disease, and lung cancer are common and often overlooked. Diagnosis and treatment are important components of COPD care.
- *Exercise* is beneficial, sometimes available as part of a pulmonary rehabilitation program. Elements should include aerobic conditioning with supplemental oxygen and upper-extremity strength training. A self-directed exercise program is important for maintaining benefits of formal rehabilitation.
- *Pacing and energy conservation* are taught as part of pulmonary rehabilitation, but should also be taught and reinforced in the outpatient setting.

## Assisted ventilation

Indications for this include respiratory arrest, acute respiratory acidosis (pH <7.2), delirium, exhaustion, or deteriorating respiratory function despite full treatment. Severe agitation or pain requiring sedation or narcotics may also indicate assisted ventilation.

If excessive oxygenation ($PaO_2$ >65) is associated with an acute respiratory acidosis, mechanical ventilation can sometimes be avoided by reducing the oxygen concentration.

In an acute exacerbation, noninvasive mask ventilation can sometimes prevent the need for intubation, pending response to bronchodilators, steroids, and antibiotics.

The decision to provide mechanical ventilation should take into account the patient's advance directives, the patient's preferences as expressed by the family and surrogate decision-makers, and the overall prognosis for meaningful recovery. Age, by itself, should not be a criterion of whether to provide life support.

## Social and practical interventions

Provide appropriate mobility aids including wheelchairs and stair lifts. Rolling walkers that support the arms during ambulation are often helpful to patients with severe emphysema.

Social isolation and fear of loss of independence are common psychological burdens of COPD patients who live in the community and need to be addressed by the treating physician and other caregivers.

## Palliative interventions

Reassurance is important. Some patients who experienced dyspnea fear that they will die of slow suffocation or strangulation. They can be reassured that this is not likely, and that effective medication is available to alleviate suffering. Moreover, the prognosis in COPD is very difficult to assess, and prolonged survival is often the result of avoiding complications such as intercurrent infections.

Involve the palliative care team. Their advice and support is often valuable and can continue into the community if discharge occurs.

## Long-term oxygen therapy (LTOT)

This improves prognosis in severe hypoxemia ($PaO_2$ ≤55 mmHg) and in moderate COPD ($PaO_2$ ≤60 mmHg) with features of cor pulmonale. To reduce pulmonary hypertension, arterial $pO_2$ should be raised above 60 mmHg for at least 18 hours each day.

Flow rates of 1–4 L/min by nasal cannula usually achieve adequate oxygenation without respiratory depression in patients with stable respiratory failure. In patients with acute respiratory failure who are prone to acute respiratory acidosis, fixed concentrations of oxygen delivered by a Venturi mask is preferred. With a nasal cannula, the concentration of oxygen will increase as hypoventilation occurs, which can exacerbate the hypercarbia.

The most convenient and cost-effective method of long-term home oxygen delivery is an electrically powered concentrator. Compressed oxygen tanks should be available for emergency power outages.

Portable oxygen for ambulation is important for those who are not bedbound. Devices include liquid oxygen systems, small compressed tanks, and portable oxygen concentrators.

Oxygen supplementation during exercise training is a helpful adjunct regardless of the level of resting hypoxemia, but is often not paid for by Medicare so it is often underutilized.

Cigarette smoking or use of an open flame while using oxygen is a common cause of burns and house fires and thus should be avoided. In cases where a patient continues to smoke while using oxygen, it is in the best interests of the patient and family members to withdraw the oxygen from the household.

# Gastroenterology

## Franklin Herlong

# The aging gastrointestinal system

**Mouth** (see Chapter 29, Dental and Oral Health)

### Esophagus

- Slight changes in innervations produce clinically insignificant changes in swallow and peristalsis.
- The misnamed presbyesophagus is a distinct disease, not a universal age change.
- Hiatal hernias and reflux are very common—probably related to anatomical and postural changes.

### Stomach

- There is an increased incidence of atrophic gastritis (with reduced acid production) but in the absence of disease; most older patients maintain normal pH levels.
- Delayed gastric emptying is common.
- Increased mucosal susceptibility to injury.
- There is increased *Helicobacter pylori* colonization, but this is less likely to cause ulceration.

### Small intestine

- Function is well preserved except for calcium absorption, which is decreased.
- There is an increased incidence of bacterial overgrowth, with malnutrition and diarrhea.

### Large intestine

- Decreased rectal sensation contributes to high incidence of constipation.

### Pancreas

- Structural changes include atrophy, but function is well preserved.

### Liver

- Hepatic weight and volume decrease by around 25% and there is brown (lipofuscin) pigment buildup, but liver function (and, therefore, liver function tests) are not affected.
- Some older patients have a slightly lower albumin level but results still remain within the normal range.

### Gallbladder

- Incidence of gallstones increases (40% females over age 80), probably related to a reduced rate of synthesis and excretion of bile salts.
- Most gallstones are asymptomatic.

# Nutrition

With normal aging the following occur:
- Calorie requirement falls because of reduced activity and lower resting metabolic rate (decreased muscle mass).
- Appetite diminishes (anorexia of aging).
- There are lower reserves of both of macro- and micronutrients (vitamins and minerals).

In the presence of disease, older patients quickly become malnourished, and malnutrition is a powerful predictor of outcome (increased functional dependency, morbidity, mortality, and use of health-care resources).

Malnutrition is extremely common in the older frail or institutionalized population, and studies have shown that once in the hospital most patients' nutritional status actually declines further. Protein energy undernutrition affects the following populations:
- 15% of community-dwelling older patients
- 5%–12% of housebound patients with multiple chronic problems
- 35%–65% of patients acutely admitted to hospital
- 25%–60% of institutionalized older persons

## Nutritional assessment
- Body mass index (BMI; weight in kg/(height in m)$^2$) is often impractical, as height cannot be accurately measured in immobile patients or those with abnormal posture.
- Simple weight is still useful, especially if patients know their usual weight—rapid weight loss (>4 kg in 6 months) is always worrisome even in obese patients.
- Nutrition screening tools are often employed to target interventions, but many have not been well validated.
- More complex tools (e.g., Mini Nutritional Assessment) are helpful but time consuming and rarely used outside research.
- Biochemical measures, including hypoalbuminemia, anemia, and hypocholesterolemia, develop at a late stage and are confounded by acute and chronic illness.

## Nutritional support
- Involve a dietician if possible.
- Record food intake carefully.
- Make mealtimes a priority and provide assistance with feeding.
- Offer tempting, high-calorie foods.
- Prescribe oral high-caloric supplements, but be aware that compliance is often poor.
- Consider the role of enteral feeding.

# Enteral feeding

Consider enteral feeding early if there is dysphagia (e.g., stroke, myopathy) or failure of oral feeding (e.g., severe anorexia, intensive care unit) with an intact gastrointestinal (GI) tract. Enteral feeding of patients with dementia but without dysphagia is controversial and lacks evidence of benefit. In most instances careful hand feeding suffices.

The burdens and risks of enteral must be carefully considered and discussed with caregivers.

There are three common methods:

1. **Fine-bore nasogastric (NG)** tubes are simple, quick, and inexpensive; they are the preferred method for short-term feeding. Some patients (usually confused or drowsy) repeatedly pull out NG tubes. Interference with the tube increases the risk of aspiration. Persistence, supervision, and careful taping can sometimes help but often a PEG or RIG is required. There are promising early studies using NG tubes that are held in place via a nasal loop. Trained practitioners can insert these by the bedside and removal by the patient is very rare.

2. **Percutaneous endoscopic gastrostomy (PEG):** The risks of insertion include perforation, bleeding, and infection for a patient who is usually already frail. The patient has to be fit to undergo sedation. Problems obtaining consent from a competent patient and "agreement" from next of kin for an incompetent patient are not uncommon. Once established, this method is discreet and better tolerated than NG tubes and is the method of choice for medium- or long-term enteral feeding.

3. **Radiographically inserted gastrostomy (RIG)** is useful if gastroscopy is technically difficult (e.g., pharyngeal pouch) and sometimes if small bowel feeding is preferred over gastric feeding. It has a similar complication rate to that of PEG.

## Complications for all methods

### Aspiration pneumonia

There is a common misconception that enteral feeding eliminates aspiration in dysphagic patients. This is not true—reflux of food into the esophagus is common and this along with salivary secretions and oral intake may still be aspirated. Always check the position of the tube if the patient develops a fever, dyspnea or, cough.

If aspiration is ongoing despite correct tube position slow the feed, feed with patient sitting upright (i.e., not at night), and add promotility drugs, e.g., metoclopramide 10 mg each day or erythromycin 250 mg with meals. A nasojejunal tube or jejunal extention to a PEG tube can also reduce aspiration rates.

### Refeeding syndrome

This occurs when the patient has been malnourished for a long time. When feeding commences, insulin levels cause minerals (especially phosphorus) to move rapidly into intracellular space and fluid retention occurs, causing hypophosphatemia, hypomagnesemia, and hypokalemia. This in turn can cause life-threatening heart failure, respiratory failure, arrhythmias, seizures, and coma.

Avoid this syndrome by "starting low and going slow" when introducing feeding. It is important to check and correct any abnormal biochemistry before feeding starts and then monitor frequently (check Ca, Mg, Phos, and glucose and K potassium daily for a few days, then weekly). Supplementation of minerals may be done intravenously or by adding it to NG feeding.

### Fluid overload and heart failure
Decrease volume infused and add diuretics.

### Diarrhea
Exclude infection (especially *Clostridium difficile*). Try slowing the feeding rate or changing the feeding to one containing more or less fiber.

# Parenteral feeding

This should be considered when the gut is not functioning. It requires central venous access and should only be undertaken when supervised by an experienced nutrition team. It is usually a temporary measure, e.g., post-gastrointestinal surgery.

Complications such as fluid overload, electrolyte disturbance, and intravenous catheter sepsis are common in older patients.

### How to insert a fine-bore nasogastric feeding tube

1. Get the patient's consent—if they refuse, come back later. They may well have just had several uncomfortable failed attempts. Obtain consent from a family member if the patient can not give informed consent.
2. Have the patient sitting upright with chin tucked forward (patients often hyperextend their neck, which makes it harder). Draw the curtains (this can be an unpleasant procedure to have done or to watch).
3. Leave the guide wire in the tube and lubricate with lots of jelly.
4. Feed the tube down one nostril about 20cm (until it hits the back of the throat).
5. If there is a proximal obstruction try the other nostril.
6. If possible, ask the patient to swallow and advance the wire.
7. Check the back of the throat carefully—you should be able to see a single wire going down vertically. Start again if there is a loop.
8. Secure the tube immediately with tape to both nose and cheek.

Once you believe the tube is in place you need to check if it is in the stomach by one or both of the following methods BEFORE you use the tube.
- A chest X-ray. If you leave the guide wire in, the tube shows more easily. The tip of the tube should be clearly below the diaphragm.
- Aspiration of gastric fluid that is clearly acidic.

The method of blowing air down the tube and listening for bubbles has now been discredited, as a bubbling sound can be generated from saliva and pulmonary secretions.

### Further reading

Potter J, Langhorne P, Roberts R (1998). Routine protein energy supplementation in adults: systemic review. *BMJ* **317**:495–501.

# The ethics of artificial feeding

Feeding is a highly emotive issue. It is viewed by many (especially relatives) as a basic need, hence failing to provide adequate nutrition is seen as a form of neglect or even euthanasia. In contrast, others feel that artificial enteral feeding is a cruel and futile treatment performed on incompetent patients which only postpones a "natural" death that involves anorexia or dysphagia.

There are numerous high-profile legal cases regarding feeding (usually withdrawal of). Controversial cases should always involve consultation with an ethics service. The key to steering a course through this minefield is good communication.

### Initiating treatment

- Establish if the patient has decision-making capacity—even dysphasic patients may understand a little with nonverbal cues, etc.
- If the patient has decision-making capacity ensure that they understand the chosen method (and its risks) and projected duration of feeding. Patients with dysphagia must realize that they will be expected to dramatically decrease, or stop, oral feeding.
- For patients without decision-making capacity be sure you have communicated with all interested caregivers and family. There is sometimes disagreement between interested parties; these are best detected and negotiated early. A caregiver or family conference is often helpful.
- Establish that everyone accepts the indications for feeding and the aims of treatment and set a date for review, e.g.,
  - 2 weeks of NG feeding in a patient with dysphagia following a stroke, which is hoped will resolve.
  - PEG insertion in a patient with neurological diseases causing malnutrition with recurrent aspiration pneumonia, to be reviewed if the patient requests or enters a terminal phase of disease.
- Don't be afraid of a therapeutic trial (e.g., if you don't know whether the patient's lethargy, drowsiness, or depression is related to malnutrition). Always be sure that everyone understands and agrees on review dates and criteria for reassessment. Patients and relatives can be reassured that PEG tubes can be removed if improvement occurs.
- Record discussions and plan carefully in the medical record.
- If there is still dispute, obtain an ethics consult.

### Withdrawing treatment

Withholding treatment is not morally different from withdrawing it. There are, however, technical and emotional differences, which is why many more ethical problems arise with withdrawing treatment and why some doctors are resistant to trials of treatment.

Artificial feeding can be withdrawn for the following reasons:
- It is no longer required (rarely controversial).
- A therapeutic trial has failed (see How to manage weight loss in older patients; sometimes a trial is controversial).
- Although feeding is successful, the patient's quality of life is felt to be unacceptable (this is nearly always controversial).

An ethics consult should be obtained prior to withdrawal of long-term feeding if there is any disagreement.

## How to manage weight loss in older patients

Peak body mass is reached at age 40–50 and weight loss can occur after this due to decreased lean mass, although the proportion of fat is relatively increased so overall weight is often remarkably stable.

As a rule of thumb, unintentional weight loss of more than 5 lb (2.3 kg) or 5% of body weight in a month or 10 lb (4.5 kg) or 10% body weight in 6 months is worrisome.

Always try and get recorded weight (rather than relying on the patient's or caregiver's memory)—a search of old outpatient clinic and primary care records can help. Record weight regularly while you investigate to look for ongoing trends.

Dramatic weight loss should always prompt a search for remediable pathology. It is important to consider the following:
- Dementia (p. 214)
- Depression (p. 238)
- Malignancy (p. 674)
- Chronic infection or disease, e.g., COPD, heart failure, TB
- Inflammatory conditions, e.g., giant cell arteritis (p. 500)
- Malabsorbtion (p. 386)
- Drug causes e.g., digoxin, theophyllines
- Metabolic disorders e.g., hyperthyroidism, Addison's disease
- Swallowing problems
- Persistent nausea or abdominal pain or reflux (p. 377)
- Social causes, e.g., inability to cook, poverty, social isolation, alcoholism

A careful history (including dietary history and mental state), examination and routine blood test, and chest X-ray will usually give clues of significant underlying pathology. If preliminary investigations are negative a "watch and re-weigh and wait" plan is reasonable—be reassured if weight is actually stable or rising, reexamine, and rescreen if further loss occurs.

Obviously if a remediable cause is found and treated, weight loss may be halted or reversed. When no such cause is found or it is not reversible, interventions are still possible.
- Prioritize and help with feeding (this sounds obvious but often neglected in hospital). Involving relatives at mealtimes can be beneficial.
- Offer high-fat or high-calorie food (e.g., substitute whole milk and yogurt if patient is on the lower-fat variety).
- Refer to a dietician, especially if anorexia is prominent.
- Keep a diet diary—this highlights deficiencies in intake and helps identify where interventions might help.
- Prescribe dietary supplements between meals.
- Appetite stimulants (e.g., megasterol) are of unproven benefit and risk serious side effects.

# Esophageal disease

### Gastroesophageal reflux disease (GERD)

The symptoms (retrosternal burning, acid regurgitation, flatulence, atypical chest pain) correlate poorly with the pathology (normal mucosa to severe esophagitis).

Dangerous features that might suggest malignancy include sudden or recent onset, dysphagia, vomiting, weight loss, and anemia. They should guide management.

- In the absence of dangerous features a "blind" trial of treatment is given.
- If there are dangerous features then endoscopy should be arranged.

Esophageal pH monitoring is rarely necessary.

**Barrett's esophagus** is where glandular gastric mucosa replaces the esophageal squamous cell mucosa. It is associated with an increased risk of malignancy and should have regular endoscopic surveillance regardless of symptoms.

### Treatment

Check if the patient is taking prescribed or over-the-counter NSAIDs, steroids, or bisphosphonates and stop or minimize the dose. Proton-pump inhibitors (PPIs) have revolutionized treatment, making antacids and H2 blockers such as ranitidine almost redundant. They are very effective (for symptoms and healing) and safe. They are used for prophylaxis as well as treatment. Rarely, older patients can have side effects of diarrhea or confusion.

### Hiatal hernia

- Very common in older patients, occurring to a degree in almost all
- Laxity of structures at the gastroesophageal junction allows esophagogastric junction or portions of stomach to move up (permanently or intermittently) into the thorax.
- It may be asymptomatic but often presents with GERD symptoms and occasionally with dysphagia.
- Very large intrathoracic hernias can impair respiratory function and strangulate or perforate.

### Diagnosis

Diagnosis is on CXR (stomach or fluid level behind heart), at endoscopy, or on contrast radiology.

### Treatment

To reduce reflux suggest losing weight, avoiding alcohol, caffeine, and nicotine, eating small meals often, avoiding eating before bed, and elevating the head of the bed on blocks. PPIs will nearly always relieve symptoms; consider investigations if they don't. Prokinetic agents, e.g., metoclopramide 10 mg each day, sometimes help.

Younger patients with intractable problems can be assessed for surgery—laparoscopic surgery is now available.

## Achalasia

- This is an idiopathic neurological degeneration causing impaired peristalsis and a lack of lower esophageal sphincter relaxation.
- A dilated esophagus and aspiration can develop but gastroscopy may be normal.
- Barium swallow may show abnormalities, but 24-hour manometry is the gold standard.
- Despite the lack of anatomical abnormality, endoscopic balloon dilation can relieve dysphagia.

## Esophageal candidiasis

- This condition can present with dysphagia or odynophagia.
- Consider it in frail or immunosuppressed patients, especially if oral candidiasis is present.
- Characteristic appearance is on endoscopy (biopsy confirms) or barium swallow.
- Treat with fluconazole 50–100 mg each day for 2 weeks.

# Dysphagia

Dysphagia, difficulty in swallowing, is a common symptom in older patients.

## History
- Ask what type of food is difficult (solids or liquids) and the level at which food sticks (mouth, throat, retrosternal, or epigastric).
- Distinguish dysphagia from early satiety and regurgitation (when successfully swallowed food returns after seconds or minutes), which usually occurs with gastric outlet obstruction.
- If swallowing fatigues through a meal, consider myasthenia.
- Cough, wheeze, or recurrent aspiration pneumonia can be a presentation of swallowing problems that cause aspiration.

## Signs
Look for weight loss, oral thrush (may be associated with esophageal candida), supraclavicular lymphadenopathy, and a gastric splash (implies gastric outlet obstruction). Watch the patient swallow some water and food—the diagnosis might be clear.

## Causes
These can be divided into two categories.

### 1. Structural lesions (worse with solids)
- Esophageal or gastric cancer
- Benign strictures—scarring following, e.g., esophagitis, scleroderma, polymyositis, radiotherapy
- Pharyngeal pouch
- Esophageal candida or severe esophagitis
- Hiatal hernia can produce obstruction symptoms
- External obstruction, e.g., bronchial tumor, aortic aneurysm, or cervical osteophyte
- Foreign bodies (e.g., hair balls) are more common in demented patients.

### 2. Functional problems (often worse with fluids)
- *Pharynx or throat:* The most common neurological cause is stroke but can occur in advanced dementia. Rarer neurological conditions include myasthenia gravis, inclusion body myositis, multiple sclerosis, and Parkinson's disease.
- *Esophagus:* Dysmotility problems are relatively common in older patients and include achalasia and diffuse esophageal spasm.

## Investigations
Endoscopy is now the primary investigation and is well tolerated even in frail patients. Sometimes a barium swallow is performed first if there is a high risk of perforation with an endoscope, but gastroscopy allows biopsy and therapy, e.g., dilation. Videofluroscopy provides functional imaging and is useful diagnostically, but the correlation between observed aspiration and clinically significant problems is poor.

### Treatment of dysphagia

- An empirical trial of PPI can be used in the very frail and those who are deemed unfit for investigation.
- If oral thrush is present, try fluconazole 50–100 mg each day for a week.
- Esophageal dilation ± stenting can be very successful for benign or malignant strictures.
- For functional problems consult a speech therapist. Changing the consistency of food and fluids, and positioning patient correctly can minimize problems.
- For esophageal dysmotility try a PPI and calcium-channel blocker (e.g., nifedipine) or a nitrate (e.g., isosorbide mononitrate).
- Gastoparesis causes early satiety and vomiting. It can be very hard to treat—try metoclopramide 10 mg each day or erythromycin 250 mg three times a day.
- Nutritional support: Older patients with dysphagia are usually malnourished to start with and are then put NPO for investigations. Refer to the dietician and consider dietary supplements and early enteral feeding (p. 346).

**Aspiration pneumonia** is largely a chemical rather than infective insult treated by the following:

- Preventing or minimizing aspiration (NPO, NG feeding)
- Oxygen therapy
- Chest physiotherapy
- Intravenous antibiotics (Augmentin® or cefuroxime and metronidazole) are given to prevent superinfection (also see Pulmonary aspiration in Chapter 11, Pulmonary medicine, p. 325).

There is a group of patients who have dysphagia, weight loss, and recurrent aspiration due to progressive neurological conditions such as dementia who merit palliative treatment. It is not always appropriate to aggressively manage such patients who are frequently incompetent and derive pleasure from eating normally.

Adopting a palliative policy is impossible unless everyone, including the whole multidisciplinary team and relatives, understands and sympathizes with the aims of management.

# Peptic ulcer disease

This disease is becoming much rarer with the advent of effective medical treatment. It remains predominantly a disease of the older population. NSAID use (see p. 126) is the most common cause, followed by *Helicobacter pylori*.

*H. pylori* is a spiral gram-negative bacterium that colonizes the gastric mucosa, causing gastritis. Carriage rates increase with age—40% at age 50, 75% at age 70. Infection is usually asymptomatic but is the most common cause of dyspepsia in older patients. *H. pylori* is strongly associated with duodenal ulcers and their recurrence and may have a link with NSAID-associated ulceration.

### Presentation

Patients present with acute bleeding, pain (epigastric, retrosternal, or back), indigestion, "heartburn," dysphagia, perforation (peritonitis), iron deficiency anemia, or an incidental finding (e.g., on endoscopy).

### Investigation

- Upper GI endoscopy is very safe and well tolerated in older patients. It can often be performed without sedation using local anesthesia in the throat only. *H. pylori* can be detected with gastric biopsy and histology or with a test for urease activity.
- Serological tests remain positive but titers gradually decline after eradication.
- Breath tests can detect *H. pylori* colonization but obviously don't demonstrate pathology.

### Treatment

Dietary restriction is unnecessary (it is worth mentioning because older patients can remember harsh or bizarre anti-ulcer diets). Stop any NSAIDs. When there is *H. pylori* and ulceration or gastritis, treat with one of the many "triple-therapy" antibiotic PPI regimens (e.g., Amoxil®, clarithromycin *or* metronidazole, and omeprazole 20 mg for 6 weeks). In the absence of *H. pylori* just a PPI will suffice.

Arrange a repeat endoscopy at 6 weeks to check healing of all gastric ulcers and malignant-looking duodenal ulcers.

#### *For bleeding*

- Resuscitation with blood product is life saving.
- Early interventional endoscopy with epinephrine injection (or other modalities, e.g., heater probes or clips) into the bleeding point is suitable for almost all patients. Don't delay because of age or comorbidity.
- Postendoscopic intervention omeprazole 80 mg IV stat followed by infusion of 8 mg/hr for 72 hours reduces rebleeding.
- Continued bleeding or rebleeding despite endoscopic treatment is an indication for surgical intervention. These patients have a high mortality but overall do benefit from operative intervention.

*For perforation* (p. 390)
Remember "silent" perforation (without signs of peritonitis) is more common in older patients. Mortality is high due to delayed diagnosis, reluctance to perform surgery, and postoperative complications.

## How to investigate and manage persistent unexplained nausea and vomiting (N+V)

This group of patients can be very challenging, but you should actively manage them from an early stage because they are often very uncomfortable and bed-bound. There is often reversible disease and they are at high risk of dehydration or malnutrition and complications of immobility.

N+V can be the major presenting feature of illnesses as diverse as pneumonia, myocardial infarction, intracerebral hemorrhage, and constipation.
- Start with a careful history (especially drug history).
- Thorough examination (including rectal examination and neurological assessment)
- Regular observations of vital signs (looking for intermittent fever, arrhythmia, etc.)
- Screening blood tests (including calcium, thyroid function, CRP), urinalysis, CXR, and ECG

### Drugs

Look very carefully at the patient's drug history—almost any drug can cause N+V but digoxin (even with therapeutic serum levels), opiates, tramadol, entacapone, antidepressants, NSAIDs, and PPIs are some of the more common candidates. New drugs are the most likely, but remember there may be poor adherence for drugs at home that are prescribed in the hospital. If there is polypharmacy, try stopping the drugs one at a time. Some drugs can take days to wash out.

### Central causes

Raised intracerebral pressure can occasionally present this way. A CT scan is needed if there is drowsiness, focal neurologic signs, or a past history of intraventricular blood (exclude hydrocephalus). If there is vertigo or tinnitus consider labyrinthitis or posterior circulation stroke (p. 166).

### Gut causes

Constipation is a very common cause of nausea, even without obstruction. An abdominal x-ray should be done early on to exclude obstruction. Consider repeating this if symptoms persist and you remain suspicious. Plain radiology will remain normal in high obstruction and a small bowel follow through may help.

Severe gastritis or peptic ulceration can present with N+V without pain and bleeding. Gastroparesis is most common in diabetics and is very hard to treat—try metoclopramide or erythromycin.

# The liver and gallbladder

### Abnormal liver function tests

These can be transiently elevated, e.g., with sepsis, drugs (e.g., statins, antibiotics, analgesics—can occur up to 6 months after exposure to drug), and viruses (cytomegalovirus [CMV], Epstein–Barr, and adenovirus). Persistently elevated LFTs should always prompt investigations (ultrasound, CT scan).

An isolated elevated alkaline phosphatase is often from a bone source (commonly Paget's disease) but don't assume this—liver metastases can present this way.

### Cirrhosis

Chronic liver disease can present for the first time in older people. The presentation is often nonspecific. The prognosis is worse than for a younger person with the same degree of liver damage. Common causes include alcohol, hepatitis C, autoimmune hepatitis, and nonalcoholic fatty liver. A proportion is cryptogenic (thought to be "burnt out" autoimmune hepatitis or nonalcoholic fatty liver disease).

- **Hepatitis C** may have been transmitted from blood products received before 1991 when screening was introduced. Alcohol consumption is known to increase the percentage of those infected with hepatitis C who develop cirrhosis.
- **Alcohol excess** can present with falls, confusion, and heart failure at any age but older patients are less likely to volunteer (or be asked!) their alcohol history.

Always enquire about alcohol!

- **Nonalcoholic fatty liver disease** is not always a benign condition (half will be progressive and 15% develop cirrhosis). Obesity, hyperlipidemia, and type 2 diabetes are risk factors, so this condition is more common in older patients.

If you suspect cirrhosis your initial investigations should include alpha-1-antitrypsin, autoimmune profile (ANA, SMA, LKM, antimitochondrial antibody, and immunoglobulins), ferritin and transferrin saturation, hepititis B and C serology, and ultrasound, including Doppler imaging of portal and hepatic vein.

### Gallstones

- These are very common (1:3 elderly females) and mostly asymptomatic, although troublesome symptoms are often misdiagnosed as gastroesophageal reflux or diverticulitis in older age groups.
- Management is largely as for younger patients but the risks of surgical intervention are higher, so conservative or less invasive approaches are often adopted.
- Acute cholecystitis in older patients may present atypically (e.g., without pain) and is not always associated with gallstones. It has a 10% mortality rate and should be aggressively treated with IV antibiotics and supportive care. Failure to improve should prompt early surgical evaluation.

## Further reading

American Gastroenterological Association medical position statement: evaluation of liver chemistry tests. *Gastroenterology* 2002: **123**:1364.

# Constipation

The term *constipation* is used in different ways, indicating one or more of the following:

- The time between bowel evacuations is longer than normal.
- The stool is harder than normal.
- The total fecal mass present is increased.

The most precise definition may be delayed alimentary tract transit time: this is delayed in age, in the institutionalized, and in those eating a Western or low-fiber diet.

There are said to be three types of constipation:

1. Hard feces present in the rectum (often in massive amounts)
2. The whole distal large bowel filled with soft, putty-like feces that cannot be evacuated
3. High (proximal) impaction that may be due to obstructing pathology (e.g., diverticular disease, carcinoma)

### Diagnosis

The diagnosis is largely clinical (based on history and examination alone).

▶▶Ask specifically about constipation, as some patients are embarrassed to trouble doctors with bowel symptoms. Constipation may rarely be the primary cause of delirium but commonly contributes to the presentation of the frail older patients with other pathology such as sepsis or renal failure.

Rectal examination may be diagnostic, and sometimes the rectum will barely admit the examining finger. If the rectum is empty, consider high impaction. In a thin patient, high impaction is unlikely if the loaded colon cannot be felt during abdominal examination. In more obese subjects a plain abdominal X-ray will be necessary to confirm high impaction, but is insensitive in the very obese.

▶▶Do not exclude constipation as the cause of fecal incontinence until there has been an adequate therapeutic trial for high fecal impaction.

### Causes

- *Reduced motility of the bowel:* chronic laxative abuse, drugs (e.g., opiates, iron, anticholinergics, antidepressants), immobility, constitutional illness, electrolyte disturbances, dehydration, hypothyroidism, lack of dietary fiber, hypercalcemia
- *Failure to evacuate the bowels fully:* any painful condition of the rectum or anus, difficulty in access to the toilet, lack of privacy, altered daily routine
- *Neuromuscular:* Parkinson's disease, diabetic neuropathy, pseudo-obstruction.
- *Mechanical obstruction of the bowel:* carcinoma of the colon, diverticular disease

### Prevention and treatment

Precipitating causes such as dehydration, hypothyroidism, hypercalcemia, and drugs should be identified and reversed.

**Nonpharmacological** measures including regular exercise, improving access to the toilet, adequate dietary fiber, and adequate hydration are effective.

**Laxatives** should be used in combination with nonpharmacological measures.

- Unless there are reversible factors, always prescribe laxatives on a regular schedule. Waiting for constipation to occur, then using prn doses is far less effective.
- Titrate the laxative dose with time and changing patient circumstances.
- Stimulant laxatives such as senna (1–4 tabs/day) or bisacodyl (5–20 mg/day), or stimulant suppositories may be appropriate for those with bulky, soft fecal overloading.
- Avoid stimulant laxatives in patients with rock hard feces, as this may produce abdominal pain. Use a stool-softening laxative instead such as lactulose (10–40 mL/day) or docusate sodium.
- Long-term use of stimulant laxatives has been said to cause "bowel tolerance" or neuronal damage leading to a dilated, atonic colon that requires even more laxatives. There is very little evidence to support this, and stimulant laxatives are now considered safe, in moderate doses, for long-term use.
- Sometimes stimulant and osmotic laxatives are used in combination, typically in severe constipation (e.g., opiate-induced) that has been unresponsive to a single drug.
- Stool-bulking agents such as methylcellulose (Citrucel) are useful in prophylaxis but are less effective in treating established constipation; both fiber and other bulking agents will increase stool volume and may increase problems.
- Costs of laxatives vary enormously, and there is no correlation between cost and patient acceptability. Try cheaper preparations first (fiber, senna).

Fecal retention severe enough to cause incontinence nearly always needs a determined effort to clear the colon (see p. 565).

### Further reading

Lock GR III, Pemberton JH, Phillips SF (2000). American Gastroenterological Association Medical Position Statement: guidelines on constipation. *Gastroenterology* **119**(6):1761–1776.

Muller-Lissuer SA, Kamm MA, Scarpignato C, et al. (2005). Myths and misconceptions about chronic constipation. *Am J Gastroenterol* **100**:232–242.

# Diverticular disease

Narrow-necked pockets of colonic mucosa occur adjacent to blood vessel penetrations of the muscle bands, like "blow-outs" on a tire. They occur anywhere in large bowel but most commonly in the sigmoid colon.

- *Rare* below age 40, increasing frequency with age and almost universal over age 85
- *Cause:* thought to be raised intraluminal pressure due to low-fiber Western diet
- *Investigation:* colonoscopy, flexible sigmoidoscopy, or barium enema are usually diagnostic and rule out other pathology. Abdominal CT with oral contrast is increasingly used as a better-tolerated test in frail patients.

## Treatment

Most cases are asymptomatic most of the time. On other occasions innocent diverticulae are blamed for symptoms that arise from other pathology, e.g., constipation, irritable bowel disease, or gastroenteritis. The previous diagnosis of diverticular disease should not stop the careful evaluation of new bowel symptoms to exclude important diagnoses such as colitis or cancer.

The treatment depends on presentation:

- **Pain,** especially if associated with constipation, can be improved by a high-fiber diet with or without extra stool bulking drugs (e.g., Citrucel).
- **Diverticulitis** should be thought of as "left-sided appendicitis." Infection occurs within a pocket and may be due to a fecolith blocking the neck, so avoiding constipation is key to prevention. Abdominal pain and tenderness, diarrhea, and vomiting occur with fever and raised inflammatory markers. Treat with antibiotics (include anaerobic coverage, e.g., ciprofloxacin 500 mg twice a day with metronidazole 400 mg three times a day). For mild cases give oral antibiotics at home, severe cases may need admission for intravenous rehydration, antibiotics, and with surgical consultation.
- **Hemorrhage:** Selective angiography can be used to demonstrate bleeding point with therapeutic embolization.
- **Diverticular abscess:** Perform ultrasound or CT for diagnosis and radiographically guided drainage under local anesthetic.

## Perforation/peritonitis (see p. 390)

**Fistula:** most commonly to bladder causing urinary infection and bubbles in urine (pneumaturia). Cystoscopy or CT scan is used for diagnosis. Surgery is required but simple colostomy is often sufficient.

# Inflammatory bowel disease

Ulcerative colitis (UC) and Crohn's disease (CD) are chronic, relapsing conditions caused by inflammation of the bowel wall. Inflammatory bowel disease is idiopathic and has an increasing incidence in the population as a whole.

Initial presentation is usually in adolescence but there is a second peak of incidence in older patients. Diarrhea and urgency in this age group can be particularly disabling and may result in incontinence and social isolation.

## Features

- Diarrhea (often with blood), malaise, weight loss, and abdominal pain. Delayed presentation may result from embarrassment or fear of cancer. Delayed diagnosis is more common in older adults because symptoms are ascribed to one of the common differential diagnoses such as diverticular disease, colonic carcinoma, and ischemic colitis.
- Associated conditions include arthritis, iritis, sclerosing cholangitis, ankylosing spondylitis, and skin disorders (pyoderma gangrenosum, erythema nodosum).
- Complications include thromboembolism, malabsorbtion and malnutrition, perforation, stenosis with obstruction, fistula formation, and colonic and biliary malignancy.

## Investigations

- Exclude infection with stool culture and examination for leukocytes ova, cysts, and parasites and *Clostridium* toxin (if patient was in the hospital or has had recent antibiotics).
- ESR and CRP are usually elevated but may be normal in localized disease.
- A normochromic, normocytic anemia is common but if there is excessive bleeding, iron deficiency can develop.
- Plain abdominal X-rays are usually normal but contrast studies are often diagnostic.
- Sigmoidoscopy or colonoscopy and biopsy have high diagnostic yield.

## Treatment

Confirmed cases are best managed by gastroenterologists who have specialist nurses and dieticians working with them. Treatment in older patients is not greatly different from that in younger patients and is aimed at obtaining and then maintaining remission. There are many new treatments (e.g., cyclosporin, infliximab) that are beyond the scope of this text. Some principles for treating older patients are as follows:

- Exacerbations of distal colitis are usually treated with topical mesalazine and steroids given as enemas. This may be impractical in older patients unless a caregiver can help; oral steroids can be a better option.
- Budesonide is a steroid with high topical potency (poor absorption and rapid first-pass metabolism); equivalent doses cause fewer side effects.

- Side effects, drug interactions, and polypharmacy may be more problematic in older patients, thus always consider bisphosphonates with oral steroids therapy.
- Look for and treat proximal constipation, which can impair the efficacy of treatment of a distal colitis.
- Oral 5-aminosalicylic acid preparations (e.g., slow-release mesalazine such as Pentasa®) are often successful (for exacerbations and maintenance) and well tolerated.
- The risk of malignancy is higher the longer the patient has active disease, so theoretically many older patients should be under surveillance by a gastroenterologist. Unfortunately, the risk of colonic perforation during colonoscopic screening is higher in the elderly population; many screening programs stop at age 75.
- For failure of medical management elective colectomy is well tolerated and may give the best quality of life. In contrast, emergency surgery in older patients has high mortality.

# Diarrhea in the older patient

### Acute

Short-lived bouts of diarrhea are most commonly due to viral gastroen-teritis. Supportive management (rehydration, light diet) is usually suffi-cient for this self-limiting condition. However, if diarrhea persists, always send samples for fecal leukocytes culture and parasite examination and *Clostridium difficile* toxin (p. 650).

### Chronic

There is a group of older patients who suffer chronic or recurring episodes of diarrhea that merit active investigation. Untreated they suffer high morbidity (especially if diarrhea induces fecal incontinence) and many causes are treatable. How to investigate and manage chronic diarrhea (next page) gives a suggested plan of investigation.

### Malabsorbtion

Patients do not always have diarrhea. Look for low BMI and falling weight despite reasonable oral calorie intake. Biochemical markers of malnutri-tion, e.g., hypoalbuminemia, may be present. Anemia is caused by malab-sorbtion of iron, $B_{12}$, or folate and can be therefore microcytic, macrocytic, or normocytic.

The common causes of malabsorption in older patients often coexist and include the following:
- **Celiac disease or gluten-sensitive enteropathy**
  - Peak incidence is at age 50 but can manifest for the first time in old age with weight loss, bone pain (osteoporosis), fatigue (anemia), and mouth ulcers.
  - Duodenal biopsy should be performed in all who present with iron deficiency.
  - Antiendomysial antibodies have very high specificity (100%) and reasonable sensitivity (around 85%). False negatives can occur with low IgA, so always check serum immunoglobulins at the same time.
- **Pancreatic insufficiency** can occur without history of pancreatitis, alcoholism, or gallstones.
- **Bile salt malabsorbtion**, ileal resection, or disease allows bile salts to reach the colon, which causes diarrhea.
- **Bacterial overgrowth** is particularly common in any person with anatomical abnormality of the gut (e.g., post-gastrectomy, small bowel diverticula, scleroderma, diabetes) but can also occur with normal gut architecture.

### Further reading

Fine KD, Schiller LR (1999). AGA technical review on the evaluation and management of chronic diarrhea. *Gastroenterology* **116**(6):1464–1486.

Guerrant RL, Van Gilder T, Steiner TS, et al. (2001). Practice guidelines for the management of infectious diarrhea. *Clin Infect Dis* **32**(3):331–351.

## How to investigate and manage chronic diarrhea

Diagnoses to consider in the elderly population include the following:
- Inflammatory bowel disease
- Malabsorption
- Colonic tumor
- Diverticular disease
- Chronic infections
- Constipation with overflow diarrhea

### History

Ask about foreign travel, antibiotic exposure, full drug history, previous bowel surgery or pancreatitis, and family history of inflammatory bowel disease. Ask patient or caregiver to make a record of stool frequency and texture.

### Examination

Conduct abdominal and digital rectal examination. If rectum is full, be highly suspicious of overflow diarrhea.

### Investigations

1. Stool: culture, *Clostridium difficile* toxin, ova, fecal leukocytes and parasites
2. Blood tests: (anemia) (iron, $B_{12}$, folate deficiency) endomysial antibody (and IgA levels), CRP, and ESR
3. Radiology: plain abdominal X-ray is rarely diagnostic (except unexpected, left-sided fecal impaction)
4. Sigmoidoscopy: biopsy in several places even if mucosa looks normal to exclude microscopic colitis (p. 388)

More complex investigations:
5. Colonoscopy or barium enema

### Treatment

This obviously depends on the cause, but for patients in whom the diagnosis is not clear and they are not fit for or refuse more complex investigations, there is a place for a trial of empirical treatment. One such strategy is at least 2-week trials of the following:
- Metronidazole (for overgrowth/diverticular disease)
- Creon® (pancreatic disease)
- Questran® (bile salt malabsorption)
- Steroids (inflammatory bowel disease)

Pick the most likely or try each in turn for a few weeks.

# Other colonic conditions

### Irritable bowel syndrome (IBS)

IBS is a chronic, noninflammatory condition characterized by abdominal pain, altered bowel habit (diarrhea or constipation), and abdominal bloating, but with no identifiable structural or biochemical disorder.

- This diagnosis should not made de novo in older patients without very careful exclusion of structural disease (particularly colonic tumors and diverticulitis).
- Lifelong sufferers may continue with symptoms in later life, but if the symptoms change the patient should also undergo investigations.
- Pain or diarrhea that wakes a patient at night, blood in stool, weight loss, or fever are NEVER features of IBS.
- Some drugs used to treat IBS (e.g., tricyclic antidepressants) are less well tolerated in older patients. Bentyl may be better tolerated for spasm.
- Dietary advice should be given (low fiber for bloating or flatulance, high fiber or Citrucel for diarrhea or constipation).

### Angiodysplasia

Tiny capillary malformations (like spider nevi) that can occur anywhere in the gut are important only because they bleed.

- Slow blood loss leads to unexplained recurrent iron deficiency anemia, brisk loss may produce life-threatening hemorrhage.
- Unless they are inherited in a syndrome (e.g., hereditary hemorrhagic telangiectasia) they are acquired and thus have increased prevalence with age (most cases are age over 70).
- Asymptomatic angiodysplasia in older patients is common. Diagnosis is often by exclusion of other causes of iron-deficiency anemia.
- Sometimes colonoscopy can visualize lesions (which can then be treated by cauterization).
- Selective mesenteric angiography can demonstrate lesions that are actively and rapidly bleeding.
- Estrogens and thalidamide are sometimes successful in controlling chronic blood loss.

### Microscopic colitis

Also known as collagenous colitis or lymphocytic colitis, this is an idio-pathic condition causing chronic or episodic watery, non-bloody diarrhea but with no gross structural changes seen at colonoscopy.

- Biopsy changes are diagnostic with collagenous thickening of the subepithelial layer and infiltration with lymphocytes.
- Peak incidence is in the 50s.
- There is no increased risk of cancer.
- Keep treatment as simple as possible—start with diet and antidiarrheal drugs, mesalazine, then steroids.

### Ischemic colitis

This is an underdiagnosed cause of acute diarrhea ± blood in dehydrated, hypotensive older patient with vascular disease. It is often self-limiting if volume depletion corrected.

# The "acute surgical abdomen"

Peritonitis or perforation often presents in a nonspecific or nondramatic way. Patients often go to internists rather than directly to surgeons. The diagnosis is easily missed, so always have a high index of suspicion and examine the abdomen carefully and repeatedly in sick older patients without a diagnosis.

Common causes in older patients include the following:
- Complications of diverticular disease or appendicitis
- First presentation of tumor (gut, pancreatic)
- Ischemic bowel (emboli in patients with atrial fibrillation)
- Strangulated hernias (always remember groin examination)
- Ruptured abdominal aortic aneurysm
- Duodenal ulcer perforation (becoming less common)
- Biliary stones, sepsis (stones), and pancreatitis.

### Signs

Peritonitis or perforation may not have guarding or rigidity, particularly in the very old, those on steroids, or diabetics. Lack of bowel sounds can be helpful. Signs may develop with time, so repeated assessments are helpful.

### Investigations

Upright CXR can reveal air under the diaphragm (this is sometimes the only indication of a "silent" perforation). Ultrasound or CT imaging will often reveal the cause.

### Management

Always involve the surgical team even when patient is unsuitable for operation as they can advise on conservative management and future management (e.g., gallstone surgery once cholecystitis has settled). Ensure that surgical decisions are made on the basis of health status (i.e., frailty, comorbidity, or patient-centered goals) and not just age alone.

Medical management involves the following:
- Broad-spectrum intravenous antibiotics (e.g., cefuroxime 750 mg three times a day or ciprofloxacin 500 mg twice a day with metronidazole 500 mg three times a day)
- Resting the bowel (NPO, NG tube if vomiting)
- Careful monitoring of fluid balance—heart failure from fluid overload or renal failure from dehydration is often the mechanism of death. A urinary catheter and central venous pressure monitoring are sometimes necessary.
- Consider prophylactic low-molecular weight heparin.

It is surprising how often patients survive with conservative measures, so continue to monitor the patient and adjust treatment carefully. Once the signs and symptoms recede, try to get the patient eating, on oral antibiotics, and mobilizing as soon as possible to avoid the complications of malnutrition, pressure sores, venous thromboembolism, and *Clostridium difficile* colitis, which may be more lethal than the initial peritonitis!

# Reference

De Dombal FT (1994). Acute abdominal pain in the elderly. *J Clin Gastroenterol* **19**(4):331–335.

Hendrickson M, Naparst TR (2003). Abdominal surgical emergencies in the elderly. *Emerg Med Clin North Am* **21**(4):937–969.

Lyon C, Clark DC (2006). Diagnosis of acute abdominal pain in older patients. *Am Fam Physician* **74**(9):1537–1544.

# Obstructed bowel in older patients

As with peritonitis, this often presents in a nonspecific or nondramatic way. Common causes in older patients include the following:

- Constipation
- Colonic tumors
- Sigmoid volvulus
- Strangulated hernias (remember to examine groins)
- Adhesions (look for old abdominal scars)
- Complications of diverticular disease (abscess, localized perforation, stricture)

### Signs

Consider excluding obstruction (with plain X-ray) in any patient with persistent vomiting and/or abdominal bloating (ask the patient if their tummy is a normal size for them). Pain and colic, absence of defecation, tinkling bowel sounds, and gastric splash are helpful diagnostically when present, but often are not.

Always examine the groin in both sexes for obstructed hernias.

### Investigations

Plain abdominal X-ray shows dilated bowel—standing X-rays have fluid levels but are often impractical in older patients and rarely add diagnostic information to a supine film.

Ultrasound or CT imaging may localize a cause. Contrast radiology and endoscopy are sometimes useful.

### Management

Always involve the surgical team, who can advise on diagnosis and conservative management, e.g., insertion of a rectal tube for sigmoid volvulus.

General management usually involves the following:

- Resting the bowel (NPO and wide-bore NG tube)
- Careful monitoring of fluid balance—heart failure from fluid overload or renal failure from dehydration is often the mechanism of death.
- Consider broad-spectrum antibiotics if there is fever or features of coexistent perforation.
- Consider prophylactic low-molecular-weight heparin.

When conservative management fails and an operation is necessary, less invasive or palliative procedures are often more appropriate (e.g., defunctioning colostomy rather than anterior resection).

*Pseudo-obstruction* presents with vomiting and dilated bowel on X-ray but is due to an atonic bowel, so bowel sounds are absent or decreased rather than increased. This can occur with electrolyte abnormality (especially low potassium), any severe illness (e.g., septicemia), or narcotic analgesics and reverses with correction of the underlying abnormality.

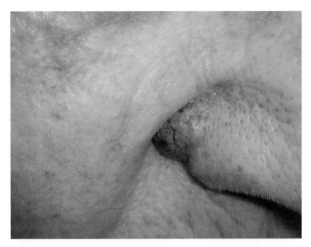

**Plate 1.** Nodular basal cell carcinoma of the alar crease of the nose. This is a pearly papule with overlying telangiectasia. The location is considered high risk because of tendency to extend deep between the cartilage/bone interface.
(Eric Ehrsam MD, Dermatlas; http://www.dermatlas.org. Used with permission).

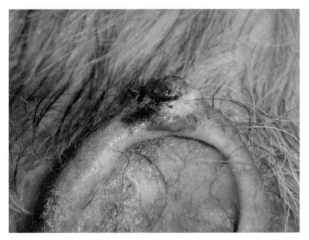

**Plate 2.** Squamous cell carcinoma of the helical rim of the ear. The surface of this tumor is friable. (Eric Ehrsam MD, Dermatlas; http://www.dermatlas.org. Used with permission).

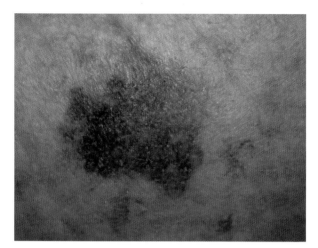

**Plate 3.** Lentigo maligna of the left cheek. The borders are often indistinct in this reticulated macular growth. (Eric Ehrsam MD, Dermatlas; http://www.dermatlas.org. Used with permission).

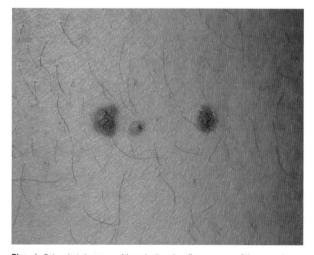

**Plate 4.** Seborrheic keratoses. Note the "stuck on" appearance of these papules. (Bernard Cohen MD, Dermatlas; http://www.dermatlas.org. Used with permission).

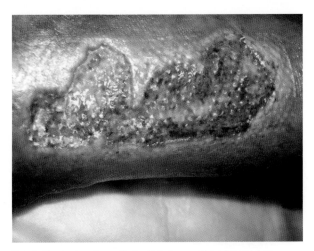

**Plate 5.** Venous ulceration on the leg. Note the smooth borders and clean base. The surrounding skin is brawny. Indentations on the ulcer are from wound dressings.

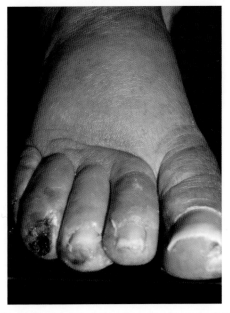

**Plate 6.** Arterial ulceration. Note distal location and overlying eschar. Pulses are barely palpable in this patient. There is exquisite pain and tenderness.

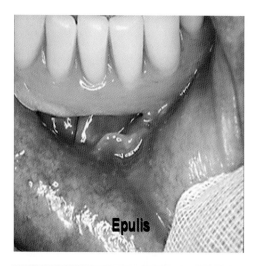

Epulis

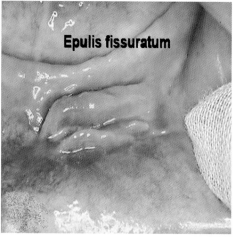

Epulis fissuratum

**Plate 7.** Loose dentures resulting in folds of fibrous tissue (epulis fissuratum).

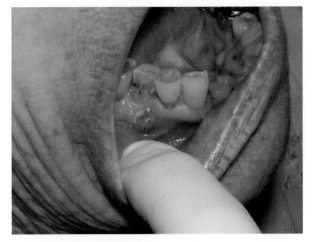

**Plate 8.** Apical abscess pointing below a broken tooth.

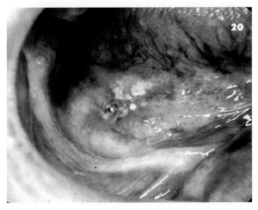

**Plate 9.** Precancerous mixed erythroplakia and leukoplakia.

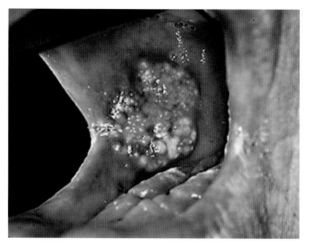

**Palte 10.** Squamous cell carcinoma.

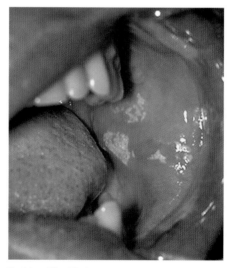

**Plate 11.** Candida or "thrush" infection.

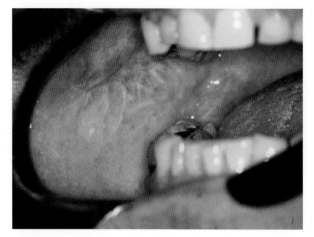

**Plate 12.** Lichen planus.

# Nephrology

**Derek Fine**

# The aging kidney

Kidney function tends to decline with age, but unless there is additional renal disease, function is usually sufficient to remove waste and to regulate volume and electrolyte balance. It is only when stressed that the lack of renal reserve becomes apparent. The relative contribution of cumulative exposure to risk factors (extrinsic aging), disease acquisition (often occult), and intrinsic aging is unknown, but not all the changes described are universal in an older population.

### Falling renal reserve

Glomerular filtration rate (GFR) falls steadily after the age of 40 in most healthy older people, in part due to the following age-related changes:

- Rise in blood pressure within the "normal" range
- Decrease number of glomeruli (~50% fewer at age 70 than at age 30)
- Increase in sclerotic glomeruli
- Renal blood flow decreases by around 10% per decade (cortex more than medulla, leading to patchy cortical defects on renal scans).

Lower GFR and renal blood flow are the major causes of reduced renal reserve, with the following clinical implications:

- Renally excreted substances are likely to be retained longer (especially drugs), making drug dose adjustments necessary (see Chapter 6, Pharmacology and medication use, p. 111).
- Reduced threshold for damage from ischemia or nephrotoxins

The normal range for plasma urea and creatinine levels does not change with age. However, as production of urea and creatinine decreases with falling body muscle mass, renal function may be substantially diminished in an older person with apparently normal blood chemistry.

▶▶Estimation of GFR, therefore, is a better measure of renal function than plasma urea and creatinine (see p. 403).

### Blunted fluid and electrolyte homeostasis

The following changes occur with age:

- A blunted response to sodium loading and depletion, so balance is achieved more slowly
- Less ability to dilute and concentrate urine (falls by 5% every decade)
- Lower renin and aldosterone levels (30%–50% less than in younger people)
- Diminished sensation of thirst, even when plasma tonicity is high, for reasons that are unclear (may relate to altered osmoreceptor function, or altered mental capacity)
- Reduced response to antidiuretic hormone (ADH)
- In addition, many commonly prescribed drugs interfere with kidney function (diuretics, NSAIDs, ACE inhibitors, lithium, etc.)

Hyponatremia (excess water intake relative to sodium intake) is therefore common, but in times of acute illness (increased fluid demand and decreased intake) the slower adaptive mechanisms make hypernatremic dehydration more common. Etiologies are otherwise similar to those in other adults.

Hypokalemia may occur because of poor intake and frequent diuretic use, but lower GFR and hypoaldosteronism lead to a vulnerability to hyperkalemia, especially when exacerbating drugs (ACE inhibitors, NSAIDS, spironolactone) are used.

With age, there is a change in the circadian rhythm of ADH and aldosterone secretion, which, combined with diminished response to these hormones, leads to altered sodium and water handling. Therefore, in those over the age of 60, the proportion of water and sodium excretion occurring at night increases, causing nocturia.

## Structural changes
- Renal mass falls by 20%–30% between age 30 and 90 years, making kidneys appear smaller on ultrasound scanning, without necessarily implying disease.
- Distal nephrons develop diverticulae (3 per tubule by age 90) that may become benign cysts.

## Other changes
Renal 1-hydroxylase activity decreases with age, leading to decreased 1,25-hydroxy vitamin D production. Combined with low phosphate intake, this can mildly elevate parathyroid hormone (PTH) levels.

## Further reading
Mühlberg W, Platt D (1999). Age-dependent changes of the kidneys: pharmacological implications. *Gerontology* **45**:243–253.

# Acute renal failure

This is more common in older people, but with a similar prognosis if occurring de novo and then treated correctly.

▶▶Do not deny treatment on he basis of age alone—even anuric patients can make a full recovery.

### Etiology

Eighty percent of cases of acute renal failure (ARF) are a result of prerenal causes and acute tubular necrosis (ATN).

#### Prerenal causes

These are due to poor kidney perfusion, which may be caused by the following conditions:
- Dehydration
- Sepsis
- Volume loss (e.g., bleeding, excessive diuresis)
- Volume redistribution (e.g., with low-serum albumin)
- Poor cardiac output (e.g., congestive heart failure or cardiogenic shock)
- Aggravation by many drugs (e.g., diuretics, ACE inhibitors, NSAIDs, IV contrast)

Older patients are prone to infections, have less capacity to maintain circulating volume under stress, and are more likely to be on aggravating medications, making this a very common problem (e.g., urinary sepsis in a patient taking diuretics and NSAIDs can often cause prerenal renal impairment, and responds well to antibiotics, fluids, and drug cessation).

All ill elderly patients should have renal function assessed routinely and repeatedly. Consider stopping diuretics and ACE inhibitors and avoid use of NSAIDs during an acute illness.

#### Renal causes

These are most often ATN, less frequently acute interstitial nephritis (AIN) or glomerulonephritis (GN). The patient may need to be assessed by a nephrologist promptly to make management decisions (often after biopsy).

Older people are more susceptible to ATN, which may be
- Ischemic (occurs when prerenal failure is not corrected quickly, e.g., with sepsis, surgical procedures, prolonged hypotension, etc.)
- Nephrotoxic (usually medication such as aminoglycoside antibiotics, e.g., gentamicin)
- Due to pigment deposition (e.g., myoglobin in rhabdomyolysis)

Drug-induced AIN is an important diagnosis to make in the elderly, who are frequently exposed to multiple medications. The diagnosis can be made by symptoms of fever, flank pain or rash in the presence of some combination of urine white blood cells or casts, urine eosinophils, or high blood eosinophils associated with initiation of a medication. Importantly, however, AIN occurs even in the absence of any of these features and must be considered with unexplained acute renal failure. Simple discontinuation of the culprit drug may be sufficient for resolution.

*Postrenal causes*

Although anuria is a strong clue suggesting a postrenal cause, one must keep in mind that patients with partial obstructions resulting in renal failure may present with normal or even excessive urine output.

- Obstruction of the urinary tract, e.g., prostatic enlargement, renal stones, urethral strictures, pelvic tumors
- Urinary retention (e.g., bladder or urethral dysfunction, sometimes due to medications such as narcotics or tricyclic antidepressants)
- Ultrasound shows a dilated collecting system (hydronephrosis). Hydronephrosis may be absent if obstruction is acute (up to 36 hours of onset) or incomplete.
- These conditions are all more common in older people and may be very responsive to treatment if found early, often with full recovery of renal function.

## Further information

Cheung CM, Ponnusamy A, Anderton JG (2008). Management of acute renal failure in the elderly patient: a clinician's guide. *Drugs Aging* **45**:455–476.

# Acute renal failure: management

### Is this acute renal failure?

Older people are more likely to have underlying chronic kidney disease, and this confers both a higher risk and worse prognosis. Make sure an increase in creatinine (decrease in estimated GFR) is new by reviewing the patient record and asking the patient, family, and health-care provider about known history.

### Investigations

See Table 13.1.

### Treat cause

Generally, management and response to it does not differ significantly from that for younger patients.

### Monitor meticulously

- Pulse and blood pressure, cardiac monitor, input (IV and oral) and output (urine, stool, emesis, drains). Note level of insensible losses (sweat).
- Aim for euvolemia (assessed clinically), then maintain by matching input to output on an hourly basis initially.
- Fluid balance may be more difficult in older people because of comorbidities (especially heart failure).
- The presence of peripheral edema does not necessarily indicate intravascular volume overload. Circulating volume is best assessed by blood pressure, pulse, JVP, and skin turgor.
- The patient may need central venous pressure (CVP) monitored and urinary catheter initially, but remove as soon as possible because of infection risk.
- Document daily weight and total fluid balance summary.
- Be prepared for polyuria in the recovery phase, and ensure that the patient does not become fluid depleted.

### Treat complications

Importantly, treat hyperkalemia, acidosis, and pulmonary edema.

Refer early to nephrology for further renal support (ultrafiltration or dialysis)—a patient can remain oliguric for some time while renal recovery is occurring. Indications for renal replacement therapy are as follows:

- Refractory pulmonary edema (older people are particularly prone to this after excessive initial fluid replacement)
- Persistent hyperkalemia (K >6 mEq/L) that cannot be controlled with dietary restriction, diuretics, or sodium polystyrene resin (Kayexlate)
- Worsening acidosis (pH <7.2)
- Uremic pericarditis
- Uremic encephalopathy

### Further reading

Longmore M, Wilkinson I, Rajagopalan S (2004). *Oxford Handbook of Clinical Medicine*, 6th ed, Oxford: Oxford University Press, pp. 272–275.

**Table 13.1** Acute renal failure: investigation

| Investigation | Rationale | Special points for older people |
|---|---|---|
| Urea and creatinine | Elevated in renal failure. Urea:creatinine ratio can be useful—elevated in prerenal failure, acting as a marker of dehydration | Older people with very little muscle mass will have lower baseline creatinine levels, so a creatinine of 1.2 in a small elderly woman may reflect significant renal impairment. |
| Electrolytes | Potassium may rise dangerously in ARF | More prone to cardiac complications of electrolyte disturbance—monitor carefully |
| Arterial blood gases | Monitor pH, which falls in ARF | pH can also be checked on a venous sample. |
| Inflammatory markers (ESR, CRP, WBC with diff) | Check for infection or inflammation. | Common precipitant of ARF in older people (may be occult) |
| Urine dipstick | Check for leukocyte esterase and nitrites (infection), blood and protein (active renal lesion) | High rate of positive urine dipstick in older people—does not always imply infection |
| Urine microscopy | Looking for casts (red cell casts in glomerulonephritis, white cell casts in infection or AIN, granular in ATN) and blood cells | Always send for culture, even when the dipstick is negative. |
| Blood and urine cultures | Identify microbes | Ensure these are sent on all patients (who may have occult infection) prior to starting antibiotics. |
| Creatine kinase (CK) | Elevated in rhabdomyolysis | Always check after falls (especially after a long period on the floor before being found). Even if there is not myoglobin-induced ARF, an elevated CK level indicates the need for hydration and monitoring of renal function |

| Urinary sodium/Fractional excretion of sodium (FeNa) | Helps distinguish between prerenal failure (urinary Na <20 mmol/L, FeNa <1% as kidney still functioning to preserve sodium) and ATN (urinary Na >40 mmol/L, FeNa >2%; tubule not functioning, so losing Na) | Particularly useful in older people in whom clinical assessment of fluid balance may be harder because of peripheral edema, etc. FeNa is generally better. Not helpful if the patient has taken diuretics (increases sodium excretion). Fractional excretion of urea more useful in this situation. |
|---|---|---|
| Chest X-ray | Looking for evidence of cardiac disease, source of infection, pulmonary edema, or pulmonary infiltrates (vasculitis) | More prone to pulmonary edema—use extra caution with fluid replacement if there is cardiomegaly, even where there is no history of cardiac failure |
| ECG | Looking for evidence of cardiac disease and monitoring for effects of hyperkalemia | May identify occult cardiac disease if ECG is abnormal |
| Renal ultrasound | Assess kidney size and look for evidence of hydronephrosis. | Diagnosis of treatable obstructive disease is common in this patient population. May suggest presence of CKD (small kidneys). Asymmetric kidneys may suggest underlying atherosclerotic renovascular disease. Ultrasound can be used to asses for excessive post-void residual urine suggestive of lower obstruction (e.g., prostate or bladder dysfunction) |
| Other tests | All should have CBC and LFTs Usually also send autoantibodies (ANA, ANCA), complement, and electrophoresis of blood and urine | See sections on nephrotic syndrome and glomerulonephritis |

# Chronic kidney disease

Chronic kidney disease (CKD) is an irreversible, long-standing (>3 months), and often progressive loss in renal function. Although anyone with GFR <60 mL/min/1.73 m$^2$ for more than 3 months has CKD, CKD can be diagnosed in those with GFR ≥60 based on the presence of kidney damage (pathological abnormalities or markers of damage such as proteinuria).

CKD is more common in older people; the incidence in those over 75 is 10 times higher than in those under 40. Half of all renal replacement therapy is started in patients over 65. This does not represent the true burden of renal impairment, as most die with and not of renal failure.

CKD is often discovered incidentally by finding elevated urea and creatinine levels (i.e., it is asymptomatic). There are adaptive mechanisms that maintain reasonable health with failing renal function until severe damage has occurred.

Most frequently CKD is due to diabetes and hypertension (>70% cases). Obstruction (usually due to prostatic enlargement), primary kidney disease, and renovascular disease are also important causes.

When abnormal renal function is discovered, first assess the setting: Is the patient acutely ill? Are they being overdiuresed? Are they on new drugs? Correct all potential causes, and recheck renal function in a stable clinical state. If CKD is confirmed, manage disease as follows:

- Estimate GFR (see next page), even with normal creatinine levels.
- Most patients benefit from early renal workup (i.e., as soon as renal disease is recognized) to clarify diagnosis, optimize management, and discuss renal replacement therapy (see p. 406, 407). Late referral for dialysis is associated with a poor outcome.
- Identify and treat any modifiable factors (e.g., diabetes, hypertension and obstructive uropathy).
- Delay disease progression by controlling diabetes and hypertension and by using an ACE inhibitor (or an ARB). Lipid lowering with statins and correcting anemia may also help.
- Avoid exacerbating factors such as volume depletion, intravenous contrast, and nephrotoxic drugs.
- Try to establish the rate of decline, using previous creatinine measurements. Deterioration tends to be steady and so it is often possible to estimate when interventions are likely to be needed.
- Identify and treat complications as they arise (see p. 420).
- Prepare for the end stage in those with stage IV or beyond.
- Dose drugs appropriately. The patient may need to avoid renally cleared drugs if alternatives are available (e.g., change atenolol to metoprolol, avoid phosphate-based bowel preparations, use sulphonylureas with caution, may need to discontinue metformin).
- Avoid gadolinium-based contrast agents in those with estimated GFR <30 mL/min/1.73 m$^2$ (including those on dialysis) to prevent nephrogenic systemic fibrosis.

## Further reading

Stevens LA, Levey AS (2005). Chronic kidney disease in the elderly—how to assess risk. *N Engl J Med* **352**:2122–2124.

## How to estimate the glomerular filtration rate

Although elevated urea and creatinine levels often alert the clinician to renal impairment, they give a poor estimate of extent, as the levels are determined by many factors other than GFR. Creatinine is made by muscle and thus has levels directly related to muscle mass, which tends to fall with age.

This means that
- A small rise in urea and creatinine in an elderly person may be significant, and should be taken seriously.
- A creatinine within the "normal range" may represent renal failure in a small old patient.

GFR is the best measure of kidney function, but is hard to measure. Creatinine clearance (CrCl) by 24-hour urine collection approximates GFR. The Cockcroft–Gault formula can be used to estimate CrCl. The GFR estimating modification of diet in renal disease (MDRD) formula is increasingly popular due to its increased accuracy. However, the MDRD formula tends to overestimate GFR in low-body-weight patients. For this reason, the Cockcroft–Gault is generally preferred for older adults and especially for those with <50 kg body weight.

$$\text{Cockcroft–Gault estimated CrCl (mL/min)} = \frac{[(140 - \text{age [years]}) \times \text{weight (kg)}]}{\text{Plasma creatinine (mg/dL)} \times 72}$$

Result needs to be multiplied by 0.85 for women.

$$\text{MDRD estimated GFR (ml/min/1.73m}^2) = 186 * \text{SCr}^{-1.154} \times \text{Age}^{-0.203} \times (0.742 \text{ if female}) \times (1.210 \text{ if Black})$$

Using the estimated GFR, CKD can be classified according to the National Kidney Foundation/Kidney Disease Outcomes Quality Initiative (NKF/KDOQI) guidelines as follows:

| GFR (mL/min) | GFR stage | Degree of renal failure |
|---|---|---|
| >=90 | I | Normal GFR with other kidney damage |
| 60–89 | II | Mild failure with other kidney damage |
| 30–59 | III | Moderate failure |
| 15–29 | IV | Severe failure |
| <15 | V | End-stage renal failure |

## Further information

National Kidney Foundation (2002). *Am J Kidney Dis* **39**(Suppl 1):S1–S266.

Stevens LA, Coresh J, Greene T, et al. (2006). Assessing kidney function—measured and estimated glomerular filtration rate. *N Engl J Med* **354**:2473–2483.

# Chronic kidney disease: complications

### Hypertension
- This is a cause and consequence of CKD.
- Monitor blood pressure regularly in all patients.
- Treat with an ACE inhibitor (preserves renal function).

### Hyperlipidemia
- This may contribute to renal damage.
- Treat with a statin.

### Atherosclerosis
- Accelerated atherosclerosis occurs with renal impairment.
- Ensure that all vascular risk factors are addressed.

### Salt and water retention
- Onset is with moderate impairment.
- Restrict dietary sodium intake (ideally <2 g/day)
- Consider loop diuretics for edema (e.g., furosemide—high doses may be required, but start low and increase as needed).
- Fluid restriction may be necessary with more severe renal impairment.

### Secondary hyperparathyroidism
- Onset is usually with moderate impairment (> stage III).
- Low calcium, high phosphate, and low 1, 25-hydroxy vitamin D and appropriately high intact parathyroid hormone (iPTH) occur.
- Measure calcium, phosphate, and iPTH.
- Consider dietary phosphate restriction (milk, cheese, eggs, etc.), phosphate binders (e.g., calcium carbonate, calcium acetate, Sevelamer), calcium supplements, and 1,25-hydroxy vitamin D supplementation (calcitriol).
- Risk of renal bone disease (renal osteodystrophy)

### Anemia
- Onset is usually with moderate impairment.
- Check for alternative causes of anemia (iron deficiency, chronic disease, etc.).
- If none are found, consider erythropoietin injections to keep hemoglobin between 11 and 12 g/dL (usually initiated by nephrologist).

### Central nervous system
- Onset is with severe impairment.
- Complications include peripheral neuropathy, autonomic neuropathy, and encephalopathy.

### Acidosis and hyperkalemia
- Onset is with moderate impairment.
- This may indicate the need for renal replacement therapy if not manageable by medical interventions.

### Further reading
National Kidney Foundation (2002). *Am J Kidney Dis* **39**(Suppl 1):S1–S266.
www.kidney.org/professionals/kdoqi

# Renal replacement therapy: dialysis

This includes hemodialysis (HD; usually done at a dialysis center and accounting for around 80% of dialysis in the older age group) and peritoneal dialysis (PD; mainly managed at home).

## Survival

Older patients have a shorter survival on dialysis than do younger patients, probably because of an increase in complications (see below), yet can still expect a 20%–40% 5-year survival (mean life expectancy 3–5 years).

Those over 80 on dialysis have a median survival of 26 months, irrespective of the age at onset of treatment.

## Effectiveness

Dialysis adequacy (clearance of solute) may be more effective in older patients because of their lower body mass. Some older patients may be underdialyzed due to intolerance of dialysis (see below). In addition, dialysis sessions are more frequently stopped early because of hypotension. Optimizing adequacy through frequent assessments and providing nutritional support, erythropoietin, and appropriate buffer selection can improve effectiveness in older people.

## Complications

In older people the following complications can occur:
- Nausea, vomiting, and hypotension during dialysis are more common (due to autonomic dysfunction and decreased cardiac reserve).
- Malnutrition occurs in up to 20%.
- There is increased risk of infection (aging immune system and malnutrition), depression, and GI bleeds (from uremic gastritis, diverticulosis, and angiodysplasia).

## Quality of life

Many older patients on dialysis enjoy a high quality of life. They resent the intrusion of visits to a dialysis center less than younger patients and can find it offers positive social interaction. Many of this highly selected cohort (frailer elderly with renal impairment do not reach this service) retain their independence, with over 90% maintaining good community social contacts, and over 80% regularly going outdoors. Around 40% rate their health positively. However, for some it becomes tiring and burdensome, especially if relying on hospital transport for attendance.

## Who should be offered dialysis?

The number of elderly people with end-stage renal disease (ESRD) is large. Many elderly patients with ESRD elect to have dialysis if offered, but offering it to all is not sensible or feasible. The decision to offer it must be considered carefully and made on an individual basis.

It should not be offered to simply delay dying—rather, it should be used if the renal failure is the main threat to continued survival. Severe dementia, advanced malignancy (except, possibly, multiple myeloma), or advanced liver disease generally makes dialysis inadvisable. Caution should be exercised before offering dialysis to patients with severe heart or lung disease or to frail patients with multiple comorbidities.

## What next?

Many patients need to switch dialysis modalities for various reasons. The rate of voluntary withdrawal (overall, about 5%) increases with age and is usually because of general dissatisfaction with life or the development of significant comorbidity (often cancer). Forty percent of patients would like to proceed to transplant.

# Renal replacement therapy: transplantation

This is the gold standard of renal replacement therapy for ESRD, as it improves survival and quality of life over that with dialysis. It also releases the patient from the burden of regular dialysis sessions.

Transplant recipients are getting older—10% of transplants in 2002 were performed for patients over 65, compared with only 5% a decade earlier. However, because the majority of ESRD occurs in the elderly population, this still represents an imbalance.

Donated kidneys are in short supply and tend to be given to those who will get the most use out of them—namely, younger patients with a longer natural life expectancy.

The most common cause of graft failure in older people is death of the host with a functioning graft. This is due to a number of factors:

• The most common cause of death after transplantation is cardiovascular disease. Risk of cardiovascular disease is much higher in older persons than in the general population.
• Older people have altered immune responses—this makes it less likely that they will reject a donated kidney, but it also increases the risk of serious infection.
• Older people have increased side effects to immunosuppressive medication, particularly steroids.
• Other common conditions make the transplant procedure more complicated, e.g., peripheral vascular disease (technical surgical problems), diverticular disease (predisposes to post-transplant perforation), and cholelithiasis (predisposes to biliary sepsis).

There are limited outcome data for older patients, but the following is known:

• Patients over 60 have 70%–80% 5-year patient survival post-transplant, compared with >90% 5-year survival for younger patients.
• Graft survival (up to 90% 5-year post transplant) is similar to that for younger patients.
• Transplant carries a greater chance of survival than dialysis, in older and in younger patients (around 10 years compared with 6 years on dialysis for those aged 60–74).
• Dialysis is often well tolerated by older people and may be less intrusive, as there are fewer work and domestic commitments.

Each individual must be considered separately, taking into account biological and not chronological age. Careful screening for comorbidity will reveal those most likely to benefit, regardless of age. The use of older donors for older recipients could partially redress the imbalance, as the grafts themselves will have a limited life span and thus be most appropriate for an age-matched recipient.

# Nephrotic syndrome

Increased glomerular permeability to protein causes proteinuria (> 3g/day considered nephrotic), hypoalbuminemia, generalized edema, and hyperlipidemia. There is an increased susceptibility to infection, thrombosis, and renal failure.

▶▶This syndrome is more common in older people but is often missed, as edema may be attributed to cardiac failure, or a low-serum albumin to poor nutrition. Always obtain dipstick urine for protein analysis (or measure with quantitative testing) in an edematous patient.

## Causes

Diabetes, membranous and minimal-change nephropathies, glomerulonephritides, and amyloid are common pathologies. Look for associated conditions, including malignancy (e.g., carcinoma, lymphoma, myeloma), infection (e.g., hepatitis B), and systemic disease (e.g., SLE, rheumatoid arthritis, chronic infection). NSAID use may be the only cause.

## Presentation

Patients may have frothy urine, anorexia, malaise, muscle wasting, edema (dependent—moves from sacrum and eyelids at night to legs during day), and effusions (pleural, pericardial, ascites). Blood pressure varies. Patients are prone to intravascular depletion with increased total body water, especially when overdiuresed due to assumed cardiac failure.

## Investigations

- Routine blood screen (CBC, BUN, creatinine and electrolytes, liver function)
- Complete urinalysis
- 24-hour urinary protein
- Antinuclear antibody (ANA), anti-neutrophil cytoplasmic antibody (ANCA), complement
- Urine and serum electrophoresis
- Hepatitis serology
- HIV testing
- Renal ultrasound
- Refer to renal team for possible biopsy.

## Treatment

- Monitor proteinuria and electrolytes, fluid balance, blood pressure
- Fluid and salt restriction
- Diuretics (e.g., furosemide 80–360 mg daily)
- Prophylactic heparin SC in immobile patient
- Monitor closely for infection
- Specific treatment with steroids and immunosuppressants after histology is known (specialist advice)
- Control of hypertension in all patients

# Glomerulonephritis

- An inflammatory process involving the glomeruli
- Presents with renal failure, hypertension, edema, hematuria, red cell casts, and/or proteinuria
- Older people often present nonspecifically (e.g., with nausea, malaise, arthralgia, and pulmonary infiltrates due to vasculitis).

▶▶GN is often misdiagnosed initially, causing delay in treatment. In ill older people, always assess for proteinuria (urine dipstick, albumin- or protein-to-creatinine ratio or 24-hour collection). Think of glomerulonephritis if there is hematuria, especially in the presence of proteinuria, elevated creatinine, or systemic signs and symptoms.

## Causes

*Postinfectious*
- In adults only ~25% streptococcal; ~25% staphylococcal
- Most often upper respiratory; also with cellulitis, endocarditis and pneumonia
- Occurs 2–6 weeks after exposure

*Systemic disease*
- ANCA related: Wegener's granulomatosis (usually C-ANCA), micropolyangiitis (usually P-ANCA), Churg–Strauss syndrome (high blood eosinophils)
- Anti-glomerular basement membrane (GBM) related: Goodpasture's disease if there is pulmonary involvement, anti-GBM disease if isolated to kidney
- Immune complex related: lupus nephritis, membranoproliferative (usually hepatitis C related); Henoch–Schönlein purpura

*Primary renal disease*
- IgA nephropathy

## Investigations

See above for nephrotic syndrome.

## Treatment

- Immunosuppression
  - Refer early to a renal team to confirm diagnosis (usually by renal biopsy)
  - Varying choices, dependent on disease and other individualized patient factors
- Supportive—see previous section on nephrotic syndrome
- Many patients require dialysis.

## Outcome

Outcome is worse in older people. More die, and more progress to CKD and ESRD.

# Renal artery stenosis

This condition is more common with increasing age. It is usually due to atherosclerosis, so occurs in patients with known vascular disease in other areas. Consider diagnosis in a hypertensive patient in the following circumstances:

- Deterioration of renal function after starting an ACE inhibitor. Stopping the drug promptly should reverse the changes.
- New-onset hypertension in a person older than 50 years
- Sudden worsening of blood pressure in a person with existing hypertension
- Difficult-to-control blood pressure despite multiple antihypertensives
- Unexplained hypokalemia (due to high aldosterone levels)
- Renal bruit heard on clinical examination
- Unilateral small kidney seen on imaging
- Person who develops flash pulmonary edema

## Diagnosis

Digital subtraction angiography is the gold standard and may be accompanied by angioplasty stenting.

Noninvasive imaging is best with magnetic resonance angiography or CT angiography. Ultrasound Doppler is used when gadolinium-based contrast is contraindicated (GFR <30 mg/min/1.73 $m^3$) and radiocontrast is avoided due to low GFR (reasonable cutoff of 50 mL/min/1.73 $m^2$).

## Management

As there are often no symptoms, conservative management with blood pressure control, optimizing vascular secondary prevention but avoiding ACE inhibitors, is often appropriate. If, however, renal function declines or blood pressure cannot be controlled, then percutaneous angioplasty or stent insertion is well tolerated even in very old people.

## Further reading

Garovic VD, Kane GC, Schwartz GL (2005). Renovascular hypertension: balancing the controversies in diagnosis and management. *Cleve Clin J Med* **72**(12):1135–1147.

# Homeostasis

### Samuel C. Durso

# Volume depletion and dehydration

This combination constitutes losses of water and sodium that may be isotonic or hypotonic. It is an important, common, easily missed clinical condition, especially in older people. It is highly prevalent among acutely ill older people admitted to the hospital due to a combination of increased fluid loss (fever, GI loss) and decreased intake (nausea, anorexia, weakness).

There is no sensitive biochemical marker of volume depletion—urea and creatinine may be in the normal range because of malnutrition and small muscle mass. True dehydration (water deficit) is evidenced by elevated serum sodium.

## Causes
- Blood loss
- Diuretics
- GI losses (e.g., diarrhea, nasogastric drainage)
- Sequestration of fluid (e.g., ileus, burns, peritonitis)
- Poor oral intake
- Fever

## Symptoms and signs
- Thirst is reduced in older people.
- Malaise, apathy, weakness
- Orthostatic symptoms (lightheadedness or syncope) and/or hypotension
- Nausea, anorexia, vomiting in severe uremia; oliguria
- Tachycardia, hypotension (late signs, and seen also in fluid overload)
- Absence of visible jugular venous waves when patient is supine
- Decreased skin turgor, sunken cheeks, and absence of dependent edema are nonspecific and unreliable.

The symptoms and signs of clinically important dehydration may be subtle and confusing. It is therefore underrecognized. Continual clinical assessment, assisted by basic tests (urinalysis; urea, creatinine, and electrolytes) is essential. Invasive monitoring or other tests are rarely needed. Older patients commonly become dehydrated for the following reasons:
- Poor oral intake, or kept NPO awaiting tests, or inadequate maintenance intravenous fluid administration for fear of precipitating volume overload
- Intravenous infusions often run more slowly than prescribed, or cannot run for periods if IV access is lost
- Moderate leg edema is not specific for heart failure—don't use diuretics simply on the basis of edema alone, in the absence of other evidence of volume overload.
- Poor urine output on the surgical (or medical) unit is more often a sign of dehydration than of heart failure. Diuretics are the wrong treatment.

## Management
- Treat the underlying cause(s).
- Continually reassess clinically, assisted by urinalysis and BUN, creatinine, and electrolytes (basic metabolic panel [BMP]) levels. Measure and document intake, output, and weight.

- If the condition is mild, oral rehydration may suffice (see How to make simple oral rehydration solution). Older frail people need time, encouragement, and physical assistance with drinking. Encourage relatives and friends to help.
- More severe dehydration, or mild dehydration not responding to conservative measures, will require other measures—usually parenteral treatment, either subcutaneous (SC) or intravenous (IV).

The speed of parenteral fluid administration should be tailored to the individual patient, based on volume of fluid deficit, degree of physiological compromise, and perceived risks of fluid overload. For example, a hypotensive patient who is clinically volume depleted with evidence of end-organ failure should be fluid resuscitated briskly, even if there is a history of heart failure.

In the absence of end-organ dysfunction, rehydration may proceed more cautiously, but continual reassessment is essential, to confirm that the clinical situation remains benign and that progress (input > output) is being made.

### How to make a simple oral rehydration therapy (ORT) solution

A simple ORT solution can be made at home by mixing 1 level teaspoon of table salt and 8 level teaspoons of table sugar in 1 liter of water. A half-cup of orange juice or other unsweetened fruit juice can be added to supplement potassium and enhance taste. The patient should drink several ounces every 10 minutes until they are urinating 4–5 times per day.

### How to administer subcutaneous fluid

This method (hypodermoclysis) was widely used in the 1950s, but fell out of favor following reports of adverse effects associated with very hypo- or hypertonic fluid. Fluids that are close to isotonic are a safe and effective substitute for IV therapy.

- A simple, widely accessible method for parenteral fluid and electrolytes
- Fluid is administered via a standard giving set and fine (21–23 G) butterfly needle into SC tissue, then draining centrally via lymphatics and veins.
- SC fluid administration should be considered when insertion or maintenance of IV access presents problems, e.g., difficult venous access or persistent extravasations.
- Intravenous access is preferred if rapid fluid administration is needed (e.g., GI bleed) or if precise control of fluid volume is essential.

**Sites of administration** Preferred sites include abdomen, chest (avoid breast), thigh, and scapula. In agitated patients who tear out IV (or SC) lines, try sites close to the scapulae.

**Fluid type** Any crystalloid solution that is approximately isotonic can be used, including normal (0.9%) saline, 5% dextrose, and any isotonic combination of dextrose–saline. Potassium chloride can be added to the infusion, in concentrations of 20–40 mM/L. If local irritation occurs, change site and/or reduce the concentration of added potassium.

**Infusion rate** Typical flow (and absorption) rate is 1 mL/min or 1.5 L/day. Infusion pumps may be used. If flow or absorption is slow (leading to lumpy, edematous areas):
- Change site.
- Use two separate infusion sites at the same time.

Using these techniques, up to 3 L of fluid daily may be given. For smaller volumes, consider an infusion of 500–1000 mL, or two daily boluses of 500 mL each (run in over 2–3 hours), leaving the patient free of infusion lines during the daily rehabilitation and activity. Some patients need only 1 L on alternative nights to maintain hydration.

**Monitoring** Patients should be monitored clinically (hydration state, input/output, weight) and biochemically as they would if they were receiving IV fluid. Be responsive and creative in your prescriptions of fluid and electrolytes—one size does not fit all.

**Potential complications** are rare and usually mild. They include local infection and local adverse reactions to hypertonic fluid (e.g., with added potassium).

### Contraindications

- Exercise caution in thrombocytopenia or coagulopathy.
- SC infusion is not appropriate in patients who need rapid volume repletion.

# Hyponatremia: assessment

This is a common problem. It may be safely be monitored rather than treated if modest in severity ([Na] >125 mM), the patient is stable and without side effects, and if there is an identifiable (often drug) cause.

## Clinical features

- Subtle or absent in mild cases
- Typically [Na] = 115–125 mM: lethargy, confusion, and altered personality are present.
- At <115 mM: delirium, coma, seizures, and death can occur.

## Causes

Iatrogenic causes are most common. Acute onset, certain drugs, or recent intravenous fluids make iatrogenesis especially likely.
  Important causes include the following:

- Drugs. Many are implicated
- Excess water administration—either nasogastric (rarely oral) or intravenous (5% dextrose)
- Failure of heart, liver, thyroid, kidneys
- Stress response, e.g., after trauma or surgery, exacerbated by IV colloid or 5% dextrose
- Adrenal insufficiency: steroid withdrawal or Addison's disease
- Syndrome of inappropriate ADH secretion (SIADH)

In older people, multiple causes are common, e.g., heart failure, diuretics, and acute diarrhea.

## Approach

Take a careful drug history. Examine to determine evidence of cause and volume status (JVP, postural BP, pulmonary edema, ankle/sacral edema, peripheral perfusion).

## Investigations

Clinical history and examination and urine and blood biochemistry are usually all that are needed. Ensure that the sample wasn't delayed in transit or taken from a drip arm. If it is genuine hyponatremia, take the following:

- Blood for creatinine, osmolarity, TFT, LFT, glucose
- Spot urine sample for sodium and osmolarity

Consider a short ACTH test to exclude adrenal insufficiency, particularly if the patient is volume depleted and hyperkalemic (though hyperkalemia is not always present).

# Hyponatremia: treatment

**Treatment** (see Fig. 14.1)
- Combine normalization of [Na] with correction of fluid volume and treating underlying cause(s).
- The rate of correction of hyponatremia should not be too rapid. Usually, correction to the lower limit of the normal range (130 mM) should be achieved in a few days. Maximum correction in any 24-hour period should be <10 mM. Full correction can reasonably take weeks.
- Rapid correction risks central pontine myelinolysis (leading to quadriparesis and cranial nerve abnormalities) and is indicated only when hyponatremia is severe and the patient critically unwell.

▶▶ By definition, hyponatremia is a low blood sodium concentration. Therefore, a low level may be a result of low sodium, high water, or both. Dehydration and hyponatremia may coexist if sodium depletion exceeds water depletion. This is common—don't worsen the dehydration by fluid restricting these patients!

### Drugs and hyponatremia
- Most commonly diuretics (especially in high dose or combination), SSRIs, carbamazepine, or NSAIDs are involved.
- Other drugs include opiates, other antidepressants (MAOIs, TCAs), other anticonvulsants, e.g., valproate, oral hypoglycemics (sulphonylureas e.g., chlorpropamide, glipizide) and barbiturates.
- Combinations of drugs (e.g., diuretic and SSRI) are especially likely to cause hyponatremia.

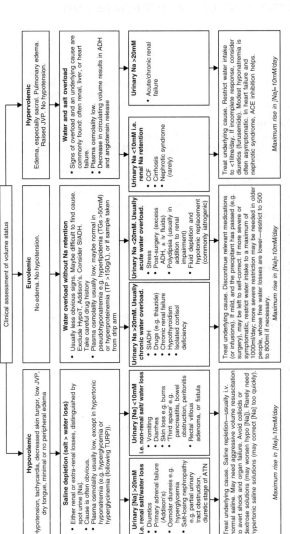

**Fig. 14.1** Hyponatremia: etiology and treatment

# Syndrome of inappropriate ADH

### Definition
Less than maximally dilute (i.e., inappropriately concentrated) urine is in the presence of subclinical excess body water.

▶▶ Syndrome of inappropriate antidiuretic hormone secretion (SIADH) is often overdiagnosed, especially in older people, leading to inappropriate fluid restriction. Consider it a diagnosis of exclusion—drugs or organ impairment causes a similar clinical syndrome.

### Diagnosis
Essential features include the following:
- Hypotonic hyponatremia ([Na] <125 mM and plasma osmolarity <260 mOsm/L).
- Normal volume status, i.e., euvolemia—there is slight water overload, but not clinically identifiable.
- Normal renal, thyroid, hepatic, cardiac, and adrenal function.
- Inappropriately concentrated, salty urine: osmolarity >200 mOsm/L and [Na] >20 mM
- No diuretics or ADH-modulating drugs (opiates, anticonvulsants, antidepressants, NSAIDs, barbiturates, and oral hypoglycemics). Drug effects may take days or weeks to diminish.

### Causes
Common causes include the following:
- Surgical stress
- Neoplasms (especially bronchogenic, pancreatic)
- CNS disease (especially trauma, subdural hematoma, stroke, meningoencephalitis)
- Lung disease (TB, pneumonia, bronchiectasis)

### Treatment
- Treat underlying cause.
- If the condition is mild and the precipitant has passed (e.g., surgery), it may be left to self-correct.
- If it is more severe and/or symptomatic, restrict water intake to a maximum of 1000 mL/day; more severe restriction may be needed in older people, whose free water losses are lower—restrict to 500–800 mL if necessary.

## How to do a short ACTH stimulation test (short Cortrosyn® stimulation test)

The diagnosis of adrenocortical insufficiency is made when the adrenal cortex is found not to synthesize cortisol despite adequate stimulation. Within 30 minutes of ACTH stimulation, the normal adrenal releases several times its basal cortisol output.

### Performing the test
- The test can be done at any time of day.
- Take blood for baseline cortisol. Label tube with patient identifiers and time taken.
- Give 25 mcg Cortrosyn® (synthetic ACTH, 1–24 amino acid sequence). Give intravenously if IV access is present; otherwise IM.
- 30 minutes after injection, take more blood for cortisol. Label tube with patient identifiers and time taken.

### Interpreting the test
A normal response meets three criteria:
- Baseline cortisol level >150 nmol/L
- 30-minute cortisol >500 nmol/L
- 30-minute cortisol greater than baseline cortisol by 200 nmol/L or more.

The absolute 30-minute cortisol carries more significance than the baseline 30-minute increment, especially in patients who are stressed (ill) and at maximal adrenal output.

A normal Cortrosyn® test excludes Addison's disease. If the test is not normal:
- Consider further tests such as the prolonged ACTH stimulation test, usually after specialist advice, e.g.:
  - ACTH level (elevated in primary and low in secondary adrenal insufficiency)
  - The prolonged ACTH stimulation test
- If the patient is very unwell, give hydrocortisone 100 mg IV pending confirmation of adrenal insufficiency.

# Hypernatremia

## Causes
- Usually due to true "dehydration," i.e., water loss > sodium loss
- Not enough water in, or too much water out, or a combination e.g., poor oral intake, diarrhea, vomiting, diuretics, uncontrolled diabetes mellitus
- Rarely due to salt excess—iatrogenic (IV or PO), psychogenic, or malicious (poisoning)
- Very rarely due to diabetes insipidus (urine osmolarity low) or mineralocorticoid excess (Conn's)

Hypernatremia is commonly seen in septic older people: increased losses (sweating) + reduced oral intake + reduced renal concentrating (water conserving) mechanism.

## Clinical features
- Hypotension (supine and/or orthostatic)
- Sunken cheeks
- Urine output low and concentrated
- Lethargy, confusion, coma, and seizures

## Tests
Urea and creatinine are often high, but may be in the high normal range; the patient is still water depleted. Hemoglobin and albumin are often high (hemoconcentration), correcting with treatment.

## Treatment
- Encourage oral fluid.
- Usually intravenous fluid is required; rarely subcutaneous fluid will be sufficient.
- Fluid infusion rates should not be too cautious: e.g., 3–4 L over 24 hours is reasonable, guided by clinical and biochemical response. Too-rapid infusions risk cerebral edema, especially in the more chronically hypernatremic patient.
- Ensure that the patient becomes clinically euvolemic as well as eunatremic. Most dehydrated patients have a normal [Na], and [Na] will correct into the normal range before the patient is fully hydrated.
- Many patients are Na-deplete as well as water-deplete; therefore, consider alternating normal saline with 5% dextrose infusions.

# Hypothermia: diagnosis

This is a common medical emergency in older people, occurring both in and out of the hospital.

### Definition
- Core temperature is <35°C, but <35.5°C is probably abnormal.
- Mild: 32–35°C; moderate: 30–32°C; severe: <30°C
- Fatality is high and correlates with severity of associated illness.

### Causes
- Cold exposure (clothing, defective temperature discrimination, climate, poverty)
- Defective homeostasis (failure of autonomic nervous system–induced shivering and vasoconstriction; decreased muscle mass)
- Illness (drugs, fall, pneumonia)

In established hypothermia, thermoregulation is further impaired and is effectively poikilothermic (temperature varies with environment).

▶▶ Hypothermia is a common presentation of sepsis in the hospital in older people, and probably an indicator of poor prognosis. Don't ignore the temperature chart.

### Diagnosis
Rectal temperature is the gold standard but well-taken oral or tympanic temperature will suffice.

Ensure that the thermometer range includes low temperatures.

### Presentation
Presentation is often insidious and nonspecific. Multiple systems are affected.

#### Skin
The skin may be cold to touch (paradoxically warm if defective vasoconstriction). Shivering is unusual (this occurs early in the cooling process). There may be increased muscle tone, skin edema, erythema, or bullae.

#### Nervous system
Signs can mimic stroke with falls, unsteadiness, weakness, slow speech and ataxia. Reflexes may be depressed or exaggerated with abnormal plantar response and dilated sluggish pupils. Conscious level ranges from confused and sleepy to coma. Seizures and focal signs can occur.

#### Cardiovascular system
- Initially there is vasoconstriction, hypertension, and tachycardia.
- Then myocardial suppression, hypotension, and sinus bradycardia occur.
- Eventually extreme bradycardia, bradypnea and hypotension occur. These may lead to a false diagnosis of death; however, the protective effect of cold on vital organs means survival may be possible.
- Dysrhythmias include atrial fibrillation (early), ventricular fibrillation, and asystole (late).

### Renal
There is early diuresis with later oliguria and acute tubular necrosis.

### Respiratory
Respiratory depression and cough suppression occur with secondary atelectasis and pneumonia. Pulmonary edema and ARDS occur late.

### Gastrointestinal
Hypomotility may lead to ileus, gastric dilation, and vomiting. Hepatic metabolism is reduced (including of drugs). There is a risk of pancreatitis with hypo- or hyperglycemia.

### Other
Disseminated intravascular coagulation (DIC) and rhabdomyolysis occur.

## Investigations
- CBC, ESR
- BMP
- Glucose
- Amylase
- CRP
- LFT
- TFT
- Blood culture
- Drug or toxin screen
- Chest X-ray

### CK, urinalysis
This may show rhabdomyolysis.

### Arterial blood gases (ABG)
Look for metabolic and respiratory acidosis, lactate acidosis. Do not correct for temperature.

### ECG
Abnormalities include prolonged PR interval, J waves (peak between QRS and T in leads V4–6) at <30°C, and dysrhythmia.

### Serum cortisol
Consider if there are features of adrenal insufficiency or if hypothermia is unexplained or recurrent.

▶▶ It is important to repeat key investigations during rewarming, e.g., BMP, ECG, and ABG.

# Hypothermia: management

### Monitoring

Monitor regular blood pressure, pulse, temperature, respiratory rate, oxygen saturation, and glucose; run continuous ECG; and consider a urinary catheter. Consider admission to ICU.

### Treatment principles

- The features of severe hypothermia may mimic those of death. In these cases, begin resuscitation while gathering information that permits a decision as to whether further intervention is likely to be futile or not in the patient's interests. Stop resuscitation according to clinical judgment; generally don't declare the patient dead until rewarmed or rewarming fails.
- System support: maintain airway, ventilate as necessary. Provide good IV access. Warm IV fluid: The patient may need large volumes as warming causes vasodilatation. Treat organ dysfunction as appropriate. Cardiac pacing is indicated only if the bradycardia is disproportionate to the reduced metabolic rate.
- If severe, or if there is multiple organ failure, consider ICU admission. Handle the patient carefully—rough handling and procedures (including intubation) may precipitate ventricular fibrillation.
- Rewarming: rate should approximate that of onset (0.5–1°C per hour if not critically ill). Use caution, as rewarming may lead to hypotension. A combination of the following modalities is usually sufficient:
  - Passive external: surround with dry clothes, blankets, space blankets
  - Active external: warm blanket, hot air blanket
  - Active internal: heated oxygen, fluid, and food

### Drug treatment

Consider the following:
- Empirical antibiotics (most have evidence of infection on careful serial assessment)
- Adrenal insufficiency (prescribe hydrocortisone 100 mg/day)
- Hypothyroidism (prescribe levothyroxine 50 mcg then 25 mcg/day IV, always with hydrocortisone)
- Thiamine deficiency (malnourished or alcoholic) (B vitamins oral or IV)

Drug metabolism is reduced and accumulation can occur. Efficacy at the site of action is also reduced. Exercise caution with SC or IM drugs (including insulin) that may accumulate and be mobilized rapidly as perfusion improves.

### Prevention

Before discharge, establish why this episode occurred—is recurrence likely? (Consider housing, cognition, hypoglycemia, sepsis, etc.) Consider how further episodes may be prevented or terminated early.

# Heat-related illness

This is an important cause of morbidity and mortality in older people. The contribution of heat stress to death is rarely mentioned on death certificates, but epidemiological studies indicate significant excess morbidity and mortality during heat waves. There is an increased incidence of acute cerebrovascular, respiratory, and, especially, cardiovascular disease.

## Risk factors

Consider older people as being relatively poikilothermic, i.e., lacking close control of body temperature in some circumstances. Homeostasis is weakened due to raised sweating threshold, reduced sweat volume, altered vasomotor control, and behavioral factors (e.g., lessened sensation of temperature extremes).
- Climate: high temperature, high radiant heat (indoors or out), high humidity
- Drugs, e.g., diuretics, anticholinergics, psychotropics
- Comorbidity: frailty, cerebrovascular and cardiovascular disease

## A spectrum of illness

The presentation is usually different in older people, typically occurring not after extreme exertion but during heat waves in temperate zones.
- *Prickly heat ("miliaria"):* itchy, erythematous, papular rash. Treat with cool, wash, antifungal cream for intertrigal areas (heat rash).
- *Heat edema:* peripheral edema, usually self-limiting
- *Heat syncope:* increased syncope risk due to fluid depletion and vasodilation
- *Heat exhaustion* is a potentially catastrophic illness. Dehydration and heat stress lead to nonspecific presentation with collapse, immobility, weakness, vomiting, dizziness, headache, fever, and tachycardia. However, treatment should result in rapid improvement.
- *Heat stroke* occurs when untreated heat exhaustion progresses to its end stage (hyperthermic thermoregulatory failure). Core temperature is generally >40°C, mental state is altered (confusion coma), circulatory and other organ failure is common, and sweating is often absent. CNS changes may be persistent and severe. Prognosis reflects pre-existing comorbidity, severity, and complications and is often poor.

## Management

### Individual response
Emergency inpatient treatment is required. Identify and reverse precipitants. Cool patient rapidly until temperature is 38–39°C—use a fan and tepid sponging and remove patient's clothing. Monitor (temperature, BP, P, saturation, urine output) patient closely; consider CVP. Give cool IV fluids according to assessment of fluid and electrolyte status.

### Community response
Modify the local environment with fans, air conditioning, shades, opening windows at night, seeking cooler areas, avoiding exercise, maintaining or increasing cool fluid intake, and wearing light and loose clothing. Educate the patient and caregivers. Governments should have public health measures in place to reduce the impact of heat waves.

## How to monitor temperature

No method is absolutely precise.
- Digital electronic and infrared thermometers can provide reliable results when used correctly and in accordance with the manufacturer's instructions.
- Thermochromic (forehead) thermometers are imprecise, although they may be useful for screening or with uncooperative patients.

### Digital electronic thermometers

These may permit oral, axillary, or rectal measurement. They typically require a small (1–2 seconds) period of equilibration and a degree of patient compliance.

### Infrared ("tympanic") thermometers

These measure the temperature of tissue within and close to the eardrum, returning a value rapidly. Ensure that the earlobe is gently pulled posteriorly and superiorly, straightening the external ear canal, before inserting the probe fairly firmly.

Ear wax has only a slight effect, reducing measured temperature by <0.5°C.

Tympanic thermometers may offer a choice of displaying temperature as either "true tympanic" or the derived value "oral equivalent." Ensure that you are familiar with the thermometers in use in your hospital and what output they give: tympanic or oral equivalent.

### Measurement in practice

- Precise temperature measurement is fundamental in detecting and monitoring disease.
- Fever may be due to infection, malignancy, inflammation, connective tissue disease, or drugs.
- A reduced or absent fever response to sepsis is seen in some elderly patients. Do not dismiss modest fever (<37.5°C) as insignificant or rule out infection because the patient is afebrile.
- Hypothermia occurs inside and outside the hospital and may be missed unless thermometers with an appropriate range (30–40°C) are used.
- Temperature varies continuously: lowest in peripheral skin, highest in the central vessels and brain. No site truly represents "core" temperature. Typically, when compared to oral temperature, axillary temperatures are 1.0°C lower, and rectal and tympanic temperatures 0.5–1.0°C higher (but see notes on tympanic thermometry, above).
- When clinical suspicion is high, make measurements yourself. Body temperature changes continuously and a fever may manifest only after the patient has rewarmed following a cooling ambulance journey.

# Endocrinology

**Amit Shah**

# The aging endocrine system

### Aging and hormone levels and function

The basal levels of most hormones remain essentially unchanged with normal aging. Compensation to maintain homeostasis does occur—e.g., pituitary luteinizing hormone levels will increase to offset reduction in testicular testosterone secretion. However, when stressed, the aging endocrine system shows a decreased ability to maintain homeostasis. For instance, healthy older patients demonstrate a greater rise in the serum glucose level in response to a glucose challenge than do healthy younger patients.

### Aging and thyroid function

Normal thyroid function is preserved in healthy older people. Median thyroid-stimulating hormone (TSH) level may drift slightly upward with increasing age, but remains within normal limits in the absence of disease. The diurnal variation of TSH secretion is diminished in older adults. There is an increased prevalence of thyroid autoantibodies with aging. There is also a high prevalence of hypothyroidism in patients older than 65, and so testing is warranted if there is any suspicion.

### Aging and glucose metabolism

- Glucose-induced insulin release is delayed and reduced in amount.
- Insulin-induced suppression of hepatic glucose production is delayed.
- Insulin-mediated peripheral (muscle and fat) glucose uptake is reduced.

In addition to reductions in physical activity and lean muscle mass, the above factors lead to higher frequency of impaired glucose tolerance (IGT) with age. IGT is associated with macrovascular disease but not with specific diabetic complications. A minority of people with IGT progress to diabetes.

### Aging and adrenal function

- Cortisol secretion is decreased, matched by decreased clearance of cortisol; therefore, cortisol levels and ACTH levels are normal.
- Cortisol response to stress differs between young and old subjects, with older patients having a prolonged rise in cortisol after a stressor such as surgery

# Diabetes mellitus

Diabetes is more common with advanced age. It is estimated that about one-eighth of all people over the age of 70 in the United States have diabetes. The prevalence is even higher for some ethnic groups, such as Mexican Americans.

## Comparing type 1 and type 2 diabetes

- Both type 1 (insulin dependent; IDDM) and type 2 (non-insulin dependent; NIDDM) diabetes can occur in older people. The onset of type 2 is much more common.
- In overweight older people, diabetes is mostly due to peripheral tissue insulin resistance (type 2). Glucose-induced insulin secretion is normal.
- Lean older people with diabetes often have impaired insulin secretion and may have islet cell antibodies more typical of type 1 diabetes. They respond poorly to oral hypoglycemic agents.
- There are increasing numbers of older people with type 1 diabetes who developed diabetes in early or mid-life and have survived decades on insulin, sometimes with few complications.
- Many people with type 2 diabetes progress to requiring insulin to achieve acceptable glycemic control. However, they are unlikely to develop ketoacidosis if insulin is withdrawn.
- When assessing a patient on insulin, determine whether they are insulin dependent (type 1; must always have background insulin) or insulin requiring (type 2; in which insulin may safely be withheld for a time, without risk of ketosis).

## Secondary diabetes

This is more common in older people. Causes include the following:

- Drugs, e.g., steroids, thiazide diuretics, antipsychotics, and niacin
- Pancreatic disease, e.g., chronic pancreatitis
- Other endocrine disease, e.g., Cushing's, hyperthyroidism

## Presentation

- Diabetes often presents atypically (e.g., less thirst, polyuria) or late.
- Many older people with diabetes are undiagnosed (up to 10% in some studies). This is at least partly due to physiological age-related changes, e.g., the renal threshold for glucose increases (glucosuria and polyuria occur later) and the thirst mechanism is impaired (polydipsia occurs later).
- The diagnosis is often made by screening blood or urine tests, or during intercurrent illness.
- Think of diabetes in many clinical circumstances, e.g., coma, delirium, systemic stress (e.g., pneumonia), oral or vaginal candida infection, vulvar itch (subclinical candida), cellulitis (and necrotizing fasciitis), weight loss, urinary incontinence, polyuria, malaise, vascular disease, or peripheral neuropathy.
- Steroid administration may reveal a diabetic tendency—always monitor, especially when high doses are used.

## How to diagnose diabetes in older people

- Confirm the diagnosis with a random blood sugar or fasting blood sugar. Criteria are the same as for younger patients (see below).
- In general, the diagnosis is confirmed with a second measurement unless the diagnosis is clear (e.g., severe hyperglycemia with metabolic decompensation).
- In some older diabetic people, fasting sugars may be normal. This is more common in lean older people, who have only postprandial hyperglycemia. If the diagnosis will impact patient management, do an oral glucose tolerance test
- Elevated glycosylated hemoglobin ($HbA_{1c}$) levels are only moderately specific and sensitive to diabetes and are not currently recommended to diagnosis DM. $HbA_{1c}$ is used for monitoring established disease.
- The U.S. Preventive Services Task Force recommends screening for DM in asymptomatic adults with treated or untreated sustained blood pressure >135/80. The balance of benefit and harm of screening for diabetes mellitus in asymptomatic adults with blood pressure ≤135/80 is not clear. Note, however, that the intensity of management in older adults should take the patient's preferences, functional status, comorbidities, and life expectancy into account.

### Diagnostic criteria

At least one of the following criteria must apply:
- Symptoms + **random plasma glucose** ≥200 mg/dL
- Fasting plasma glucose ≥126 mg/dL
- 2-hour plasma glucose ≥200 mg/dL during **oral glucose tolerance test** (75 g anhydrous glucose or the equivalent)

### Obtaining a fasting blood sugar

There must be no caloric intake for at least 8 hours before the blood test.
- Tell the patient to go for the blood test before breakfast.
- Non-calorie-containing clear fluids (water; coffee without milk or sugar, diet soda, etc.) may be taken.
- Patients should take all of their medications.

# Diabetes: treatment

Control of cardiovascular risk factors (i.e., hypertension, lipids) reduces morbidity and mortality. The average time to benefit from managing these risk factors is approximately 2–3 years.

The benefit of intensive glycemic management in older adults is unclear and the risk of hypoglycemia (e.g., falls with injury) is significant. Intensive management for those without existing microvascular complications may be considered for robust patients with an average life expectancy of >10 years who are capable of monitoring blood sugar safely and willing to do it. It may also reduce complications in those with existing renal or retinal microvascular disease.

In all patients, aim to avoid symptoms of hyperglycemia.

For robust older patients (life expectancy greater than 8–10 years) for whom intensive glycemic control is desirable and feasible, treatment targets are the same as for young patients. Aim for HbA$_{1c}$ levels close to normal (7.0%) and fasting sugar of 80–120 mg/dL. Note, however, that lower HbA$_{1c}$ levels are associated with an increased incidence of falls.

The frail, and the very old (>80 years) have not been included in most prospective treatment studies. There is doubt whether tight glycemic control improves long-term outcome. Treating symptomatic hyperglycemia may lead to improved cognition, functional status, mood, and vitality.

- Balance the potential benefits of intensive management with the risk of drug-induced symptomatic hypoglycemia, falls, and fractures.
- Symptoms of hypoglycemia may go unrecognized or be considered an aging change by caregivers.
- A reasonable target for the frail elderly patient is a HbA$_{1c}$ 8% and avoidance of all low fasting sugars.

## Diet

- Dietary change and weight reduction may be the only treatment needed in obese people with type 2 diabetes.
- Severe dietary restrictions are not appropriate for frail older adults. Beware the strict diet that takes enjoyment from the last months of life while giving little back.

## Education

- Educate and work as a team with the family, caregiver, and nursing home staff to implement a plan.
- Provide simple, written information and instructions.
- The approach must be tailored to the individual, taking note of cognitive and sensory impairments.

## Other interventions

- Exercise, especially endurance exercise (e.g., walking, cycling), improves insulin sensitivity.
- Weight loss—even modest reductions are beneficial
- Reduction of other vascular risk factors, including smoking
- Patient-worn alarm system so patients can call for help if they become hypoglycemic or suffer a fall

## Disease surveillance and prevention

Patients should be reviewed at least annually. Especially in the very frail or dependent person, regular reviews remain vital to ensure that treatments remain appropriate and that adverse effects are not occurring.

- Assess diet and drug concordance; check weight.
- Assess glycemic control and optimize cardiovascular risk factors including blood pressure and lipids consistent with patient goals.
- Finger-stick blood glucose testing, supplemented by 6-monthly $HbA_{1c}$ estimation is the preferred method.
- Urine glucose testing is less reliable and not recommended.
- Examine for evidence of complications, including microalbuminuria, an early signs of nephropathy and retinopathy.
- Check feet and refer to podiatrist as indicated.
- If there are no contraindications, consider daily aspirin (81–325 mg).
- Patients with DM should be encouraged to quit smoking and given resources to do so (counseling, pharmacological treatments).
- Screen for depression, cognitive impairment, urinary incontinence, and falls, which are common in older patients with DM.

## Control of hypertension

See Chapter 10, Hypertension, p. 274.

## Control of lipids

In the non-frail older diabetic, aggressive control of lipids can reduce cardiovascular events. The primary treatment target is the low-density lipoprotein (LDL) level:

- LDL <100 mg/dL: recheck lipids every 2 years
- LDL 100–129 mg/dL: dietary changes, exercise, and check lipids annually. Consider treatment with medications if goal of LDL <100 mg/dL not achieved in 6 months. Recheck annually.
- LDL ≥130 mg/dl start pharmacological treatment (i.e., with a statin) and lifestyle modification. Recheck at least yearly.
- High-density lipoprotein (HDL) goal: >40 mg/dL
- Triglycerides goal: <150 mg/dL. If patient has normal LDL and only elevated triglycerides, prescribe fibrate along with lifestyle modification.
- Be alert to muscle pain and soreness secondary to statin medication.

## Further reading

Durso SC (2006). Using clinical guidelines designed for older adults with diabetes mellitus and complex health status. *JAMA* **295**:1935–1940.

# Diabetes: oral drug treatment

### Sulfonylureas

These include, e.g., glipizide (start at 2.5 mg daily).

- Beware as they can cause hypoglycemia, especially with erratic eating patterns (e.g., frequent skipping of meals). Avoid long-acting drugs (chlorpropamide, glyburide), which can cause prolonged hypoglycemia.
- Commonly cause weight gain (2–5 kg)

### Biguanides

These include, e.g., metformin (start at 500 mg daily).

- Commonly used as first-line drug therapy in obese (BMI >25) patients (where insulin resistance predominates)
- Rarely cause hypoglycemia when used alone
- Common side effects are nausea, diarrhea, anorexia, and weight loss. Less common if the drug is introduced slowly (500 mg daily, increased incrementally each week to max. 850 mg three times a day).
- Lactic acidosis is rare, unless the patient has hepatic or renal impairment, or when tissue hypoxia increases lactate production.
  - Age itself is not a contraindication.
  - Do not use in patients with renal impairment (for women, creatinine >1.4 mg/dL; men, creatinine >1.5 mg/dL).
  - Stop metformin in acutely sick patients (especially with sepsis, respiratory failure, heart failure, or myocardial infarction).
  - Discontinue before anesthesia or administration of radiographic contrast media.

### Alpha-glucosidase inhibitors

These include, e.g., acarbose (start with 25 mg taken with the first mouthful of food).

- Moderately effective (HbA$_{1c}$ reduction 0.5%–1%) for patients with mild DM and reduce postprandial hyperglycemia. Hypoglycemia is never a problem.
- GI side effects (flatulence, bloating, diarrhea) usually improve with time and are lessened by starting low and increasing slowly.

### Thiazolidinediones

These include, e.g., rosiglitazone (start with 4 mg daily).

- May cause fluid retention and worsen congestive heart failure
- Does not cause hypoglycemia and may be used in renal impairment

### Dipeptidyl peptidase IV inhibitors

These include, e.g., sitagliptin (100 mg daily if normal renal function; decrease dose to 25–50 mg if renal function is impaired).

- Modestly effective, but do not cause hypoglycemia

## How to manage older diabetic people in nursing homes and assisted living facilities

### Overall approach

- The prevalence of diabetes is approximately 25% for short-stay (<6 months) and long-stay (> 6 months) residents combined.
- Hypoglycemia and other medication side effects are frequent in patients who are treated for diabetes. Remember: short-stay residents admitted for respite or rehabilitation may need relaxed glycemic goals during transition to avoid hypoglycemia due to changing activity or food intake.
- Life expectancy, quality of life, and comorbidities often favor relaxed glycemic control.
- Exercise and weight control are often limited by cognitive and functional impairments.

### To enhance quality of care

- Most residents should be screened for diabetes on admission to the nursing home and as determined by clinical course.
- Every resident with diabetes should have an individual care plan including at least diet, medications, glycemic targets, and monitoring schedule.
- Frequency of monitoring should be tailored with care goals. Checking finger-stick blood glucose can cause unnecessary patient discomfort and use significant staff effort. Monitor patient consistent with goals of care.
- An annual diabetes review should be performed with focus on preventative care.
- An annual ophthalmic screening assessment should be performed when consistent with quality-of-life goals.
- There should be easy access to specialist services including podiatry, optometry, diabetic foot clinic, and diet and nutrition.
- Each facility with diabetic residents should have a diabetes care policy with established protocols for the care of common occurrences, e.g., hypoglycemia and hyperglycemia.

Cayea D, Durso SC (2007). Management of DM in the nursing home. *Ann Long-Term Care* **15**(5):27–33.

# Diabetes: insulin treatment

- Insulin is essential for the treatment of type 1 diabetes.
- Insulin is started in type 2 diabetes when oral agents fail to achieve adequate control, if hyperglycemia is severe (especially if the patient is lean and insulin deficiency likely), or if oral drugs are contraindicated (e.g., hepatic or renal impairment).
- Quality of life and symptoms such as fatigue or urinary incontinence may improve substantially with insulin treatment

Side effects include the following:
- **Weight gain** is common. It is lessened if metformin is co-prescribed.
- **Hypoglycemia** is more common with insulin than with oral drugs.

## Initiating insulin

- Patients may be reluctant to begin treatment because of fear about injections or adverse experiences of relatives or friends.
- Consider burden on the caregiver if involved in implementing regimen.
- Consider whether the patient is physically and cognitively able to administer insulin, monitor blood glucose, and recognize and treat hypoglycemia.
- Use a diabetic nurse educator where available.
- There are a number of insulin delivery devices that can be used to make things easier (e.g., insulin pen with preloaded vial).
- Premixed insulin should be used to avoid having to draw up multiple types of insulin if that is the patient's insulin regimen.
- Some patients are able to self-inject but cannot safely draw up insulin into syringes or use an insulin pen. In this case, doses may be drawn up in syringes and stored in a refrigerator until needed.

## Insulin regimens

- Consider long-acting NPH insulin started once daily at bedtime, perhaps supplemented by oral hypoglycemic medication during the day.
- Very long-acting insulins (insulin glargine and insulin detemir) are effective if given just once daily (but costs more than NPH insulin) and are helpful in those who
  - Require assistance with injections.
  - Are frequently hypoglycemic on other regimes, especially at night.
  - Would otherwise need twice-daily insulin injections plus oral drugs.
- If eating is very erratic, consider giving short-acting insulin after each meal based on what has been eaten—a simple sliding scale.

Complicated regimes based on rapid-acting insulin alone or a basal-bolus structure is rarely appropriate unless the patient's lifestyle (meals and activity) is especially chaotic and the patient has the cognitive and physical ability to manage dosing and desires very tight control.

## Further reading

Cayea D, Boyd C, Durso SC (2007). Individualizing therapy for older adults with diabetes mellitus. *Drugs Aging* **24**(10):851–863.

# Diabetes: complications

In general, these are more common in older people, especially vascular complications. Evidence for risk reduction in the very old diabetic is weak. In practice, evidence from younger age groups is extrapolated to apply to older groups. For the very frail and those with very poor life expectancy a more conservative approach may be appropriate. Make an individualized decision and do not blindly follow guidelines.

## Cardiovascular

This type of complication is a very common cause of morbidity and mortality. The risk of myocardial infarction is as high in diabetics without known coronary disease as it is in nondiabetics who have had an infarct.

- Treat hypertension (see p. 274).
- The drug class used is less important than the reduction in blood pressure achieved. Beta-blockers are not contraindicated but may blunt ability to sense hypoglycemia. ACE inhibitors may reduce risk of nephropathy.
- Treat hyperlipidemia except in those with very limited life expectancy (e.g., <2–3 years) (see p. 260).
- The patient should stop smoking. Health benefits begin in 3–6 months.
- Low-dose aspirin should be offered to all older patients with diabetes unless there is a contraindication. Control hypertension beforehand.

## Neuropathy

- More than 50% of patients with diabetes over the age of 60 have diabetic neuropathy. Most common is distal symmetric polyneuropathy, but sudden, painful mononeuropathy (diabetic tabes), autonomic neuropathy, and diabetic amyotrophy producing pelvic girdle and thigh wasting are also seen.
- Many patients are asymptomatic and may not complain of numbness.
- More than 30% of older diabetics cannot see or reach their feet, making foot self-care problematic.
- Older diabetic patients should have their feet examined at every visit—check pinprick, vibration sense, light touch (with monofilament), and reflexes.
- The patient should be instructed on routine self-examinations of feet; it they are unable, a family member, friend, or caregiver should be trained to do so.
- Regular preventative visits to podiatrist can be useful.
- Treatment of all the above is to exclude other causes of neuropathy, to optimize glycemic control, and control pain.

## Nephropathy

- Diabetes mellitus is a leading cause of end-stage renal failure requiring dialysis in older adults.
- A test for urine microalbumin should done at diagnosis and, if absent, then checked yearly.
- Microalbuminuria indicates a group at high risk of progression. Microalbuminuria, however, may not be as predictive of progression to renal failure in older patients with type 2 DM as it is for those with type 1 DM.

- If consistent with health status, treat hypertension aggressively (preferentially with ACE inhibitors or ARBs), target blood pressure (≤130/80), and optimize glycemic control.
- If renal failure is developing rapidly, rule out other causes such as obstruction or glomerulonephritis.

## Eyes

- Glaucoma and cataracts are much more common causes of visual impairment than retinopathy in older patients with DM.
- The ability to see is a key aspect of quality of life regardless of health status.
- All diabetics should have annual screening ophthalmic assessment that includes retinal examination (fundoscopy with dilated pupils) and visual-acuity testing. This is usually provided by an ophthalmologist with expertise in diabetic eye disease.
- Preventing blindness depends on early diagnosis of diabetes, effective retinal screening, and early treatment of retinopathy. Tight glycemic control reduces the incidence of visual impairment in type 1 DM; evidence is suggestive, though weaker, for type 2 DM.

## Ears

Malignant otitis externa, manifesting as severe ear pain, is more common in DM.

## Teeth

Gum disease and caries are more common. Unsuspected or asymptomatic dental abscess may lead to worsening glycemic control. Good oral hygiene and regular dental assessment are essential.

## Feet: peripheral vascular disease and neuropathy

Along with diabetic neuropathy, severe peripheral vascular disease can lead to injury, ulceration, infection, and ischemia. Outcomes include chronic pain, chronic ulceration, immobility, and amputation.

## Immune system

All patients with DM should be vaccinated for influenza (unless contraindicated) annually and *Streptococcus pneumoniae* every 5 years.

# Diabetic emergencies

Two presentations are especially common—hyperosmolar hyperglycemic state and hypoglycemia. However, older patients can present with any diabetic problem, including diabetic ketoacidosis (DKA).

## Hyperosmolar hyperglycemic state (HHS)/ hyperosmolar nonketotic coma (HONK)

- A complication of type 2 diabetes, and may be the first presentation. It is most common in older people.
- Often severe. Mortality is very high (10%–20%).
- There is often underlying sepsis, particularly pneumonia. Leukocytosis is common, with or without infection. Have a low clinical threshold to beginning antibiotics, after blood and urine cultures.
- There is usually enough endogenous insulin to suppress ketogenesis but not hepatic glucose output. Thus there is usually only a mild metabolic acidosis (pH >7.3), and ketoacidosis is absent or mild. Blood glucose is often very high (even >1000 mg/dL).
- Subacute deterioration occurs, along with impaired thirst and an impaired "osmostat" contributing to severe dehydration with high serum osmolarity, hypernatremia, and uremia. The fluid deficit is large, even >10 liters.
- Neurological problems are common and include delirium, coma, seizures, or focal signs, e.g., hemiparesis. Only a small proportion is in a coma.

### Treatment
*Fluid volume resuscitation*
Frequent and careful clinical assessment and fluid prescription are usually sufficient to determine rate and volume, but consider insertion of a central line in those with cardiac or renal disease or who are in shock. In general, fluid administration should be slower than in the younger patient with diabetic ketoacidosis. For the patient who is sick but not moribund, 2 liters in the first 3 hours and a total of 3 or 4 liters in the first 12 hours is often optimal. The exception is the patient in shock, where filling should be more aggressive, with treatment in an ICU.

*Correction of electrolyte abnormalities*
Initially, give normal saline. Once fluid status is improved, switch to 5% dextrose with half normal saline when sugars are under control (<200 mg/dL). Maintain serum potassium in the range 4–5 mmol. Give potassium with fluid even if the patient is normokalemic, as patients are usually total-body potassium depleted, and insulin will drive potassium into cells. Hypokalemia is a major cause of arrhythmias and sudden cardiac death in patients with DKA and HHS.

*Hyperglycemia*
This often responds well to volume replacement and treatment of underlying cause (e.g., sepsis). Intravenous insulin is often needed, but modest doses (e.g., 1–3 units per hour) are usually enough. Patients with HHS are usually more insulin sensitive than those with diabetic ketoacidosis.

*Thromboprophylaxis*

Anticoagulation with low-molecular-weight heparin (LMWH) can be justified because the thromboembolic complication rate is very high.

Although mortality rates are high, many patients recover promptly. The severity of presentation does not correlate closely with the severity of underlying disease, and in some, the diabetes may subsequently be controlled with diet alone.

## Hypoglycemia

Risk of severe hypoglycemia increases greatly with age. In older people:
- The physiological response to hypoglycemia is weaker (e.g., reduced glucagon secretion).
- Autonomic warning symptoms (e.g., sweating, tremor) are less marked.
- Psychomotor response may be slow, even if symptoms are recognized.
- Other risk factors include frailty, comorbidity, renal impairment, nursing home residency, transitions in care (e.g., hospital to home), social isolation, and previous hypoglycemia.
- Clinical features are often not recognized or are atypical
- Check a sugar in an ill-appearing patient with known DM.
- Focal neurological signs or symptoms may be misdiagnosed as stroke. Signs may persist for some time after correction of blood sugar.
- Acute severe or chronic hypoglycemia can cause a dementia-like syndrome.

*Prevention*
- Assess each patient's risk of hypoglycemia and individualize therapy.
- Balance the lifetime risk of hypoglycemic attacks with reduction in long-term complications.
- If altering medications, monitor sugars closely afterward.
- Educate patient and caregivers about signs and symptoms, and the therapeutic response.
- Put in place alarm systems—necklace alarms.
- Accept higher target glucose levels (e.g., fasting glucose 120–140 mg/dL, evening glucose ≤180 mg/dL, target $HbA_{1-C}$)

*Treatment*
- Hypoglycemia can persist for hours or days and can recur late, especially if a long-acting insulin or oral drug (especially sulfonylurea) is responsible. If severe, monitor closely (if necessary by admission) for 2–3 days.
- Post-event, explore why the hypoglycemic event occurred. How might the next be prevented or better treated? Reassess medications and social situation.

## How to manage diabetes in the terminally ill patient

This includes end-of-life situations in all disease, not just cancer. The sole aim of therapy is to minimize symptoms of hypoglycemia and hyperglycemia.

Ensure that family and caregivers understand the changed aims of treatment and the rationale for medication changes.

*Drug treatment*
- As weight declines and oral intake falls, lower doses of insulin and oral drugs are usually needed.
- Dose reductions will also be needed as renal function declines.
- Make stepwise reductions in drug(s) and assess response.
- In some cases, drugs may be phased out completely. For example, type 2 patients on insulin may now manage on oral drugs alone; those on oral drugs may be asymptomatic off them.
- Type 1 patients require insulin until the very latest stages of dying (e.g., coma). Simplification of an insulin regime (e.g., a move to once daily insulin) is often helpful.

*Diet*
Encourage food and fluid of whatever type is acceptable and attractive to the patient. Rigidly imposed diabetic diets are futile and unkind—it is usually better to encourage food of whatever type can be taken, and to accept the (usually modest) consequences for glycemic control.

*Blood glucose monitoring*
- Monitoring should be tailored to the individual patient. In general, testing can be relaxed and often made only as needed (i.e., mental status changes or other symptoms)
- In all cases, test if symptoms suggest hypo- or hyperglycemia.
- In patients who are clinically stable or slowly deteriorating, testing can be infrequent (perhaps once on alternate days).
- In patients whose condition is deteriorating, or in those who have begun steroids, or where diabetes treatment has recently been changed, testing should be more frequent.
- In the patient who is moribund or comatose due to terminal illness, testing is pointless and only adds pain.

# Hypothyroidism: diagnosis

Hypothyroidism is common, with up to 5% prevalence in older men and 15% in older women. Incidence increases with age.

## Causes

Primary autoimmune disease (Hashimoto's disease, usually without goiter) is by far the most likely cause, unless iatrogenic causes are present (e.g., drugs—amiodarone, antithyroid drugs; previous hyperthyroidism treatment—radioiodine or surgery; head and neck radiotherapy).

## Presentation

- Onset is usually insidious: over months, years, or decades.
- It is very variable presentation, often unmasked by intercurrent illness. In older people, symptoms and signs are more often mild and non-specific.
- Classic signs of hypothyroidism such as cold intolerance, weight gain, and muscle cramps are less frequent in older than in younger hypothyroid patients.
- In older patients, weight loss and decreased appetite are reported by 13% of patients in some studies.

### Symptoms

- Hypothermia, cold intolerance
- Dry skin, thinning hair
- Weight gain or loss, constipation
- Malaise
- Falls, immobility, weakness, myalgia, arthralgias
- Bradycardia, heart failure, pleural or pericardial effusion, non-pitting edema (feet and hands)
- Depression or cognitive slowing. Frank dementia is very rare.
- Hyporeflexia with delayed relaxation phase; ataxia or nonspecific gait disturbance
- Anemia. Often normocytic; less commonly macrocytic or microcytic (reduced iron absorption)
- Hyponatremia, hypercholesterolemia, hypertriglyceridemia.

Symptoms of hypothyroidism are very common in the euthyroid older population. Often, only treatment reveals which symptoms were due to hypothyroidism.

## Investigation

- *Have a low threshold* for thyroid function testing, in view of high disease incidence, poor sensitivity of clinical assessment alone, and the ease and effectiveness of treatment.
- *Frequent screening* of older people in primary care (e.g., at yearly health assessment) is advocated by some, but balance of benefit to harm is unclear. But beware of abnormal TFTs due to sick euthyroid syndrome.
- *Overt primary (thyroid gland failure) hypothyroidism* is confirmed when TSH is high and free T4 low. TSH elevations may be less marked in older people.

- *Subclinical or "compensated" hypothyroidism* is suggested when TSH is high, but free T4 is normal (although often toward the lower end of normal range). The patient is often asymptomatic, but may have higher risks of atherosclerosis and myocardial infarction. Careful screening often reveals symptoms consistent with hypothyroidism.
- Thyroid masses are sometimes found on examination. Ultrasound can help characterize them.
- Antithyroid antibodies have reasonable sensitivity and specificity in confirming autoimmune hypothyroidism and may help management in subclinical disease.
- Patients may be persistently lethargic despite successful treatment. Consider the presence of other autoimmune disease, e.g., celiac disease, Addison's disease, or pernicious anemia.

# Hypothyroidism: treatment

*Overt (or "clinical") hypothyroidism*
This should always be treated. Typically the TSH is >10 mIU/L. The patient might believe themselves to be asymptomatic due to gradual and subtle nature of symptoms, but could feel better with treatment.

*Subclinical hypothyroidism*
Consider treatment if:
- The patient is asymptomatic and TSH is >10 mIU/L or
- TSH is between 4.5 and 10 mIU/L and symptoms are present, or
- Thyroid autoantibodies are positive, since risk of transformation to overt hypothyroidism is much higher or there is another coexisting autoimmune condition.

Note: adults older that 85 years with subclinical hypothyroidism and TSH 4.5–10 mIU/L should probably not be treated. In other cases, monitor clinically and biochemically every 6–12 months, but have a low threshold for starting what is a very safe treatment.

## Starting treatment
- Begin levothyroxine (T4) at low dose—usually 25 mcg daily. More rapid initiation risks precipitating angina, insomnia, anxiety, diarrhea, and tremor.
- Dosing is optimized using laboratory data alone—symptoms and signs alone are very misleading.
- Repeat TFTs every 6 weeks, increasing the dose of T4 in 25-mcg increments based on the TSH until a stable dose is reached.
- TSH levels guide dosage; T3 and T4 levels are **not needed**.
- For individuals age 70 and older, aim for a TSH around 4–6 mU/L.
  - Overtreatment risks atrial fibrillation and osteoporosis.
  - Undertreatment risks physical and cognitive slowing, weakness, and depression.
- Older people usually require slightly less T4—usually 50–125 mcg daily is sufficient.
- Heavier people require proportionately more T4 than lighter people.
- T4 half-life is around 1 week. Therefore, if fine-tuning of dosing is needed, simply alternate higher and lower doses, e.g., 100/125 mcg on alternate days.

## Long-term management
- Tell the patient that treatment is for life.
- Check thyroid function every year and if clinically indicated (e.g., addition of medications that may alter metabolism).
- In the long term, thyroxine requirements may rise, fall, or remain unchanged.

## Administration
- Foods reduce absorption—take on an empty stomach, usually first thing in the morning.
- If a dose is missed, take it as soon as remembered and the next dose on the usual schedule.

- If adherence is a problem, twice-weekly or weekly administration (of proportionately higher doses) gives acceptable control.

**Drug interactions**

- **Antiepileptics** (e.g., phenytoin and carbamazepine), **barbiturates**, and **rifampin** are among the drugs that increase thyroid hormone metabolism, so a higher T4 dose may be needed.
- **Iron, calcium, and antacids** (e.g., aluminium hydroxide) reduce T4 absorption. Give T4 at least 2 hours beforehand.
- **Amiodarone** has complex effects. Monitor TFTs regularly.
- **Beta-blockers** may reduce conversion of T4 to T3.
- As thyroid disease is controlled, dose changes of the following may be needed: **diabetic drugs** (insulin and oral hypoglycemics), **digoxin, warfarin, theophylline**, and **corticosteroids**.

# Hyperthyroidism: diagnosis

Hyperthyroidism is much less common that hypothyroidism but is also a significant problem in the geriatric population.

## Causes

### Toxic nodular goiter

This is the most common cause of hyperthyroidism in older people. There is often slow (years) progression from smooth goiter (euthyroid) to multi-nodular goiter (euthyroid). Then nodule(s) begin autonomous function, with subclinical and then clinical hyperthyroidism. It does not remit, but may be relatively mild and indolent.

### Graves' disease

The thyroid is stimulated by autoantibodies. Exophthalmos and diffuse goiter are less common than in younger people; no goiter is palpable in 40%. Many remit within a year, perhaps more so than in younger patients.

### Exogenous levothyroxine

Overtreatment of hypothyroidism usually occurs insidiously when age-related slowing in T4 metabolism is not paralleled by reductions in the dose of T4.

### Less common causes

- **Amiodarone** and other sources of excess iodine
- **Subacute thyroiditis and Hashimoto's thyroiditis**. There is transient thyroid hormone excess due to gland destruction. Suspect this if acute hyperthyroidism occurs with a sore throat or tender neck. There may be an associated viral syndrome or upper respiratory tract infection.
- **Single autonomous nodules**
- Malignant T4-secreting thyroid tumors and pituitary/non-pituitary TSH-secreting tumors

Distinguishing between the two very common causes (toxic nodular goiter and Graves' disease) is relatively unimportant, as treatment is similar. However, always consider the possibility of drugs or subacute thyroiditis, for which treatment is clearly different.

## Presentation

In older people with overt hyperthyroidism:
- Presentation may be more subtle, with fewer symptoms and signs.
- Diagnosis is often delayed. Features are attributed to comorbidity or suppressed by beta-blockers.
- "Negative" symptoms may dominate ("apathetic hyperthyroidism"), e.g., anorexia, weight loss, fatigue, weakness, and depression. Nonspecific symptoms are more common e.g., nausea, weakness, functional decline.
- More classical symptoms of sympathetic overactivation may be absent e.g., tremor, restlessness, sweating, tachycardia, and hypertension.
- Cardiovascular complications are more common, e.g., angina, heart failure, atrial fibrillation (although ventricular response may be slow) (see Box 15.1).
- Constipation is more common than diarrhea.
- Increased bone turnover can lead to hypercalcemia and osteoporosis.

### Box 15.1 Life-threatening thyroid emergencies

*Thyroid storm*

This is a rare but life-threatening manifestation of hyperthyroidism.

- Most commonly seen in patients with undiagnosed hyperthyroidism, often precipitated by nonthyroidal illness (including surgery, sepsis, or trauma), or administration of iodine-containing drugs
- Very rarely seen after radioiodine treatment
- Features include delirium, restlessness, coma, fever, vomiting, heart failure, tachycardia, and myocardial ischemia.
- The diagnosis is clinical—TFTs are no worse than in typical hyperthyroidism.
- Support failing organs, treat the underlying cause(s), and seek urgent specialist advice.
- Antithyroid drugs and iodide may be given intravenously to reduce thyroid hormone synthesis.
- Beta-blockers and corticosteroids reduce the peripheral activity of thyroid hormones.

*Myxedema coma*

This a rare but life-threatening manifestation of hypothyroidism.

- More common in older people, presenting as circulatory and respiratory failure, and progressive drowsiness leading to coma, often with seizures
- There is usually an acute precipitant (e.g., infection) in a patient with chronic hypothyroidism.
- Think of this also in patients who have stopped taking or absorbing levothyroxine.
- Myxedema coma is a medical emergency with up to 80% mortality if not treated and requires treatment with IV levothyroxine and IV hydrocortisone initially to cover for possible coexisting adrenal insufficiency.

### Sick euthyroid syndrome

- TFTs are often abnormal in euthyroid patients who are ill with non-thyroid systemic disease.
- Changes depend on illness severity, and when TFTs are checked (during acute illness or recovery).
- T3 levels fall first, followed by T4 levels with more severe illnesses.
- T4 levels recover more quickly than T3 levels once the underlying illness is resolved.
- In the convalescent phase following illness, TSH may be elevated as low thyroid hormone levels drive TSH production. For a time, TSH may be high and T4/T3 low, mimicking primary hypothyroidism. TFTs repeated a few weeks later are usually normal.
- Patients getting dopamine or glucocorticoids may have a low TSH level with low T3 and T4 levels. Secondary hypothyroidism (due to hypothalamo-pituitary failure) causes a similar pattern of TFTs but is rare, and other features of pituitary failure are present (e.g., hypogonadism).

# Hyperthyroidism: investigation

### Thyroid function tests

Have a low threshold for testing in older people due to the protean nature of symptoms. Screening is recommended by some authorities; at what age and frequency is controversial.

Low TSH is sensitive but not specific to hyperthyroidism.

- Drugs or nonthyroidal illness can suppress TSH below normal, but it usually remains detectable (0.1–0.5 mU/L).
- Very low TSH levels (<0.1 mU/L), indicating total suppression of TSH secretion, are more specific to hyperthyroidism.

*Overt hyperthyroidism*

- In most cases, TSH is undetectable and both T4 and T3 are high.
- Elevated T3 without T4 ("T3 toxicosis") suggests toxic nodules or relapsing Graves' disease, and is treated as hyperthyroidism.
- Elevated T4 but normal T3 (due to reduced peripheral conversion) suggests intercurrent illness.
- In severe hyperthyroidism, T4 may be normal (reduced binding globulin). Free T4 remains high.
- Acute systemic illness in euthyroid people may cause transient (days) elevation of T4. TSH will be normal or moderately low.

*Subclinical hyperthyroidism*

- This is common, with up to 5% prevalence of decreased TSH in healthy older people. TSH levels are low, with normal free T3 and T4.
- In most cases, TSH levels revert to normal within a year.
- Progression to overt hyperthyroidism occurs in up to 10% per year.
- Symptoms are few, but there is an increased risk of osteoporosis, atrial fibrillation, left ventricular hypertrophy, and possibly dementia.
- Consider the possibility that nonthyroidal illness (rather than thyroid hormone excess) may be suppressing TSH production.

### Antithyroid antibodies

- Their presence supports a diagnosis of Graves' disease, especially if a smooth goiter is also palpable, but they are not wholly specific.
- The most specific autoantibody for autoimmune thyroiditis is anti-TPO antibody (thyroperoxidase)
- Antibody tests are usually negative in toxic nodular goiter.
- Graves' and toxic nodular goiter are both common and can coexist. In that case a nodular goiter may be palpable, with positive antibodies.
- If Graves' disease is likely, screen for pernicious anemia and celiac disease (using relevant autoantibody tests and vitamin $B_{12}$ levels).

## Thyroid radioisotope scanning

This can help confirm the cause of hyperthyroidism and to determine glandular size prior to radioiodine treatment.

- In thyroiditis, uptake is low or very low. Inflammatory markers are up.
- In Graves' disease there is a diffuse pattern of increased uptake.
- In toxic nodular goiter there are multiple "hot" nodules with surrounding "cold" tissue.
- A single autonomous "hot" nodule is surrounded by "cold" tissue.
- A dominant cold nodule needs biopsy to rule out cancer.

# Hyperthyroidism: drug treatment

*Overt hyperthyroidism* should always be treated, even if mild. Several options are available for immediate and long-term treatment. Select treatment on an individual basis, depending on the likely diagnosis, severity of illness, and patient characteristics and preferences.

### Drug treatment: thioamides (methimazole or propylthiouracil)

This is suitable for initial management of Graves' disease or toxic nodular goiter, but it can take 2–3 months to achieve euthyroid state.

In **Graves' disease** this is an option for long-term therapy, as there is a greater probability of long-term remission than in younger people. Duration of treatment is usually 18 months, after which treatment is stopped and regular monitoring continues. Relapse risk is ~50% and is more likely if disease is severe, there is a large goiter, or antibody levels are high. If relapse occurs, begin thioamides again and refer for definitive treatment (usually radioiodine).

In **toxic nodular goiter**, long-term remission is less commonly achieved using thioamides. They are therefore used either
- Short term, to achieve euthyroidism prior to definitive treatment (usually radioiodine), or
- Long-term, in the frail patient in whom life expectancy is short.

Initial daily dose is methimazole 20–40 mg daily or propylthiouracil 100–150 mg 3 times daily. More is needed for severe hyperthyroidism. Full thyroid suppression takes several weeks. Continue the initial dose for 4–8 weeks, until euthyroid. Base assessment on free T4 measurements each 2 weeks. TSH may be suppressed for months despite adequate treatment. Once control is achieved, there are two options, with similar outcomes:
- *Titration regimen.* Thioamide dose is reduced gradually, guided by TFTs, to a maintenance dose of methimazole 5–15 mg or propylthiouracil 50–150 mg daily.
- *Block and replace regimen.* Thioamide dose is maintained high, entirely switching off thyroid synthetic function. Introduce levothyroxine once free T4 is suppressed.

#### Side effects
- Skin rash or pruritus. Continue treatment. Try antihistamines. Try switching thioamides.
- Fever, arthralgia, headache, and GI symptoms are usually mild.
- Agranulocytosis is uncommon, but more frequent in older people and certain ethnic groups (e.g., Japanese). It usually occurs early in treatment. Check WBC regularly. It is vital to advise patient and/ or relative that the drug must be stopped and urgent advice sought if fever, sore throat, mouth ulcers, or other symptoms of infection develop.

### Drug treatment: beta-blockers

Beta-blockers are used for rapid symptomatic treatment (tremor, anxiety, angina) and to reduce the risk of arrhythmias. There is no effect on the hypermetabolic state itself.

They may be especially useful in those with known structural or ischemic heart disease or who are tachycardic, but should be introduced cautiously, with regular monitoring. Digoxin is ineffective in controlling atrial fibrillation in hyperthyroidism.

All beta-blockers are effective. Atenolol is a good choice, as it may be given daily. Metoprolol and propranolol should be given 3–4 times daily due to increased hepatic metabolism in hyperthyroidism.

Beta-blockers have a role in treating the following:

- In Graves' or toxic nodular goiter as an adjunct to thioamides. When hyperthyroidism is only mild, beta-blockers may be the only drugs. needed prior to definitive treatment with radioiodine.
- In thyroiditis. The hyperthyroid state is transient, and beta-blockers alone may be sufficient treatment until the disease moves on to euthyroidism or hypothyroidism.

## Subclinical hyperthyroidism

If due to excess T4 in a patient with treated hypothyroidism, reduce dose by 25 mcg and recheck TFT in 6 weeks.

In other cases, to protect bone, heart, and brain, consider treatment as for overt hyperthyroidism. This is especially indicated if

- There is osteopenia or heart disease, or significant risk factors.
- Suppressed TSH is persistent, or severe, or T3/4 levels are at the higher limits of normality.

If treatment is not begun, reassess every 3–6 months.

## Atrial fibrillation (AF) and hyperthyroidism

- AF occurs in up to 20% of older patients. Most revert to sinus rhythm within weeks of becoming euthyroid, unless AF has been present for many months.
- Digoxin is usually ineffective in controlling ventricular rate. Beta-blockade is more effective and safer to use.
- Consider a trial of cardioversion if AF persists.
- Anticoagulate with warfarin to target INR 2–3. While hyperthyroid, patients are relatively hypersensitive to warfarin.

## Amiodarone and thyroid disease

Incidence of amiodarone-induced thyroid disease is high in older people because of this cumulative exposure and the drug's very long half-life.

- Clinical assessment alone is insensitive. Check TFTs before amiodarone treatment, and then every 3–6 months. If amiodarone is stopped, continue TFT monitoring for several years.

# Hyperthyroidism: non-drug treatment

### Radioiodine ($I^{131}$)

Radioiodine is effective, well tolerated, safe, and simply administered. The contraindications are as follows:

- When safe disposal of radioactive body fluids after treatment cannot be guaranteed. This can usually be overcome.
- In early treatment of hyperthyroidism, administration of the iodine load can precipitate thyrotoxic crisis.

Radioiodine is especially useful if there are drug intolerances, polypharmacy, or comorbidities. Give once initial symptomatic control has been achieved with drugs.

Thioamides must be stopped several days before administration of radioiodine (to permit uptake) and is usually restarted several days after (to prevent thyroid storm). Permanently discontinue thioamides after 3–4 months if TFTs are satisfactory.

Estimating the dose of $I^{131}$ required to render a patient euthyroid is difficult.

- On average, larger doses are needed for patients with toxic nodular goiter, larger goiters, in severe disease, and in men.
- Most centers give a single larger dose (75–200 µCi/g of estimated thyroid tissue divided by the percent of I-131 uptake in 24 hours). This controls hyperthyroidism in most cases, but leads to early hypothyroidism in up to 50%. A second dose is needed for a minority who remain hyperthyroid.

Post-treatment, TFTs should be checked every 4–6 weeks for the first year and then lifelong at reduced frequency but at least every year.

Secondary hypothyroidism may occur early (weeks, often transient) or late (years). Eventually up to 90% become hypothyroid. There may be an early (weeks) rise in TSH that is transient and does not need treatment if there are no symptoms.

If the patient remains hyperthyroid at 6 months, then repeat $I^{131}$ dosing is usually needed.

### Surgery

This is rarely performed in older people, considered only if both drug and radioiodine treatment are problematic or if a large goiter is especially troublesome. The patient must be euthyroid before surgery; beta-blockade alone is not sufficient. Lifelong postoperative thyroid function monitoring is essential.

# Adrenal insufficiency

### Presentation

This is usually insidious and often has a nonspecific onset:

- Primary adrenal insufficiency (Addison's disease) is not as common as secondary adrenal insufficiency.
- Symptoms include fatigue (helped by rest), weight loss, anorexia, abdominal pain, nausea, constipation, hypotension (orthostatic and supine), depression, delirium, and decreased functional status.
- In primary deficiency, skin and mucous membrane hyperpigmentation is common but is a late sign and may be absent. Pigmentation affects sun-exposed and unexposed areas, especially scars and pressure points.
- Electrolyte disturbance (hyponatremia and hyperkalemia) and a mild acidosis (bicarbonate 15–20 mmol) are usual. Hypoglycemia and mild anemia may be present.

In some people with impaired adrenocortical function there may be no symptoms when well, but acute stress (trauma, illness, psychological) leads to adrenal crisis with possible shock.

### Causes

- Primary: Mostly autoimmune. Often associated with other autoimmune diseases
- Tuberculosis is relatively more common in older people.
- Uncommonly due to metastases, lymphoma, hemorrhage, or infarction. Very rarely due to drugs, e.g., ketoconazole, megesterol

### Diagnosis

If the possibility of adrenal insufficiency crosses your mind, then test for it with an ACTH stimulation test (see Chapter 14, Homeostasis, p. 413).

- *Serum cortisol.* Cortisol is secreted episodically, so do not make or exclude a diagnosis on the basis of a single measurement.
  - A very low cortisol level (<3 µg/dL) makes adrenal insufficiency likely, especially if the patient is stressed or unwell at the time.
  - A moderately high (>25 µg/dL) cortisol level makes adrenal insufficiency unlikely.
  - In Addison's disease a random cortisol may be low or normal; normal level does not exclude Addison's.
  - Early morning (6–8 AM) cortisol levels should be higher—a low level is more likely to be significant.
- *Adrenal autoantibodies* are positive in many autoimmune cases.
- *KUB and CXR* may show signs of TB (e.g., calcification).
- *Adrenal CT or MRI* reveals a small gland in autoimmune disease, large if infection or tumor.

If adrenal insufficiency is diagnosed, exclude secondary adrenal insufficiency (pituitary failure).

- Check *gonadotrophins* (FSH, LH) and **TSH.**
- *ACTH* is elevated in primary adrenal insufficiency, low in secondary.

**Treatment**
- If the patient is sick, do not delay treatment pending the results of tests: fluid resuscitate with IV normal saline, normalize electrolytes, and give high-dose intravenous hydrocortisone (100 mg IV three times per day). Improvement should occur quickly.
- Long-term treatment includes glucocorticoid (usually hydrocortisone 20 mg AM, 10 mg PM) and mineralocorticoid (usually fludrocortisone 0.1 mg)
- With treatment, older people are much more likely to develop hypertension that may require mineralocorticoid dose reduction and nondiuretic antihypertensive drugs.
- Older people have a worse prognosis, due to more sinister causation (TB, malignancy) and possibly later presentation.

# Adrenal "incidentalomas"

- An *incidentaloma* is a tumor detected by scanning (ultrasound, CT, or MRI) that is unrelated to the indication for the scan.
- Adrenal incidentalomas are relatively common (0.5–1.5% of scans). They are more common in older people and hypertensive patients Key questions are if it is malignant and if it is functional.
- 80% of incidental adrenal masses are benign and nonfunctional.
- Adrenal insufficiency does not occur unless both glands are almost totally destroyed.
- Signs of a functional nodule include hypertension and hypokalemia.
- Tests for functioning nodules are as follows:
  - Urine- and plasma-free metanephrines for pheochromocytoma
  - Plasma aldosterone-to-renin ratio for primary aldosteronism
  - Overnight 1-mg dexamethasone test for Cushing's syndrome

***Adrenal adenomas*** are very common and usually small (<2 cm), benign, and nonfunctional. Fine-needle biopsy helps exclude malignancy if scan appearances are worrying, but usually only observation (periodic scanning) is needed. The larger the tumor, the higher the chance of malignancy. Large tumors should generally be excised, as biopsy may not identify foci of malignancy.

***Metastases*** are common (primary: breast, bronchus, bowel). Scan appearances are usually diagnostic.

***Cysts and lipomas*** make up most of the remainder.

***Benign adrenal cysts*** are common in older people and may be due to cystic degeneration or local infarction.

***Tuberculosis*** may seed hematogenously, causing adrenal masses, often calcified.

Nonfunctional ***adrenal carcinoma*** usually presents late, with retroperitoneal spread and distant metastases.

# Hormone replacement therapy (HRT) and menopause

Menopause (cessation of menstruation due to ovarian failure) occurs typically between ages 45 and 55. The diagnosis can usually be made clinically. If the presentation is atypical, consider alternative diagnoses, e.g., hyperthyroidism. Following menopause, the risk of osteoporosis and vascular disease increases substantially. Symptoms can occur for several years before and after menopause and can be disabling. They include

- Hot flushes
- Genitourinary atrophy
- Insomnia, depressed mood, and cognitive symptoms

***HRT with estrogen (plus progesterone in those with an intact uterus)***
- Is an effective treatment for perimenopausal symptoms.
- Does not improve well-being in those with no symptoms.
- Does not improve cognitive function or prevent dementia.
- Increases the risk of stroke, coronary events, pulmonary embolism, and breast cancer by small but not trivial amounts.
- Reduces colon cancer and osteoporotic fractures by small amounts.

In those with menopausal symptoms consider nonsystemic treatments, e.g., topical estrogens for atrophic vaginitis (vaginal cream or tablets, given daily for 2 weeks, then once or twice weekly for 6–8 weeks; sometimes needed long-term). There is some systemic absorption; the risk of endometrial cancer is unknown. In those with reduced manual dexterity, consider a slow-release vaginal ring (replaced after 90 days).

Other drugs that can help but are less effective than systemic estrogens include the following:
- Progesterones, e.g., medroxyprogesterone, megestrol
- Herbal remedies, some of which may have estrogen-like activity
- Clonidine (an alpha-adrenoceptor stimulant) may reduce hot flushes. Side effects are often problematic. Watch blood pressure.

If symptoms continue, discuss HRT, explaining risks and benefits. Start treatment at low dose, increasing gradually until symptoms are controlled.

Every few months, taper the dose of HRT, assessing whether ongoing treatment is needed. Hot flushes usually cease after a few months to a few (<5) years. A small percentage of older women experience hot flushes for many years past menopause.

Many women have taken HRT for prolonged periods and were started on HRT prior to completion of studies on risk. Risks and benefits of continuing HRT must be assessed. In most cases, advice is to stop HRT:
- Risk is probably cumulative (dose and duration).
- Risk is probably multiplicative. Because background risk of cancer and vascular disease rises exponentially in older people, the net added risk of HRT is higher in older people.
- In most cases, HRT may be withdrawn without recurrence of menopause symptoms.

# Hematology

**Brady Stein**

# Hematopoietic changes with aging

Few changes occur as the bone marrow ages.

Be very reluctant to ascribe changes seen on testing to age alone—pathology is much more likely.

## Hemoglobin

- Epidemiological studies show that population hemoglobin (Hb) concentration gradually declines from age 60.
- There is debate as to whether the reference range should be adjusted since lower Hb levels are associated with increased morbidity and mortality compared with older patients who maintain normal levels.
- Anemia is common in old age (10%–20% will have Hb less than 12 g/dL in females or 13 g/dL in males), but this is due to disease(s), not aging per se.
- The decision about whether to investigate anemia should be made not on the absolute value but the clinical scenario. Consider symptoms, past medical history, severity of anemia, rate of fall of Hb, the mean cell volume (MCV), and, finally, the patient's wish for or tolerance of investigation.
- A healthy older man with no significant past history merits investigation with an Hb of 11.5 g/dL (especially if his Hb g/dL was 13 last year or if the MCV is abnormal), whereas a patient with known rheumatoid arthritis, renal failure, and heart failure who has a normocytic anemia 10.5 g/dL for years usually does not.

## Erythrocyte sedimentation rate (ESR)

- ESR is the height of the red cells in a standard column of blood, after being allowed to stand for 60 minutes.
- This is a simple and nonspecific test. However, it is inexpensive and remains useful for screening and monitoring inflammatory conditions in older people.
- Red cells fall gradually because they are denser than plasma, but the rate of fall increases where the cells clump together.
- This occurs in disorders associated with elevated plasma proteins (fibrinogen and globulins).
- ESR rises with age and is slightly higher in women, so values up to 30 mm/hr for men and 35 mm/hr for women can be normal at age 70.
- Anemia and numerous acute and chronic disorders can elevate ESR.
- Very high levels (>90) are commonly found with paraproteinemias (p. 483), giant cell arteritis (p. 500), and chronic infections such as endocarditis and tuberculosis (p. 643, 644).

# Investigating anemia in older adults

Three general causes for anemia are found in older adults, occurring in nearly equal frequencies: blood loss or nutritional deficiencies; chronic illness or inflammation or chronic kidney disease; and unexplained. The following general approach to investigation is suggested.

In most cases, investigation is similar to that of a younger patient. Useful initial tests include the following:

- An anemia-oriented history and physical with careful consideration of underlying disease states including medications.
- Complete blood count (CBC) with differential, red blood cell (RBC) indices to characterize the mean corpuscular volume (MCV) and review of the peripheral blood smear.
- Absolute reticulocyte count to help categorize into hypoproliferative (e.g., chronic disease, hypothyroidism, renal failure, or bone marrow failure) or hyperproliferative (e.g., acute blood loss or hemolysis) states.
- Chemistry panel with attention to the creatinine clearance (CrCl).
- Assays for iron stores and nutritional deficiencies such as cobalamin or folate.
- A decision to refer to a hematologist for bone marrow aspiration and biopsy depends on individual considerations of the patient's goals of care, general health status, and how the treatment plan will be altered by this procedure.

# Nutritional deficiencies: iron deficiency anemia

Iron deficiency accounts for nearly 20% of cases of "nutritional anemia" in those over 65. Discovering the cause is usually important because of its prevalent association with gastrointestinal blood loss and malignancy.

## Causes

Most cases result from overt or occult upper or lower gastrointestinal chronic blood loss. Chronic epistaxis, uterine, or renal–urinary tract loss is far less common.

Reduced iron supply is less common but can occur from inadequate replacement due to earlier pregnancy or menstrual periods, or chronic malabsorption (e.g., celiac disease, gastric atrophy, or, rarely, *Helicobacter pylori* infection). In all cases, causes for chronic gastrointestinal (GI) blood loss should be ruled out.

## History and physical examination

History is vital. Focus on constitutional symptoms, weight loss, change in bowel habits, and GI blood loss. Patients may present without symptoms, with symptoms due to underlying disease, or with symptoms common to all anemias. Rarely, patients present with pagophagia (craving of ice) and restless legs, glossitis, angular stomatitis, blue sclera, or koilonychia (spoon nails).

## Investigations

- Microcytosis is usually found but can be absent in combined deficiency or with acute blood loss. Long-standing microcytosis with a narrow red cell distribution width (RDW) more likely reflects thalassemia.
- Serum iron levels will be low with high iron-binding capacity and the ratio of iron to iron binding will be low (<15%).
- Low-serum ferritin levels (<12 mgm/L) are diagnostic. Moderately low levels (12–45 mgm/L) may also point to the diagnosis, as ferritin levels rise with age. Ferritin is an acute-phase reactant, so normal to high levels don't rule out deficiency. However, when the ferritin level is above 100, generally, the iron stores are intact.
- If available, to distinguish IDA from the anemia of chronic disease (ACD), a serum transferritin receptor (TR) level can be sent. The TR level is a function of erythroid activity and inversely correlates with iron stores. Thus, it will be elevated in those with iron deficiency anemia (IDA). It should be normal or suppressed in those with ACD. A TR–ferritin index above 1.5 has a high sensitivity and specificity for IDA in older adults.
- The peripheral blood smear will show hypochromic, microcytic red cells with shape changes including pencil- or cigar-shaped cells.
- Low iron stores on a bone marrow biopsy are diagnostic, but this investigation is painful and rarely required.
- Hematuria sufficient to cause anemia is rare and usually severe. Urinalysis may be indicated in patients with poor vision or cognition to look for renal tract blood loss. When found, genitourinary bleeding may reflect paroxysmal noctural hemoglobinuria or intravascular hemolysis.

- Iron deficiency without anemia should still be investigated, but the lower the Hb the higher the likelihood of finding attributable pathology.
- Because most iron deficiency is caused by GI blood loss, investigation (e.g., endoscopic or barium contrast imaging) of the upper and lower GI tract endoscopically is usually indicated. However, the decision to forego diagnostic testing may be reasonable in very frail or ill individuals or when testing will not alter therapy.

# Treatment of iron deficiency anemia

### Enteral iron

- Treatment of uncomplicated iron deficiency is best done with oral iron salts. Ferrous sulfate is cheapest. A typical replacement dose is 325 mg three times daily.
- Ferrous sulfate is best absorbed on an empty stomach.
- The most common side effects are gastrointestinal, including epigastric pain, heartburn, nausea, diarrhea, and constipation. If present, advise to take iron with food.
- If symptoms persist when taken with food, reduce dosage to once-daily administration, or switch to liquid formulation.
- Ascorbic acid can facilitate absorption.
- Antacids, tannins (found in tea), calcium, and bran can hinder absorption if taken with the oral iron salts.

### Parenteral iron therapy

- Indications for IV iron include malabsorptive states, intolerance despite modification in dose or frequency, and chronic uncontrolled blood loss from a GI source or hemodialysis.
- A screening test for malabsorption involves the administration of liquid ferrous sulfate in a fasting patient; if the serum iron levels do not increase by at least 100 mg/100 mL, malabsorption is present.
- Iron dextran has the longest history of use. Advantages include low cost and the ability to administer up to 2 grams with one dose; disadvantages include anaphylaxis, and a test dose is required prior to infusion.
- Iron sucrose and ferrous gluconate are recently approved in the U.S. While they have a much lower incidence of anaphylaxis, they are more costly.

### Duration of iron therapy

A reticulocytosis should occur between 4 and 7 days following the initiation of therapy, and a hemoglobin response is usually noticed within 4 weeks. The anemia resolves in 4 months, and it is recommended that iron therapy be continued for several months following correction of the anemia to fully replenish iron stores. If a patient fails to respond, the physician should reevaluate the diagnosis, the patient's compliance, and for ongoing blood loss.

# Vitamin B₁₂ and folate deficiency

### Vitamin B₁₂ deficiency

Vitamin $B_{12}$ deficiency, as defined biochemically, is common in older adults, with a prevalence reported between 10% and 15%. Anemia due to $B_{12}$ deficiency is less common, with an estimated prevalence of 1%–2% in the older-adult population. It is unclear how many of those with sub-clinical vitamin $B_{12}$ deficiency will progress to overt symptoms, though probably a small number.

#### Causes

Malabsorption is the most common cause. In older adults, chronic atrophic gastritis is a common cause and the prevalence increases with age. Chronic *Helicobacter pylori* infection is often the etiology. Pernicious anemia, or autoimmune atrophic gastritis, usually presents around age 60, especially in women with other autoimmune diseases.

Drug-induced changes in gastric pH, due proton-pump inhibitors and H2 antagonists, also impair $B_{12}$ absorption. Anatomic changes, such as gastrectomy, blind intestinal loops causing bacterial overgrowth, and ileal disease, such as celiac disease and Crohn's disease, can all contribute to malabsorption.

Dietary insufficiency is very unlikely, though occasionally seen in strict vegans (those who do not eat meat, dairy products, or eggs).

#### History and physical examination

The most concerning findings on history and physical are neurocognitive in nature. Psychiatric symptoms such as dementia may be present. The classical neurological syndrome includes a loss of vibratory sensation in the fingers and toes, progressing to spastic ataxia, as demyelination of the dorsal and lateral columns of the spinal chord progresses. Importantly, the neurological symptoms can be irreversible and can occur in the absence of anemia.

#### Investigations

- Macrocytosis is common, often with an MCV of between 100 and 110, unless a mixed iron deficiency is present.
- Pancytopenia can be present in severe cases; elevations of the LDH and indirect bilirubin occur due to ineffective erythropoiesis.
- Neutrophils are hypersegemented with >5% having 5 or more lobes.
- Bone marrow examination shows megaloblastosis or a dyssynchrony in nuclear/cytoplasmic maturation, due to impaired DNA synthesis.
- Vitamin $B_{12}$ level below 200 ng/L is 95% sensitive for clinically overt deficiency. The specificity is somewhat lower, as folate deficiency, anticonvulsant use, HIV, and myeloma can also cause low levels.
- An elevated methlymalonic acid (MMA) confirms overt and subclinical deficiency. Homocysteine is less specific.
- Intrinsic factor antibody is sometimes obtained to diagnose pernicious anemia. Specificity is near 100% though sensitivity is only 50%–70%.
- The Schilling test is difficult to perform and rarely done.
- Clinical judgment determines how far one goes to investigate the exact cause of malabsorption. Depending on the history, pinpointing the underlying cause (e.g., bacterial overgrowth, celiac disease, etc.) may direct specific therapy.

*Treatment*

Replacement is important to prevent neurological and hematological complications. Parenteral vitamin B$_{12}$ is recommended for those with symptomatic disease. A common schedule is 1 mg IM daily (week 1), 1 mg two times per week (week 2), 1 mg/week x4 weeks, and then 1 mg/month for life.

Oral therapy can be recommended at 1–2 mg daily for those who prefer this route of administration, though this group should be followed closely to ensure repletion. The proper management of the large proportion of patients with subclinical deficiency is unclear but probably best to prescribe replacement.

Following replacement, resolution of marrow megaloblastosis and the appearance of reticulocytes are prompt, usually within 1 week. The anemia will usually correct within 2 months. Hypersegmentation often persists for 2 weeks. Progression of neurological damage is inhibited with repletion; the degree of recovery usually depends on the extent and duration of disease.

## Folate deficiency

Unlike B$_{12}$ deficiency, the primary cause of folic acid deficiency is decreased dietary intake. Folate is found in fruits and green vegetables; older adults who consume mostly alcohol or "tea and toast" can become deficient in months. Malabsorptive states (e.g., celiac disease, amyloidosis) and conditions producing chronic cell turnover (e.g., hemolytic anemia, psoriasis) or loss due to hemodialysis can lead to deficiency.

*History and physical*

Neuropsychiatric symptoms are not as common as with B$_{12}$ deficiency. Features of malnutrition, other vitamin deficiency (e.g., scurvy), or alcoholism may be more pronounced.

*Investigations*

- The red cell indices, peripheral blood, and marrow morphology are indistinguishable from those of B$_{12}$ deficiency.
- The serum folate level is the best screening test, though it is quite sensitive to recent folate intake as well as acute alcohol consumption and anticonvulsant use.
- The RBC folate level is low in 60% of patients with B$_{12}$ deficiency, limiting its sensitivity and specificity.
- The homocysteine level will be elevated, but the MMA should be normal, which can be helpful in distinguishing folate and B$_{12}$ deficiency.
- Concomitant B$_{12}$ deficiency should be ruled out prior to starting therapy, as the anemia will improve but the neurological symptoms will progress if folate is used empirically.

*Treatment*

Oral folate (1–5 mg daily) is well tolerated and absorbed and should be continued until hematological recovery.

# Anemia of chronic illness, inflammation and kidney disease

The anemia due to chronic illness, inflammation, or chronic kidney disease accounts for nearly a third of anemias. A number of conditions are causative, including acute and chronic infections, chronic inflammatory conditions, and malignancy, which are common in older adults.

## Pathogenesis

- *Impaired iron homeostasis:* When expressed, hepcidin inhibits absorption of iron from the gut and release from the reticuloendothelial system (RES). Hepcidin is markedly up-regulated in the presence of pro-inflammatory cytokines, accounting for the limited availability of iron for erythroid progenitor cells.
- *Impaired proliferation and increased apoptosis:* Inflammatory cytokines result in impaired formation of erythropoietin and down-regulation of its receptors on progenitor cells. Additionally, there is direct toxicity on progenitor cells with enhanced apoptosis, limiting red cell survival.
- *Blunted erythropoietin response:* The erythropoietin response is inappropriate for the degree of anemia, probably due to cytokine-mediated suppression of expression. Additionally, in the presence of high concentrations of pro-inflammatory cytokines, such as interferon gamma (IFN-G) or tumor necrosis factor (TNF), higher concentrations of erythropoietin are needed to induce proliferation.
- Decreased production contributes more centrally to the anemia of chronic kidney disease. The antiproliferative effects of circulating toxin, chronic immune activation due to the dialysis membrane, and episodic infection in this population also contribute to development of anemia.

## Investigation

- The anemia is often mild to moderate (hemoglobin 8–9.5 g/dL) in severity, normochromic, and normocytic.
- There are usually no specific features on the peripheral blood film or bone marrow, except the marrow can offer a confirmation of iron stores.
- The serum iron and transferrin saturation are reduced, reflecting hypoferremia due to sequestration of iron in the RES. Ferritin levels can be normal but are often increased, reflecting preserved stores.
- The use of the soluble transferrin receptor assay to distinguish IDA is discussed in section on Nutritional Deficiencies (p. 470). The transferrin receptor level should be normal in the anemia of chronic disease.
- Measurement of erythropoietin levels in anemic patients (hemoglobin <10 g/dL) may predict response to treatment. In particular, very high levels predict a failure to respond.
- Workup for underlying conditions does not always suggest an obvious etiology. In particular, a creatinine clearance should be calculated, but the exocrine function of the kidney does not correlate well with its endocrine function.

## Treatment

- When possible, management of the underlying disease is the treatment of choice.
- Patients with concurrent iron deficiency anemia should receive oral iron, but iron is not indicated in those with ferritin levels above 100 ng/mL.
- Erythropoietic-stimulating agents (ESA) are currently approved for those with chronic kidney disease and HIV patients on antiretroviral therapy.
- However, increased mortality and cardiovascular and thromboembolic events occur in patients with CKD with hemoglobin over 12 g/dL. For this reason, the Hb values should be followed carefully and ESA titrated accordingly when used.

## Further reading

Weiss G, Goodnough LT (2005). Anemia of chronic disease. *N Engl J Med* **352**:1011–1023.

# Unexplained anemia

Unexplained anemia accounts for nearly one-third of anemia in older persons. While medication and ethanol use, low testosterone, abnormal thyroid and liver function, and hemolytic anemias should be considered, myelodysplastic syndrome (MDS) probably accounts for a large proportion of unexplained cases in older adults.

## Myelodysplastic syndrome (MDS)

Myelodysplasia reflects a clinically and biologically heterogeneous syndrome with a uniform feature of ineffective production of mature blood cells. The median age of occurrence in the United States is in the mid- to late 60s. The incidence in those over 70 years is estimated to be 15 to 50 new cases per 100,000.

Most cases are idiopathic without identifiable exposures. Possible etiologies include chemical or radiation exposure or prior chemotherapy or radiotherapy.

## Diagnosis

- Many cases are discovered incidentally in asymptomatic patients found to have unexplained macrocytosis, monocytosis, or cytopenia in any or all three lineages.
- Others present with signs and symptoms of fatigue, pallor, infection, bleeding, or bruising due to quantitative or qualitative abnormalities of peripheral blood elements.
- Peripheral blood smears may reveal macrocytes, atypical monocytes, or neutrophil dysplasia (hypogranularity or pseudo-Pelger Huet cells).
- Bone marrow will often reveal hypercellularity and morphological evidence of dysplasia in at least one of three lineages. (In some instances serial bone marrow examination is required.)
- Adjunct testing may be helpful, including iron staining to identify ringed sideroblasts, flow cytometry to quantify blast percentage, and cytogenetic analysis.
- $B_{12}$ and folate deficiency, HIV, and drug exposures should be ruled out, as all can mimic the appearance of MDS.

## Prognosis and management

The karyotype, percentage of marrow blasts, and number of peripheral blood cytopenias help generate the International Prognostic Scoring System (IPSS). Low-risk patients have a favorable karyotype, a limited number of blasts, and limited cytopenias, and have a median survival of 5.7 years and a slower evolution to acute leukemia. The highest-risk patients have unfavorable karyotypes, increasing marrow blasts, and cytopenias, with survival limited to less than 6 months.

Palliative care directed toward symptom management with RBC transfusion may be best for frail older adults with other serious comorbid conditions.

Iron chelation should be considered in those with a significant transfusion history and a life expectancy greater than 1 year. Oral iron chelation with deferasirox is more convenient than prior formulations requiring IV or SC administration.

Nearly 15% of patients will respond to recombinant erythropoietin. Those with low-risk disease based on the IPSS, with infrequent transfusion needs (<2 units/month) and an erythropoietin level <500, are more likely to respond.

Granulocyte colony stimulating factor (G-CSF) may improve the neutrophil count, but there is no survival advantage. In combination with erythropoietin, G-CSF may improve anemia by an unclear mechanism in a minority of patients.

New agents approved for MDS include azacytidine, decitabine, and lenalidomide, which is most promising in those with a 5q- on cytogenetic analysis. The former agents offer a hematological response in a substantial percentage of patients, with a minority receiving a complete or partial remission. Studies also suggest a delay in transformation to acute myelocytic leukemia (AML). Multiple courses of therapy are required, often with adverse effects including myelosuppression.

Transplantation can be curative but has a high morbidity and mortality and is often poorly tolerated in those over 65.

## Further reading

Steensma DP, Bennett JM (2006). The myelodysplastic syndromes: diagnosis and treatment. *Mayo Clin Proc* **81**(1):104–130.

# Chronic lymphocytic leukemia (CLL)

CLL is the most common form of leukemia in the world, with a median age at diagnosis of 70 years. The cause is unknown, and unlike other forms of leukemia, an association between radiation, drugs, or chemicals has not been proven. An increased risk in relatives suggests some degree of genetic susceptibility.

## Diagnosis and staging

- Many patients present without symptoms and an incidentally discovered lymphocytosis
- 15% of patients will present with constitutional symptoms including night sweats, weight loss, and fatigue.
- The most common physical findings include lymphadenopathy, splenomegaly, and hepatomegaly
- Complications include an increased risk of infections, especially respiratory, autoimmune hemolytic anemia and thrombocytopenia, aggressive (Richter's) transformation, and an increased risk of secondary malignancies.
- An absolute lymphocytosis of at least $5 \times 10^9$/L is required for diagnosis.
- Peripheral blood flow cytometry can confirm the diagnosis with a characteristic immunophenotype of CD5, CD19, and CD23+ B cells. A bone marrow is not required but can offer valuable prognostic information from cytogenetic analysis.
- Clinical features are used for Rai staging. The presence of each in order of higher risk is as follows: lymphocytosis, lymphadenopathy, splenomegaly and/or hepatomegaly, anemia (<11 g/dL, not autoimmune), and non-immune thrombocytopenia (<100,000).
- Molecular or biological features also predict disease progression, including 11q-/17q- abnormalities, and unmutated IgV$_H$ status, CD38 expression, and ZAP 70 expression.

## Prognosis and treatment

The median survival for those with low-stage disease (lymphocytosis only) is 10 years; survival for higher-stage disease (anemia and thrombocytopenia) is between 1.5 and 4 years. The prognosis is very poor for those with Richter's transformation.

Criteria for treatment include non-immune-mediated anemia or thrombocytopenia, (or refractory immune-mediated cytopenias), massive or progressive adenopathy, a lymphocyte doubling time of <6 months, or constitutional symptoms. Patients with CLL are unlikely to develop hyperviscosity; therefore, the absolute lymphocyte count alone has no impact on a need for treatment.

Age, comorbidities, organ function, performance status, and preference determine specific therapies.

For the frail older patient, the focus is on palliation and limiting the toxicity of therapy.

Options for single-agent therapy in a patient with a limited life expectancy, unrelated to CLL, include fludarabine, rituximab, or chlorambucil.

For those with a good performance status, with a goal of achieving a complete or partial remission and prolonged progression-free survival, hematologists will often use combined chemo- and immunotherapy. An example is fludarabine, cyclophosphamide, and rituximab (FCR) or pentostatin, cyclophosphamide, and rituximab (PCR). These regimens offer a response in 90% of patients.

## Further reading

Yee KWL, O'Brien SM (2006). Chronic lymphocytic leukemia: diagnosis and treatment. *Mayo Clin Proc* **81**(8):1105–1129.

# Plasma cell disorders

## Monoclonal gammopathy of undetermined significance (MGUS) and smoldering myeloma

MGUS suggests the presence of a monoclonal protein in patients without features of malignancies such as multiple myeloma, systemic amyloidosis, Waldenstrom's macroglobulinemia, lymphoma, or CLL. MGUS is increasingly prevalent as the population ages, with 5% of patients over 70 years found to have a detectable monoclonal protein.

Aside from age, MGUS is often associated with AIDS, chronic liver disease, and rheumatological disease. The cause is currently unknown, but a significant percentage of patients have translocations, possibly precipitated by infection or immune dysregulation, involving the immunoglobin heavy-chain locus on chromosome 14.

### Diagnosis

- Usually detected incidentally by labs revealing an elevated total protein
- Patients are asymptomatic and should specifically deny bone pain, symptoms of anemia, neurological symptoms, or weight loss. The physical exam is often unrevealing.
- Serum protein electrophoresis detects the M protein; immunofixation characterizes the immunoglobulin (Ig) class (IgG, IgM, or IgA) and type of light chain (kappa or lambda).
- A 24-hour urine collection should be collected to evaluate for M protein in the urine.
- Workup should include a CBC, creatinine and calcium levels, and skeletal survey. Bone marrow biopsy is not recommended in those with a serum M protein <1.5 g/dL.
- By definition, MGUS is diagnosed in those with an M protein <3 g/dL, the absence of significant light chain in the urine, and a bone marrow biopsy with <10% plasma cells. Lytic lesions, anemia, hypercalcemia, and abnormal renal function should be absent.
- A monoclonal protein of >3 g/dL or >10% plasma cells in the bone marrow, without symptoms or end-organ damage, are diagnosed with "smoldering multiple myeloma."

### Prognosis and management

- The risk of progression to myeloma is 1% per year. Older patients with MGUS are more likely to die of other illness.
- The size of the M spike and specific type (IgA and IgM) predict a higher risk of progression. An abnormal free light-chain ratio of kappa to lambda chains suggests a higher risk of progression.
- The standard of care is observation alone. Patients with lower-risk MGUS should have repeat follow-up in 6 months and then every 2 years. Those with higher risk should have repeat testing 6 months from the time of diagnosis and then yearly.
- Those with smoldering myeloma require follow up every 3–4 months.

## Multiple myeloma

Multiple myeloma (MM) evolves from MGUS, though the precise mechanisms by which this occurs is unclear. Secondary genetic events and changes in the bone marrow microenvironment have been suggested. Multiple myeloma is diagnosed most commonly in those above 65 years of age. There are nearly 15,000 new cases diagnosed each year, more commonly in African Americans than in Caucasians.

### Diagnosis and staging

The most common presenting symptoms reflect end-organ damage attributable to myeloma; at least one of the following is required for diagnosis:

- Skeletal abnormalities/lytic lesions resulting in bony pain can be found in 80% of patients. In those with pain but a negative skeletal survey, an MRI is recommended, especially if spinal bony disease is suspected.
- Anemia is present in 70% of patients.
- Abnormal renal function is present in 50% of patients.
- Hypercalcemia is found in 25% of patients.
- In addition to these end-organ manifestations, a bone marrow with >10% plasma cells and an abnormal M protein in the serum or urine is required for diagnosis. The M protein is detectable by serum and urine protein electrophoresis and immunofixation techniques.
- 20% of patients lack expression of the heavy chain of the M protein and are said to have light-chain myeloma. The light chain in this case is always detectable in the urine, requiring analysis of the urine in addition to the serum in all cases of suspected MM.
- Complications can include recurrent infections, hyperviscosity, and amyloidosis in a minority of cases.
- The erythrocyte sedimentation rate is elevated and may lead to discovery incidentally.
- The International Staging System (ISS), based on the albumin and beta-2 microglobulin, stratifies patients into three risk categories based on albumin >3.5 and a beta 2 microglobulin <3.5 (stage I); a B2 microglobulin >5.5 (stage III); or neither of the above (stage II).
- The median survival by stage is 62 months for stage I, 44 months for stage II, and 29 months for stage III disease.
- Additional features contribute to prognosis and risk, including performance status and cytogenetic abnormalities. In particular, deletion of chromosome 13 or the short arm of chromosome 17, hypoploidy and immunoglobulin heavy-chain translocations, i.e., t(4;14) suggest an adverse outcome.

### Treatment

- Consideration of age, performance status, comorbidity, and disease stage and risk determines therapy.
- In those patients who are eligible, autologous stem cell transplantation prolongs survival by nearly 12 months but is not curative. Most prior studies excluded those above age 65, but some patients over 70 may tolerate this procedure. Allogeneic transplantation carries a high mortality.

- In those eligible for transplant, regimens that do not affect the ability to harvest stem cells are chosen (e.g., thalidomide/cexamethasone, lenalidomide/dexamethasone, or regimens including bortezomib).
- For patients ineligible for transplantation, including most older patients, regimens typically include melphalan and prednisone in combination with thalidomide (MPT). MPT offers improved survival over that with melphalan and prednisone.
- The hematologist must consider the use of anticoagulation (low-molecular-weight heparin, warfarin, or aspirin) in those taking immunomodulatory drugs in combination with steroids (e.g., thalidomide/dexamethasone) due to a high rate of associated venous thrombosis.
- Improvements in supportive care contribute to improved quality of life.
- Bisphosphonates reduce pain and pathological fracture, need for radiation or surgery, and spinal chord compression. Zolendronic acid or pamidronate should be used for those with at least one lytic lesion. GI side effects and osteonecrosis of the jaw may complicate therapy.
- Vertebroplasty and kyphoplasty help reduce pain and restore height and should be considered in those with compression fractures.
- ESAs can correct chemotherapy-related anemia.
- Hypercalcemia can be treated with intravenous saline, steroids, or bisphosphonates.
- Nonsteroidal anti-inflammatory agents, dehydration, and IV contrast dye should be avoided, as they can precipitate or worsen renal failure, especially in those with high levels of light chains in the urine.
- Pneumococcal and influenza vaccinations are recommended; prophylaxis against *Pneumocystis jiroveci* pneumonia should be considered in those on high-dose steroids.

### Further reading

Rajkumar SV, Lacy MO, Kyle RA (2007). Monoclonal gammopathy of undetermined significance and smoldering multiple myeloma. *Blood Rev* **21**(5):255–265.

# Musculoskeletal system

**Catherine Schreiber and Shari Ling**

# Introduction

Older adult patients commonly develop musculoskeletal disorders and diseases. An accurate diagnosis is the foundation for effective management. Not all pain is due to arthritis. The source of painful musculoskeletal symptoms can usually be ascertained through a carefully performed history and physical examination.

## Is the pain due to arthritis?
- Arthritis symptoms include pain and stiffness.
- Physical abnormalities of arthritis include joint warmth or redness, tenderness to touch at the joint line, and pain on passive motion (with the patient relaxed, visible swelling, deformity).
- If arthritis is present, knowing how many and which joints are involved will help ascertain a diagnosis.
  - Monoarthritis (one joint): infectious, crystal-related, trauma
  - Pauciarticular (2–4 joints): crystalline, reactive arthritis, spondyloarthritis, crystal-related arthritis
  - Polyarticular (4 or more joints): rheumatoid arthritis, systemic lupus, crystal-related arthritis, hepatitis C virus

Physical abnormalities not suggestive of arthritis are diffuse tenderness that is not specific to the joint line and pain exclusively on active motions.

## If pain is due to arthritis, is the arthritis inflammatory in nature?
- *Stiffness* that persists for more than an hour a day suggests an inflammatory arthritis. Stiffness upon awakening that is less than an hour in duration or that recurs after a period of inactivity that is momentary does not suggest an inflammatory arthritis.
- *Constitutional symptoms:* Unintentional weight loss, fever, loss of appetite, and a general feeling of poor health are features of a systemic illness.
- *Physical abnormalities of an inflammatory arthritis:* Normal joints are cooler than the surrounding structures. Joints that are warm or hot, red, and visibly swollen are inflamed.

## Further reading
Barlett, SJ (ed.) (2006). *Clinical Care in the Rheumatic Diseases.* 3rd ed. Altanta, GA: Association of Rheumatology Health Professionals.

# Osteoarthritis

Osteoarthritis (OA) is the most common joint disorder in older patients and can result in substantial pain and disability. Although OA is highly prevalent, it should not be considered part of normal aging. Multiple factors contribute to OA, including genetic predisposition, biomechanics, joint injury, local inflammation, and cellular and biochemical responses.

Inherited factors determine susceptibility but individual genes are not identified. Increasing age is the strongest risk factor. Obesity, trauma, and repetitive adverse loading (e.g., miners' or gymnasts' movements) are potentially avoidable factors. Congenital factors (e.g., hip dysplasia) can predispose individuals to developing OA earlier in life.

## Clinical features

- *Pain:* Assess severity and disability (difficulty with mobility and daily-activity tasks). It is usually insidious in onset and variable over time, worse with activity and relieved by rest. Chronic pain may cause poor sleep and depression.
- *Stiffness* is the earliest symptom that is most prominent in the morning but resolves within an hour of awakening and may reappear after periods of inactivity (sitting, driving, etc.).
- *Restricted movement:* e.g., bending, stooping, stair-climbing, walking, rising from a chair

Severe OA can result in difficulty dressing and performing self-care tasks and may increase the risk of falling.

## Examination

- Bony enlargement of the distal interphalangeal joints (Heberden's nodes) or proximal interphalangeal joints (Bouchard's nodes)
- Restricted range of movement
- Crepitus
- Effusions
- Deformity
- Muscle wasting
- Knees may have valgus (knees apart, feet together), varus (knees together, foot outwards) or flexion deformity
- Hip shortening/flexion (check on exam table by flexing opposite hip to see if affected hip lifts off bed—the Trendelenberg test)

## Investigations

OA is a clinical diagnosis. Symptoms correlate poorly with radiological findings. The main role of X-ray is in assessing the severity of structural change prior to surgery. Features include joint space narrowing, osteophytes, sclerosis, cysts, and deformity. Blood tests are normal even when an osteoarthritic joint feels warm. Reconsider your diagnosis if inflammatory markers (e.g., ESR or CRP) are elevated.

# Osteoarthritis: management

The goal of OA management is to alleviate painful symptoms, minimize disability, and maximize quality of life.

Always begin by implementing nonmedicinal treatments.

## Nonmedicinal treatments (in addition to general non-pharmacological recommendations)

- Weight loss can improve pain control substantially for patients with knee and hip OA.
- Encourage the patient to exercise despite some pain. Reassure them that moderate exercise will not cause their arthritis to worsen. Swimming, yoga, and Tai Chi are particularly good.
- Sensible footwear: soft soles without heels or wedge shoe insoles. Consider foot orthotics for knee OA.
- Walking aids: e.g., cane (in contralateral hand)
- Hot and cold packs: but be very careful to avoid burns in patients who may have decreased temperature awareness.

## Pharmacologic agents

- Try topical agents next.
- Topical nonsteroidal anti-inflammatory drugs (NSAIDs) (diclofenac) and salves (methylsalicylate cream) can be helpful and are lower risk than oral medications.
- Capsaisin cream is safe and has some analgesic effect for hand and knee OA.
- Oral analgesics should be recommended for patients with persistent pain.
- Acetaminophen (maximum dose 1000 mg qid) remains the first-line analgesic for older adult patients. Consider adding other agents only after maximizing acetaminophen.
- Tramadol may be effective as a secondary agent.

A short course of an oral NSAID can be useful in acute exacerbations but try to avoid long-term use.

- If NSAIDs are used for more than 2 weeks or in the presence of known dyspepsia or ulceration, reduce the gastrointestinal (GI) risk by co-prescribing, e.g., misoprostol 200 mcg three times daily, or a proton-pump inhibitor should be added.
- The COX-2 selective inhibitors may have better GI tolerability but have fallen from favor due to vascular adverse events. Furthermore, COX-2 selectivity does not prevent the development of renal insufficiency.

Intra-articular steroids (e.g., triamcinolone hexacetonide or dexamethasone) can be considered for patients with persistent symptoms despite maximal medicinal and nonmedicinal therapies. The dose will depend on the size of the joint.

Oral chondroitin and glucosamine are available unlicensed over the counter and are very widely used. They may have a slow-onset, mild analgesic action but probably do not slow the progression of disease. Fortunately, aside from their expense, significant life-threatening side effects have not been reported.

## Further reading

Conaghan PG, Dickson J, et al. (2008). Care and management of osteoarthritis in adults: summary of NICE guidance. *BMJ* **336**(7642):502–503.
Hunter DJ (2007). In the clinic. Osteoarthritis. *Ann Intern Med* **147**:ITC8-1–ITC8-16.

# Osteoporosis

Osteoporosis (OP) is a highly prevalent condition characterized by disruption of normal bone architecture and decreased bone mass. Together with falls, OP increases risk of fractures in older adults.

Due to its silently progressive course, diagnostic testing should be pursued and treatment strategies implemented early.

## Pathology

- Total bone mass increases throughout childhood and adolescence, peaks in the third decade, and then declines at about 0.5% per year.
- Loss of bone mass accelerates after menopause in women (up to 5% per year), but declines gradually in men.
- Smoking, alcohol, low body weight, hyperthyroidism, hyperparathyroidism, hypoandrogenism (in men), renal failure, low dietary intake of vitamin D and calcium, inadequate sunlight exposure, and physical inactivity accelerate loss of bone mass further.
- Steroids, phenytoin, long-term heparin, and cyclosporin cause secondary osteoporosis.
- High-peak bone mass early in life reduces risk of OP later.

## Clinical features

In contrast to traumatic fractures, fragility fractures typically occur at the wrist, hip (femoral neck or trochanter), or vertebral body that are sustained at low-energy levels.

Fractures can be sustained from a fall, but can also contribute to falls.

Vertebral body fractures can cause a wedge deformity of one or more vertebrae that can present as one of the following:
- Acute back pain
- An incidental radiographic finding (30%)
- Loss of height
- Progressive kyphosis ("Dowager's hump") that can compromise balance, thereby increasing the risk of falling, and in severe cases result in abdominal compression, esophageal reflux, and restrictive lung disease.

## Diagnosis

The World Health Organization uses dual X-ray absorptiometry (DEXA) to define osteoporosis (T score less than −2.5 below mean peak bone mass) and osteopenia (T score between −1 and −2.5).

DEXA scanning of the hip and spine provide a quantitative measure of bone mineral density that can be used to assess risk of fracture in that region. Fracture risk is assessed using bone density together with age, body mass index (BMI), known diagnosis of secondary osteoporosis, personal and family history of a fragility fracture, diagnosis of inflammatory diseases, and glucocorticoid, tobacco, or alcohol use.

Think of secondary causes if the Z score is lower than −2.5 (compares it to age- sex-, and weight-matched adults).

X-rays may show fractures and give an idea of bone quality.

Although blood tests are usually normal (except after a fracture), the following laboratory testing are considered routine:

- Chemistry profile including alkaline phosphatase, calcium, and phosphorous
- Hormonal assays: TSH, PTH, 25-hydroxy-vitamin D
- Testosterone levels in men
- If calcium or alkaline phosphate is elevated, consider alternative diagnosis, e.g., metastases or Paget's disease.

# Osteoporosis: management

### Primary prevention
- Sensible public health measures (e.g., diet, weight-bearing exercise, stop smoking, reduce alcohol) should be advised for all people at all ages.
- Prophylaxis for those taking steroid therapy (see below)
- Hormone replacement therapy (HRT) should be weighed against risk of vascular and thromboembolic complications and cancer.

### Treatment
Primary prevention strategies outlined above should be initiated.
- **Oral calcium supplementation** (1500 mg daily)
- **Vitamin D supplementation**
  - 400–600 IU daily for standard supplementation
  - 800 IU daily for older adults, homebound, chronically ill, and institutionalized people
  - 50,000–100,000 IU every 3 weeks for severe vitamin D deficiency; monitoring of calcium levels is required.

**Bisphosphonates** increase bone mass by inhibiting osteoclast-mediated bone resorption and may be added to calcium and vitamin D.
- The weekly dose regimens (risedronate 35 mg or alendronate 70 mg once weekly) are easier to remember and tolerate than daily dosing.
- Esophageal and upper gut ulceration occurs rarely. Use bisphosphonates cautiously when there is dysphagia or a history of dyspepsia. It must be taken on an empty stomach 30 minutes before breakfast or other medicines. The patient needs to swallow the tablet whole with a full glass of water while sitting or standing, then remain sitting or standing for 30 minutes after swallowing.
- Bisphosphonates are currently also recommended prophylactically at onset of "significant" steroid therapy (>7.5 mg prednisone per day for >1 month).
- Up to 15% of patients are "nonresponders" and continue to lose bone mass (measured by chemical bone turnover markers). Such patients are unlikely to be detected in a primary care clinic because bone turnover is not monitored, but consider a change in treatment if fragility fractures continue.
- This agent is contraindicated in hypocalcemia. Manufacturers advise avoiding its use in renal impairment, but it is often given if the indication is strong.

**Calcitonin**, available in nasal spray, improves pain after acute vertebral fracture.

**Raloxifene** is an estrogen-like drug that decreases bone loss without measurable effects on the uterus. It is used if bisphosphonates are not tolerated or in nonresponders.

Estrogen therapy is indicated in those patients with persistent menopausal symptoms and those who cannot tolerate other therapies. It must outweigh concerns of malignancy and thromboembolism.

The following are less commonly prescribed agents that should be considered together with a rheumatologist or endocrinologist:
- **Teriparitide** a recombinant fraction of parathyroid hormone, administered intermittently by injection, stimulates bone formation more than bone resorption, and reduces fracture risk.
- **Strontium ranelate** inhibits bone resorption and increases bone formation. It may be considered if bisphosphonates are not tolerated.

### Further reading

Clinician's Guild to Prevention and Treatment of Osteoporosis. Available at: http://www.nof.org/professionals/Clinicians_Guide.htm
Osteoporosis fracture risk tool: http://www.shef.ac.uk/FRAX/tool.jsp

## How to manage nonoperative fractures

*General principles of management*
- Fractures of the pelvis, humerus, wrist, and vertebra are preferably managed conservatively.
- Nonsurgical management may be more appropriate for older adult patients with comorbid medical conditions for whom surgical risk is substantial.
- Fractures can result in functional limitations, e.g., a Colles fracture and plaster of Paris (POP) impede self-care, and can also impede walking with a mobility aid.
- Geriatricians and physiatrists can provide necessary expertise to optimize management for older adult patients.

*Choose the most appropriate management setting*
- Assess and reassess progress in functional recovery.
- Home with outpatient rehabilitation: Is the patient safe and capable of independent self-care and toileting? What additional services are required (e.g., skilled nursing, therapy)?
- Inpatient rehabilitation: The patient has mobility and self-care limitations that require aggressive rehabilitation services (physical therapy, occupational therapy).
- Transitional care facility (e.g., while they wait to be weight bearing or for casts to be removed)

*Initiate medical management*
- Control pain
- Initiate local modalities: TENS, ice, or heat
- Analgesic agents
- A short course of NSAIDs is sometimes appropriate in low-risk patients, but remember to reduce analgesia as soon as possible.
- Consider **prophylactic heparin** to reduce risk of thromboembolic disease.
- Initiate **osteoporosis treatment** (calcitonin may be useful for painful vertebral fractures).

*Communicate with orthopedic and interventional radiology colleagues*
- Consult on when to liberalize weight bearing and other restrictions.
- Consider vetebralplasty for acute vertebral fractures in the neurologically intact patient.
- Promptly pursue surgical stabilization in patients with neurologic deficits.
- Reassessment if progress is poor, e.g., ongoing severe pain, or apparent mal-union

*Implement fall risk reduction strategies*
- Educate the patient and the patient's family.
- Consider the mechanism of the fall or injury (Chapter 5, Falls, p. 82)
- Review and eliminate risky drugs, e.g., sedating or anticholinergic medications, excessive antihypertensive use.
- Evaluate for predisposing medical illness (e.g., neurological impairment).
- Conduct a home evaluation to maximize safety and minimize risks (e.g., lighting, rugs, rails, etc.).

# Rheumatoid arthritis

Rheumatoid arthritis (RA) is inflammatory disease of the joints and multiple body systems (bones, nerves, muscles cardiovascular, eyes). Inflammation causes pain, swelling, stiffness, and eventual destruction of the joints. Functional limitations are common. People of any age can develop RA, and it is more common in women.

Patients with long-standing RA require ongoing management of deformities and functional limitations.

Elderly-onset rheumatoid arthritis (EORA) is defined as RA starting at >60 years of age and having an acute onset accompanied by constitutional symptoms.

Two incompletely overlapping subsets of RA have been recognized:

- *Classic RA* is inflammatory polyarthritis that is erosive and seropositive. The prognosis in older adults is comparable to if not more function limiting than in younger adults because of older adults' lower functional reserve and greater number of comorbid medical conditions.
- *Polymyalgia rheumatica-like* has shoulder involvement, absence of rheumatoid factor, and, usually, a nonerosive, self-limited course.
- *Remitting seronegative symmetrical synovitis with pitting edema* (RS3PE) syndrome results in self-limited puffy (boxing glove–like hands) with pitting edema.

# Rheumatoid arthritis: management

## Diagnosis of RA

- Polyarthritis (involves multiple joints) that be distinguished from systemic lupus, crystal-related arthritis, and hepatitis C virus
- Radiographic abnormalities (joint erosions, osteopenia)
- Serology: rheumatoid factor, anti-citrullinated peptide (anti-CCP) antibody

## Medicinal therapies

Medications employed for RA therapy in younger subjects (analgesics, NSAIDs, corticosteroids, disease-modifying antirheumatic drugs, anticy-tokine drugs) can be considered for older adult patients with RA. The medications listed below should be employed only with the guidance of a rheumatologist.

- Analgesic and anti-inflammatory agents should be initiated for control of painful symptoms. They must also be monitored for gastrointestinal and renal toxicities.
- Glucocorticoid therapy is most appropriate for self-limited subtypes (PMR-like, RS3PE syndrome) or at low doses as adjunctive therapy for classic RA. Toxicities (infection, glucose intolerance, osteoporosis, and body composition changes) rise with duration and dose.
- Disease-modifying agents should be initiated for patients with classic RA. Methotrexate and hydroxychloroquine are most commonly used for older adult patients, but monitoring for liver and blood effects are a must.
- Biologic agents include tumor necrosis factor alpha (TNF-A) inhibitors, which have been shown effective in management of RA, particularly when used in combination with methotrexate. These agents may be considered for older adult patients. No greater toxicity is reported for older adult patients, although evidence in older adult patients is sparse.

Rehabilitative intervention strategies should accompany medical management to maximize function for older adults with RA.

## Further reading

Majithia, V, Geraci SA (2007). Rheumatoid arthritis: diagnosis and management. *Am J Med* **120**(11): 936–939.

# Polymyalgia rheumatica

Polymyalgia rheumatica (PMR) is a common inflammatory syndrome that preferentially affects older adults. Patients experience rapid (days) onset of shoulder and then thigh pain that is worse in the mornings.

## Clinical features

- Patients are age 50 years or older.
- Shoulder, upper arm, and hip and/or thigh pain or stiffness for 4 weeks or longer is present in 25%–50% of patients.
- Constitutional symptoms are present in up to 30% (depression, malaise, weight loss, fever).
- Laboratory evidence of systemic inflammation (ESR >40 mm/hr; or elevated C-reactive protein [CRP])
- Adjust ESR for patient age: men: 17.3 + 0.18 (age); women: 22.1 + 0.18 (age)
- Subacromial or subdeltoid bursitis, arthritis, or tendonitis of the wrists or painful hip motion (about 33%)
- Dramatic response to low-dose corticosteroids

## Differential diagnosis

Other causes must be excluded (e.g., drug induced, inflammatory muscle disease, autoimmune disease, endocrinopathy, malignancy, chronic infection, neurological disease). Other diagnoses must be entertained if treatment with glucocorticoids does not result in rapid improvement in symptoms.

- Muscle enzymes and EMG are normal. Patients often have normochromic normocytic anemia, thrombocytosis, and mild abnormalities of liver enzymes (especially alkaline phosphatase) or renal function.
- MRI demonstrates inflammation of extra-articular synovial structures. Ultrasound may reveal effusions in the effected joints.

## Treatment

- Prednisone (starting dose 15 mg, more is rarely required) usually results in prompt resolution of PMR symptoms within 7 days.
- Treat until symptoms abate and ESR/CRP normalize, then reduce dose slowly (1 mg/month) checking for relapse of symptoms or blood tests.
- Some patients can be taken off steroids after 6–8 months, but some require long-term treatment (mean duration, 2–3 years).
- Always give bone protection (e.g., alendronate 70 mg once weekly with calcium and vitamin D).

## Diagnostic dilemma and steroid "dependency"

Patients on steroids chronically can have generalized aching, pain, and fatigue. They may resist steroid withdrawal or suffer symptoms as steroids are decreased or withdrawn, even if the characteristic syndrome and inflammatory responses are not displayed.

Many other diseases (even simple osteoarthritis) respond to steroids (although usually less dramatically). Steroid withdrawal itself can cause general aches, which some have called "pseudo-rheumatism."

Avoid this difficult situation through the following measures:
- Comprehensive assessment at onset with good record-keeping, so that others can reappraise the diagnosis if response to treatment is poor
- Considering the differential diagnosis carefully
- Discussing diagnosis and treatment with the patient
- Agreeing with the patient on a clear plan for reviewing steroid therapy

## Concomitant diagnosis: temporal arteritis (TA) or giant cell arteritis (GCA)

Claudication of the jaw or neck (discomfort or fatigue with use of the muscles) should raise suspicion of temporal arteritis (TA). There is overlap between PMR and TA.; that is, about 1/3 of patients with PMR have TA and vice versa. This includes those that have both conditions simultaneously, and others that have the two conditions at different points in time.

Suspicion of TA/GCA should be high with the following:
- Presence of claudication
- Poor or incomplete response to low-dose steroid therapy
- Persistently elevated inflammatory indices (ESR, CRP) despite initiation of steroid treatment
- Clinical or laboratory abnormality recurrence with steroid withdrawal

# Temporal (giant cell) arteritis

Temporal arteritis (TA) or giant cell arteritis (GCA) is a relatively common (1 in 500 over age 50) systemic vasculitis of medium to large vessels. Mean age of presentation is 70 (does not occur age <50). TA is more common in women and in Scandinavia and northern Europe.

## Clinical features

TA is characterized by headache, scalp tenderness, and various constitutional symptoms such as fever, weight loss, malaise, sweats, myalgias, and arthralgias in adults over age 50. Many patients have features of PMR. Vascular symptoms may be the first manifestation.

"Classic" symptoms (e.g., headache, scalp tenderness) are not invariably present at the start, so a high index of suspicion is warranted when exploring cause for unexplained anemia and elevated ESR.

Claudicatory symptoms vary depending on the supply of the occluded vessel (e.g., jaw claudication due to maxillary artery involvement).

Amaurosis fugax or blindness is due to occlusion of the ciliary artery, which supplies the optic nerve. Always suspect TA if amaurosis fugax involves both eyes (atheroma is more commonly unilateral).

## Laboratory investigations

- ESR is high, often >100.
- CRP also very high and falls faster with treatment than ESR.
- The patient may have normochromic, normocytic anemia, renal impairment, and abnormal liver enzymes, particularly increased alkaline phosphatase.
- Temporal artery biopsy (TAB) remains the gold-standard diagnostic test and should be pursued in all cases. Because the vasculitis may be patchy, it is advisable to obtain a frozen section of the vessel in the operating room. If the section is negative, strongly consider biopsy of the contralateral artery. This is particularly pertinent if the patient has started treatment.
- Duplex, high-resolution ultrasound shows the TA "halo," stenosis, or occlusions, but with limited sensitivity.
- Gadolinium-enhanced MRI can demonstrate vascular inflammation and assess the degree of occlusion.

## How to manage temporal arteritis

### General principles of management

- Guidance from a rheumatologist is often helpful.
- Daily corticosteroid is first-line therapy, starting with 40–60 mg daily for uncomplicated cases. However, amaurosis fugax is an ophthalmological emergency. Give 80–100 mg oral prednisone or high-dose methyl prednisolone IV.
- For suspected TA/GCA, obtain temporal artery biopsy (3–5 cm section is preferable since involvement is usually segmental).
- For suspected TA/GCA, especially if vascular symptoms are present, start steroids immediately. Do not delay steroids while waiting for biopsy results. Histological changes persist for 2 weeks after starting therapy.
- Some advocate weekly methotrexate to facilitate steroid dose reduction in patients with TA/GCA, although efficacy is inconclusive.
- Osteoporosis prophylaxis should be started at initiation of steroids (usually a bisphosphonate with calcium and vitamin D).
- Slowly taper the dose, usually on a month-by-month basis. Use symptoms and signs of inflammation as the guide.
- If rebound of symptoms or inflammatory markers occurs, take two steps back on the reduction schedule. Maintain that dose for 4 weeks before attempting dose reduction again.
- Beware a steroid-withdrawal syndrome, which can occur without arteritis recurrence. ESR and CRP are normal.
- NSAIDs may be a useful adjunct to treatment with corticosteroids to alleviate symptoms of PMR during corticosteroid tapering.
- Most patients require treatment for ≥2 years.

## Further reading

Barilla-LaBarca ML, Lenschow DJ, Brasington RD Jr. (2002). Polymyalgia rheumatica/temporal arteritis: recent advances. *Curr Rheumatol Rep* **4**(1):39–46.

Cantini F, Niccoli L, Nannini C, et al. (2008). Diagnosis and treatment of giant cell arteritis. *Drugs Aging* **25**(4): 281–297.

Salvarani C, Cantini F, BoiardiL, Hunder GG (2002). Polymyalgia rheumatica and giant-cell arteritis. *N Engl J Med* **347**(4):261–271.

# Gout

*Gout* is an inflammatory arthritis secondary to deposition of sodium rate crystals in and around the joints. Serum urate levels equate poorly with the disease manifestations. Flares can manifest as uric acid levels rise or fall abruptly. Older adults are at greater risk of gouty arthritis for the following reasons:
- Declining renal function and impaired uric acid excretion
- Use of hyperuricemic drug use, e.g., thiazide diuretics, low-dose aspirin, cytotoxic agents
- Flares are often precipitated by physiological stressors. Common acute precipitants include sepsis and surgery.

## Presentations
- **Acute monoarthritis** is very painful, and the joint is hot and red. Patients often refuse to bear weight or move the joint. The patient can look ill and some have fever and even chills. Acute gouty arthritis of the great toe represents the classic attack (podagra) but can involve any joint (knee, wrist, fingers, and toes).
- **Chronic tophaceous deposit** is most commonly in the finger joints and ears; it can occasionally open and drain white, tophaceous paste.
- **Olecranon bursitis**
- **Uric acid kidney** stones are radioluscent stones that cannot be detected on plain X-ray.

## Laboratory investigations
- During an acute attack, serum uric acid may be normal or high and is therefore an unhelpful test to obtain.
- **WBC, ESR**, and **CRP** are usually high or very high.
- **Arthrocentesis** is the definitive diagnostic procedure.
- **Synovial fluid characteristics**
  - May be cloudy or frankly purulent on visual inspection.
  - Microscopy shows many inflammatory cells.
  - Under polarized light, negatively birefringent uric acid crystals are seen in joint fluid or piercing phagocytes.
- **X-rays** are usually normal in early disease but demonstrates small erosions with an overhanging edge at the joint line in chronic gout.

The first step in managing an acute gouty flare is to exclude the possibility of an infectious arthritis (bacterial). If in doubt, initiate IV antibiotic coverage until cultures are known to be negative.

## Treatment
### For acute gout attack
- NSAIDs are first-line therapy unless contraindicated (e.g., renal impairment).
- If NSAIDs are contraindicated, steroids can be used once infection has been excluded. Local steroid injections may be tried (e.g., methylprednisolone 40 mg either intra-articular injection for a single larger joint) or IM or PO for multiple or inaccessible joints (e.g., prednisone 40 mg each day for 7 days).

### Colchicine
Colchicine given hourly to end points of symptom resolution or diarrhea and vomiting is *no longer recommended*.

### Analgesics
Patients for whom NSAIDs, colchicines, and steroids are contraindicated or anticipated to be poorly tolerated can be managed with analgesics (e.g., codeine) alone.

### Chronic gouty arthritis
For the first one or two attacks:
- Change drugs (stop thiazide and aspirin).
- Lifestyle advice:
  - Reduce alcohol.
  - Reduce dietary purines (meat).
  - Lose weight.

For recurrent flares (several attacks per year) or problematic tophacous deposits, consider urate-lowering therapy. Initiate under the protection of chronic colchicine therapy (0.5 mg daily or three times a week if renal insufficiency is present) to reduce the risk of precipitating a gouty flare. Patients on chronic colchicine should be monitored for renal insufficiency, cytopenias, and development of neuromyopathy.

A uricosuric agent (e.g., probenecid) should be tried first but is ineffective in patients with renal insufficiency and contraindicated if there is a history of renal stones.

Allopurinol (start at 100 mg/day and increase carefully to 300 mg/day) can result in hypersensitivity (fever, cytopenia, progressive renal failure), particularly in patients with renal insufficiency.

## Further reading
Eggebeen AT (2007). Gout: an update. *Am Fam Physician* **76**:801–808.
Fox R (2008). Management of recurrent gout. *BMJ* **336**(7639):329.
Keith MP, Gilliland WR (2007). Updates in the management of gout. *Am J Med* **120**:221–224.

# Pseudogout

### Features of pseudogout

This is an acute, episodic synovitis closely resembling gout, except that
- Calcium pyrophosphate rather than uric acid crystals (with positive rather than negative birefringence) are found.
- Large joints are more commonly affected (especially knees but also shoulder, hips, wrists, and elbows).
- It is not associated with tophi, bursitis, or stones.
- X-rays often show calcification of articular cartilage, "chondrocalcinosis," in the affected joint, but can also show calification in the symphysis pubis and in triangular cartilage of the wrist, hips, knees, or fingers of asymptomatic older patients.
- Pseudogout does *not* respond to allopurinol or uricosuric agents, so consider this diagnosis when recurrent attacks persist despite allopurinol treatment.

### Management

Make a confident diagnosis. This usually involves immediate synovial fluid sampling and microscopy to exclude infection and gout.

Effective treatments for acute pseudogout include the following:
- Joint aspiration confirms the diagnosis but also alleviates symptoms.
- Oral NSAIDs
- Colchicine may be useful to prevent additional attacks, as with gouty arthritis management. Monitoring is required to prevent renal insufficiency, cytopenia, and development of neuromyopathy.
- Corticosteroids as per acute gouty arthritis management
- Analgesics as per acute gouty arthritis management

### Other clinical syndromes

Pseudoseptic arthritis can cause acute confusion in older adults. Patients may be systemically ill with a fever and highly elevated inflammatory markers.

In pseudorheumatoid arthritis, calcium pyrophosphate dehydrate (CPPD) deposition can occur simultaneously in multiple joints and be responsible for chronic polyarticular synovitis reminiscent of RA.

### Further reading

Rosenthal AK (2007). Update in calcium deposition diseases. *Curr Opin Rheumatol* **19**(2):158–162.

# Paget's disease of the bone

This is a very common bone disease of old age (up to 10% prevalence, occurs equally in men and women). It is usually clinically silent—only about 5% of cases are symptomatic. Paget's disease is characterized by abnormal remodeling, which is thought to be due to slow viral infection of osteoclasts.

It most commonly affects the pelvis, femur, spine, skull, and tibia. The resultant bone is expanded and disordered and can cause pain, and pathological fracture and predisposes to osteosarcoma.

## Presentation

- Most commonly as asymptomatic elevated alkaline phosphatase (ALP)
- Often an incidental finding on a pelvis or skull X-ray

*Less common presentation*

- Pathological fracture (especially hip and pelvis). Patients whose pain worsens suddenly should be evaluated for fracture.
- Bone pain: Constant pain is commonly in the legs, especially at night. The diseased bone itself can be painful or deformity can lead to accelerated joint disease at the hip, knee, or spine.
- Deformity: Bowing of legs or upper arm is often asymmetrical. The skull can take on a characteristic 'bossed' shape due to overgrowth of frontal bones.
- Deafness: Bone expansion in the skull compresses the eighth cranial nerve, causing conduction deafness, which can be severe.
- Other neurological compression syndromes, e.g., spinal cord (paraplegia), optic nerve (blindness), brain stem compression (dysphagia and hydrocephalus)
- Osteosarcoma can result in sudden or progressive worsening of pain.

## Laboratory investigations

- ALP levels are consistently elevated.
  - The bone isoenzyme is more specific and useful when liver function is abnormal.
  - Rarely (e.g., if only one bone is involved), total ALP can be normal but the bone isoenzyme is always raised.
- Other markers of bone turnover (type I collagen turnover products) are raised.
- X-rays show areas of osteopenia mixed with sclerosis, disordered bone texture and bone expansion (a diagnostic feature).
- Radioisotope bone scans show hot spots.
- Immobile patients with very active disease can become hypercalcemic, although this is rare. If calcium and ALP are raised, there is more likely to be another diagnosis (e.g., carcinomatosis, hyperparathyroidism).

## Management

As most cases are asymptomatic often no treatment is required. Symptomatic cases may warrant referral to a rheumatologist.

Analgesia and joint replacement may be needed.

Fractures often require internal fixation to correct deformity and because they heal poorly.

Bisphosphonates (e.g., risedronate 30 mg/day for 2 months or intermittent IV infusions of pamidronate) are very useful. They have several effects:

- Reduce pain
- Reduce vascularity before elective surgery
- Improve healing after fracture
- Improve neurological compression syndromes
- Reduce serum calcium in hypercalcemia.

Calcitonin and mithramycin are now rarely used.

Alkaline phosphatase, bone turnover markers, and occasionally nuclear bone scans can be used to assess treatment response.

## Further reading

Josse RG, Hanley DA, Kendler D, Ste Marie LG, Adachi JD, Brown J (2007). Diagnosis and treatment of Paget's disease of bone. *Clin Invest Med* **30**:E210–E223.

Ralston SH, Langston AL, et al. (2008). Pathogenesis and management of Paget's disease of bone. *Lancet* **372**(9633): 155–163.

Siris ES, Lyles KW, Singer FR, Meunier PJ (2006). Medical management of Paget's disease of bone: indications for treatment and review of current therapies. *J Bone Miner Res* **21** (Suppl 2):P94–P98.

# Osteomyelitis

Osteomyelitis is infection of the bone that is most common in the very young and the very old. It is important in geriatric practice because it complicates conditions that are common in older patients, yet presentation is often nonspecific and indolent so the diagnosis may be missed.

### Vertebral osteomyelitis

- Most common in older patients
- Usually affects the thoracolumbar spine
- Patients complain of mild backache and malaise and will often have local tenderness. Always "walk" the examining fingers down the spine, applying pressure to find local bony pain.
- Vertebral osteomyelitis (commonly T10–11) may lead to
  - Perivertebral abscess with a risk of cord compression.
  - Vertebral body collapse with angular kyphosis.
- Discitis occurs when the infection involves the intervertebral disc. The patient is relatively less septic, and X-rays appear normal until disease is very advanced (at which point end-plate erosion can occur).
- Hematogenous spread is most common, often after urinary tract infection, catheterization, intravenous cannula insertion, or other instrumentation.
- It is commonly due to *Staphylococcus aureus*, less commonly gram-negative bacilli, rarely tuberculosis.

### Osteomyelitis of other bones

Susceptible individuals (e.g., diabetics with vascular disease and neuropathy) are prone to osteomyelitis of the small bones of the feet. This may be mistaken for podagra (gouty arthritis of the foot). Organisms include *Staphylococcus aureus*, *Staphylococcus epidermidis* (especially with prostheses), gram-negative bacilli, and anaerobes.

- As a complication of ulceration (venous or pressure ulcers)
- As a complication of orthopedic surgery

### Clinical features of osteomyelitis

Pain is usual but may be missed if there is a pre-existing pressure sore or the patient has peripheral neuropathy and foot osteomyelitis (e.g., diabetics). Malaise is common. Fever may be absent.

### Laboratory investigations

- Blood cultures should be taken in all patients and are positive in around half.
- Leukocytosis is variable.
- ESR and CRP are usually raised (although very nonspecific).
- MRI is the most sensitive and specific test. Changes may be diagnostic, even in early disease.
- X-ray changes lag behind clinical changes by about 10 days. X-rays are initially normal or show soft tissue swelling. Later classic changes develop: periosteal reaction, sequestra (islands of necrosis), bone abscesses, and sclerosis of neighboring bone.

- Radioisotope bone scanning will show a hot spot with osteomyelitis, but will not distinguish this from many other conditions (e.g., fracture, arthritis, noninfectious inflammation, metastases, etc.).
- Biopsy or fine needle aspiration (FNA) of bone is required to guide antibiotic therapy. This may be done through the base of an ulcer or using radiological guidance (ultrasound is useful here).
- Wound swabs reveal colonizing organisms and are often misleading.

## Treatment

- General measures such as analgesia and fluids if needed
- The joint/bone should be immobilized where possible.
- Obtaining tissue specimens permits bacterial culture and determination of antimicrobial sensitivity. After specimens are obtained but prior to results, start therapy empirically based on the most likely pathogen (e.g., *S. Aureus,* gram-negative organisms).
- Surgical drainage should be considered after 36 hours if systemic upset continues, or if there is deep pus on imaging (required in approximately 30%).
- Treatment is initially intravenous, often later converted to oral therapy. Total treatment duration is usually many weeks or months (depending on sensitivity of organism and extent and location of infection).

## Complications

- **Metastatic infection**
- **Bacterial or septic arthritis**
- **Chronic osteomyelitis** infection becomes walled off in cavities within the bone, discharging to the surface by a sinus. Symptoms relapse and remit as sinuses close and reopen. Bone is at risk of pathological fracture. Management is long and difficult—this is a miserable complication of joint replacement. Culture organisms and use appropriate antibiotics to limit spread. Surgical removal of infected bone and/or prosthesis is required for cure. Involve an infectious disease specialist if possible.
- **Malignant otitis externa** occurs when otitis externa spreads to cause osteomyelitis of the skull base. It occurs particularly in frail, older diabetics. It is caused by pseudomonas and anaerobes. Facial nerve palsy develops in half of cases, with possible involvement of nerves IX–XII. It requires prolonged antibiotics, specialist ENT input, and possible surgical debridement.

# Problems of the axial skeleton: cervical spondylosis and myelopathy

Degeneration in the cervical spine can lead to radiculopathy (compression of nerve roots leaving spinal foramina) and myelopathy (cord compression). The resulting mixture of lower (nerve root) and upper (cord) nerve damage causes pain, weakness, and numbness. Progress is usually gradual but can be sudden (especially following trauma). The disease is unusual before the age of 50.

## History

Neck pain and restricted movement may be present but are neither specific nor sensitive indicators of nerve damage. Pain may radiate to shoulder, chest or arm in a dermatomal distribution.

Arms and hands become clumsy, especially for fine movements (e.g., doing up buttons). Weakness, numbness, and paraesthesia can occur.

Leg symptoms usually occur later, with an upper motor neuron spastic weakness and a wide-based and/or ataxic gait, often with falls.

Urinary dysfunction is unusual and late. Rarely this condition can cause vertebrobasilar insufficiency symptoms (see p. 94).

## Signs

Arms have predominantly lower motor signs with weakness, muscle wasting, and segmental reflex loss. The classical "inverted supinator" sign is due to a C5/6 lesion, where the supinator tendon jerk is lost but the finger jerk (C7) is augmented—when the wrist is tapped, the fingers flex.

Legs may have brisk reflexes, increased tone, clonus, and up-going plantars. In severe cases a spastic paraparesis with a sensory level can develop.

Forward flexion of the neck produces Lhermitte's sign—an electric sensation that radiates from the neck down the spine or into the arms.

## Differential diagnosis

This is wide and includes the following:

- Syringomyelia
- Motor neuron disease (look for signs above the neck and an absence of sensory symptoms and signs)
- Peripheral neuropathy (no upper motor neuron signs)
- Vitamin $B_{12}$ deficiency
- Other causes of spastic gait disorders
- Normal-pressure hydrocephalus
- Amyotrophic lateral sclerosis

## Investigations

- **Plain X-rays** in older people almost always show degenerative changes or osteoarthritis and correlate poorly with symptoms. Plain X-rays should only be obtained to exclude other pathology or to evaluate spinal instability.
- **MRI scanning** is the imaging study of choice. Bone and soft tissue structures and spinal cord compression can be assessed.

- **Electromyographic studies** (EMG and nerve conduction velocity) confirm the diagnosis and assess neurophysiological function. The information obtained is necessary to assess need for surgical intervention and to exclude other neurological processes.
- **CT scanning** may also be useful in diagnosis and planning treatment.

## Management

### Cervical collars
- Low soft collars can sometimes help to alleviate radicular pain if consistently worn (including during sleep).
- Soft pillows can reduce nerve compression during sleep by providing proper positioning of the head and neck.
- Hard collars stabilize the cervical spine following trauma.

### Surgical stabilization
Because function is rarely restored once lost, prompt surgical consultation should be obtained for patients with the following conditions:
- Progressive neurological deterioration (especially if rapidly progressive)
- Myelopathy more than radiculopathy.

Surgery does not guarantee complete relief from pain.

## Further reading
Mazanec D, Reddy A (2007). Medical management of cervical spondylosis. *Neurosurgery* **60**(1 Suppl 11): S43–S50.

# The painful back

### Assessment

- History should include position, quality, duration, and radiation of pain as well as associated sensory symptoms, bladder, or bowel problems and a systems review.
- Undress the patient and look for bruising and deformity.
- Conduct maneuvers to determine what reproduces painful symptoms.
- Apply pressure to each vertebra, in turn looking for local tenderness.
- Look for restriction of movement and gait abnormality.
- Always evaluate for a sensory level.
- Check for impairment in bowel or bladder function.
- Examine abdominal and peripheral arterial flow (bruits, pulses).

### Causes

- **Osteoarthritis** of the facet joints becomes more common than disc pathology with advancing age (discs are less pliable and less likely to herniate) (p. 487).
- **Osteoporosis** and vertebral crush fractures can cause acute well-localized pain, chronic pain, or no pain at all (p. 490).
- **Metastatic cancer** should always be considered especially if pain is new or severe, there are constitutional symptoms such as weight loss, or pain from an apparent fracture fails to improve.
- **Vertebral osteomyelitis and infective discitis** (p. 508) should be considered in those with fever and raised inflammatory markers, especially if they are immunosuppressed (e.g., rheumatoid arthritis on steroids).
- Spinal stenosis should be considered in patients with back pain and "pseudoclaudication," which occurs when the patient walks down an incline. Symptoms are alleviated by bending forward and exacerbated on spine extension. A stationary bicycle can be useful in distinguishing this from peripheral vascular disease.

Not all back pain comes from the spine. Differential diagnoses to not miss include pancreatitis or pancreatic cancer, biliary colic, duodenal ulcer, aortic aneurysm, renal pain, retroperitoneal pathology, pulmonary embolism, Guillain–Barré syndrome, and myocardial infarction.

### Investigations

- Complete blood count, sedimentation rate (and myeloma screen if raised), C-reactive protein, ALP, calcium and PSA (in men).
- Plain X-rays comprise the initial imaging study to confirm some diagnoses but can also be misleading given the high prevalence of degenerative and osteoarthritis findings in older adults.
- MRI provides useful information on the integrity of the spinal cord and is also helpful in diagnosing spinal stenosis, osteomyelitis, infective discitis, and metastases.
- A bone scan may be useful to evaluate suspected osteomyelitis or discitis, metastatic cancer, and multiple sites of pain, but may be normal with myeloma.

- Electrodiagnostic studies (EMG and nerve conduction velocity) are required to assess neurophysiological function in patients with pain and neurological impairment.

## Treatment

In addition to cautiously prescribed analgesics and/or anti-inflammatory agents for symptom relief, the underlying diagnosis dictates what the appropriate management is. Therapies are as follows:
- Acute vertebral compression (p. 490): vertebralplasty, bisphosphonates, or calcitonin
- Radiotherapy is very effective for metastatic deposits.
- Urgent surgery or radiotherapy should be considered for cord compression, with high-dose intravenous steroids in the meantime.

General therapies for most diagnoses include the following:
- Standard analgesia
- Physiotherapy is often helpful in improving pain and function or at least preventing deconditioning.
- Exercise and weight loss (if obese) are difficult to achieve but will help.
- Transcutaneous nerve stimulators can help some and are without side effects.
- Antispasmodics (e.g., cyclobenzaprine) should be used with caution, given sedating and anticholinergic effects in older adults. Diazepam should be avoided because of its long half-life and lingering effects in older adult patients.
- Acupuncture can achieve relief from painful symptoms.
- Consider referral to a pain specialist for local injections, e.g., facet joints or epidurals.
- Once serious pathology has been excluded, a chiropractor or osteopath can sometimes help.

## Further reading

Broder J, Snarski JT (2007). Back pain in the elderly. *Clin Geriatr Med* **23**(2):271–289.

# Regional rheumatic problems: the painful hip

There are many causes of hip pain in older adults. The initial step is to determine the origin of painful symptoms: is pain truly arising from the hip or is it referred from another source?

- Referred pain from the spine. Lumbar spine disease can be the source of "hip pain" or may coexist with hip disease. The straight-leg maneuver may reproduce pain. Reflex deficits may be present.
- Referred pain from the knee
- Psoas abscess

Having ascertained that pain is arising from the hip, consider the following diagnoses.

### Hip fracture

The absence of a recent fall and ability to weight bear should not prevent you from obtaining an X-ray to evaluate acute or severe hip pain. Always

- Get two views (AP and lateral) of the pelvis and proximal femur.
- Have the X-ray films reported by a radiologist—some fractures can be subtle.
- Check for pubic ramus fractures as well as fractures of the femoral head and shaft.
- If initial films are normal but clinical suspicion is high, consider repeating X-ray in a few days (bone fragments can move apart) or proceed to an MRI or bone scan. It is important to make the diagnosis early.

Almost all hip fractures require surgical intervention no matter how frail the patient. Therefore, operative risk assessment (medical consultation) should be obtained early.

With *intracapsular fractures* (femoral neck) the affected limb will be held in external rotation and may appear shorter. Tenderness to palpation over the groin may be observed. Joint replacement is the treatment of choice because it provides prompt pain relief and immediate return to full weight-bearing status.

With *trochanteric fractures* there is tenderness to palpation over the fracture, but no appreciable change in length or positioning. Open reduction and internal fixation can repair the fracture. Long-term disadvantages might include mal-union and leg shortening if there is slippage. Weight-bearing status following surgery is limited and changes under the direction of the orthopedic surgeon.

In any bed-bound patient after a fall, look for inability to lift the leg off the bed and pain on movement (especially rotation), even if they are not fit to stand.

Low-energy pelvic fractures in older people rarely require surgery. Even with surgery the 30-day mortality for a fractured neck of femur is high (over 15%). Remember to initiate osteoporosis treatment.

## Osteoarthritis
- Pain is "boreing" and stiffness occurs after rest.
- Painful or restriction movement occurs in all planes, with internal rotation lost first.
- Total hip replacement is now widely available and very effective.

Consider referral for radiographic study for moderate to severe disease with ongoing pain or disability despite trial of conservative treatment.

There is a 1% mortality rate but older people often have a good long-term result. Revision surgery is rarely needed because activity levels are lower than in younger people (and life expectancy less).

## Avascular necrosis of the femoral head
- This should be considered in patients receiving chronic steroid therapy or who have autoimmune disease, hemoglobinopathy, or traumatic injury.
- Pain is dull and localized to the groin but does not reproduce on motion of the hip.
- Plain X-rays may reveal a "crescent" sign.
- MRI is the imaging technique of choice.
- Surgical decompression is the intervention of choice.
- Femoral head collapse with secondary OA is the feared complication.

## Other causes of hip pain
- Paget's disease (p. 506)
- Septic arthritis is a rare and difficult diagnosis to make, but consider joint aspiration under ultrasound if your patient appears septic with a very painful hip, especially after recent hip surgery.

# The painful shoulder

Shoulder pain is a common problem in older adults. Early initiation of therapy can preserve function and prevent disability associated with chronic shoulder problems. Before diagnosing one of the conditions listed below, exclude systemic problems such as polymyalgia rheumatica (p. 498) and rheumatoid arthritis (p. 497). Remember that neck problems, diaphragmatic pathology, apical lung cancer, and angina can cause pain that is referred to the shoulder.

## Common therapeutic options

Although the following conditions are anatomically distinct, they share common treatment options.

- Analgesics and nonsteroidal anti-inflammatory agents can be used
- Corticosteroid injection can alleviate pain enough to initiate therapy.
- All require evaluation by a physical therapist to guide dedicated practice of exercises.
- Physiotherapy and exercises should be initiated early to prevent development of adhesive capsulitis.

## Bicepital tendonitis

- Pain in a specific area (anterior/lateral humeral head) aggravated by supination on the forearm while elbow is held flexed against the body
- Treatment is rest and corticosteroid injection followed by gentle biceps stretching exercises.

## Subacromial bursitis

- Dull ache of the shoulder that often precludes sleeping on the affected slide
- Diffuse tenderness to palpation
- Nonpainful passive shoulder motion excludes intracapsular pathology
- Often coexists with rotator cuff pathology

## Rotator cuff tendonitis

- Dull ache radiating to upper arm with "painful arc" (pain between 60 and 120 degrees when abducting arm)
- Rest, occasionally with short-term immobilization in a sling

## Rotator cuff tear

- This may occur following trauma—can be a relatively obscure event in older adult patients.
- Tears may be partial or complete. In the case of the complete tear, the patient will be unable to actively abduct the arm or sustain its weight against gravity.
- Ultrasound and MRI are diagnostic.
- Treat with rest following injury.
- Surgical repair is possible in cases of acute injury in healthy and highly functional older adults.

## Adhesive capsulitis (frozen shoulder)

- Can develop following direct trauma, stroke, and even minor injury
- More common in diabetics without any inciting event
- Loss of rotational movement (external lost early, abduction, extension and flexion)
- Initially painful for weeks to months then stiff (frozen) for further 4–12 months
- Mainstay of treatment is physiotherapy to restore motion and function

### Further reading

Burbank KM, Stevenson JH, et al. (2008). Chronic shoulder pain: part I. Evaluation and diagnosis. *Am Fam Physician* **77**(4): 453–460.
Burbank KM. Stevenson JH, et al. (2008). Chronic shoulder pain: part II. Treatment. *Am Fam Physician* **77**(4): 493–497.

# The older foot

Foot problems are very common (>80% over 65) and can cause major disability including increased susceptibility to falls. It is a particular problem in older people for the following reasons:

- Multiple degenerative and disease pathologies occur and interact.
- Many older people cannot reach their feet, so monitoring and basic hygiene (especially nail cutting) may be limited.
- Patients think foot problems are a part of aging or are embarrassed by them and do not seek treatment.
- Health professionals often neglect to examine feet and are too slow to refer for specialist foot care. It is common to find a patient naked under a hospital gown but still with thick socks on.
- Inappropriate footwear may be worn. Many older people cannot afford or refuse to wear orthotic shoes.

Regular podiatric nail care is a Medicare benefit for patients with diabetes mellitus or peripheral vascular disease.

### Nails

- Very long nails can curl back and cut into toes.
- Nails thicken and become more brittle with age. This is worsened by repeated trauma (e.g., bad footwear), poor circulation, or diabetes. Ultimately, the nail looks like a rams horn (onychogryphosis) and cannot be cut with ordinary nail clippers.
- Fungal nail infection (onychomycosis) produces a similar thickened, discolored nail.
- Ingrown nails can cause pain and recurring infection.

### Skin

- Calluses (hard skin)
- Corns (painful calluses over pressure points with a nucleus/core)
- Cracks and ulceration
- Cellulitis

### Between the toes

Fungal infection ("athlete's foot") is very common. The skin maceration that results is a common cause of cellulitis.

### Bone or joint disease

- A *bunion* (hallux valgus) is an outpointing deformity of the big toe, which can overlap the second toe.
- *Hammer toes* are flexion deformities of proximal interphalangeal (IP) joints.
- *Claw toes* have deformities at both IP joints.
- Osteoarthritis or gout of the metatarsophalangeal (MTP) joint causes pain, rigidity, and difficulty walking.
- *Neuropathic foot:* long-standing severe sensory loss in a foot (e.g., diabetics, tabes dorsalis) with multiple stress fractures and osteoporosis disrupting the biomechanics of joints (Charcot's joint). The foot or ankle is swollen and red but painless with loss of arches (rockerbottom foot).

## Circulation impairment

- Common
- Assess vasculature if there is pain, ulceration, infection, or skin changes.

## Sensory impairment

- Touch, pain, and joint position sense are all important to maintaining normal feet.

## Other foot problems

- Obesity
- Edema
- Skin disorders

## Management

*Prevention: advice to patients*

- Instruct patients to inspect both feet frequently (at least every other day). A hand mirror assists inspection of the sole.
  If patients cannot see, reach, or feel their feet, someone else should help them.
- Examine for swelling, discoloration, ulceration, cuts, calluses, or corns.
- If these are identified, consult a health professional (podiatrist, nurse, or doctor) promptly.
- Wash feet twice daily in warm water with mild simple soap. If feet are numb, check that the water temperature is not too hot with a hand or a thermometer (35–40°C is best).
- After washing, dry feet thoroughly, particularly between the toes.
- Change socks or stockings daily.
- Dry, hard, or thick skin should be softened with emollients such as aqueous cream or liquid and white soft paraffin ointment ("50:50").
- Footwear should be supportive but soft. Take particular care with new footwear, inspecting feet frequently after short periods of wear to ensure that no sores have developed.
- Avoid barefoot walking.
- Cut nails regularly, cutting them straight across and not too short.

*Treatment*

- Podiatrists can debride calluses and corns and use dressings and pressure-relieving pads to prevent them from recurring.
- Treat athlete's foot (e.g., cotrimazole cream twice daily for 1 week).
- Properly fitting shoes and orthotics can alleviate painful symptoms and improve biomechanical efficiency.
- Surgery may be used to remove nails or correct severe bone deformity.

# Contractures

*Contractures* are joint deformities caused by damaged connective tissue. When a joint is immobilized (through depressed conscious level, loss of neural input, or local tissue damage) the muscle, ligaments, tendons, and skin can become inelastic and shortened, causing joints to be flexed.

Common causes worldwide include polio, cerebral palsy, and leprosy; in geriatric medicine common causes include stroke, dementia, and musculoskeletal conditions, e.g., fracture. Contractures are an under-recognized cause of disability—they occur to some degree in about a third of nursing home residents. It is still common to find patients who are bed-bound and permanently curled into the fetal position.

## Problems

- *Pain* occurs especially on moving a joint but can occur at rest
- *Hygiene:* Skin surfaces may oppose (e.g., the hand after stroke or groins in abduction/flexion contractures), making it difficult for care and painful for the patient to keep the skin clean and odorless.
- *Pressure areas:* Abnormal posture can put pressure areas at increased risk.
- *Aesthetics:* Although the lack of movement causes most disability, the abnormal posture or appearance can be more noticeable and distressing.
- *Function:* Chronic bed-bound patients may become so flexed that they are unable to sit out in a chair.

## Prevention

When immobilization is short term, e.g., after a fracture, passive stretching followed by exercise regimens should be initiated promptly.

All health-care staff should understand the importance of maintaining patients' mobility (including sitting out of bed for short periods) and positioning of immobile patients.

Preventative measures are rarely successful at preventing contractures in joints with long-term immobility, e.g., in residual hemiparesis after stroke. Splinting might help mold the position.

## Treatment

Periodic injection of botulinum toxin is often successful when muscle spasticity is the major problem. There are no real adverse effects, but some patients develop an antibody response after repeated treatment, which renders therapy less effective. Newer Botox® preparations are less immunogenic.

There is little point in using muscle relaxants except to help with pain. Even then, drugs such as baclofen, dantrolene, and diazepam usually cause side effects of drowsiness before they reach therapeutic levels.

Surgery (e.g., tendon division) has a place in severe cases.

Physiotherapy can, to some extent, reverse established changes, especially if not severe and of relatively recent onset.

Serial casting should not be pursued in older adult patients.

## Further reading

Huckstep RL (2007). Management of neglected joint contractures. *Clin Orthop Relat Res* **456**:58–64.

# Pressure injuries

**William Greenough, III**

# Pressure sores

*Pressure sores* are areas of skin and deep tissues necrosis due to pressure-induced ischemia found on the sacrum, heels, over greater trochanters, and shoulders, etc. They are also known as decubitus ulcers or bedsores. Their incidence is higher in the hospital (new sores form during acute illness) but prevalence is higher in long-stay community settings (healing takes months or years).

Average hospital prevalence is 5%–10% despite drives to improve education and preventative strategies. The financial and staffing resource burden of pressure sores is huge. New bed technologies have not altered the increasing incidence over the past 20–30 years.

### Risk factors

These include age, immobility (especially postoperative), low or high body weight, malnutrition, dehydration, incontinence, neurological damage (either neuropathy or decreased conscious level), sedative drugs, and vascular impairment.

Several scoring systems (e.g., Braden scale) combine these factors to stratify risk. They aid clinical judgment of individual patient risk.

### Grading

| | |
|---|---|
| 0 | Skin hyperemia |
| I | Non-blanching erythema |
| II | Broken skin or blistering (epidermis ± dermis only) |
| III | Ulcer down to subcutaneous fat |
| IV | Ulcer down to bone, joint, or tendon |

It takes less than 2 hours for a subcutaneous tissue infarction that results in a pressure ulcer to develop, and the causative insult often occurs just prior to or at the time of admission (on ambulances, intraoperatively, at home). Hypotension is a major risk factor for pressure sores.

There is considerable lag between the ischemic insult and the resulting ulcer. Grade I erythema can progress to deep ulcers over days or weeks without further ischemic insult. An eschar must be incised to be certain there is viable tissue beneath it, except in the heels.

### Mechanisms

- **Pressure:** Normal capillary pressure is 24–34 mmHg—pressures exceeding 35 mmHg compress and cause ischemia. This pressure is easily exceeded on a simple foam mattress at pressure points such as heels.
- **Shear** Where skin is pulled away from the fixed axial skeleton small blood vessels can be kinked or torn. When a patient is propped up in bed or a "geriatric chair" or dragged (e.g., during a lift or transfer), there is considerable shear on the sacrum.
- **Friction** Rubbing the skin decreases its integrity, especially at moving extremities, e.g., elbows and heels. Avoid crumbs, drip sets, and debris between the patient and sheets. Massage of pressure areas is no longer recommended.
- **Moisture** Sweat, urine, and feces cause maceration and decrease skin integrity.

## Management

Prevention demands not only awareness but also adequate hands-on staff at the bedside who are aware of the risk factor—e.g., the Braden Scale and NICE guidelines from October 2003 suggest that all patients be risk assessed within 6 hours of admission (www.nice.org.uk). Regular reassessment during hospital admission should occur especially for immobile patients.

It is not known how often immobile, high-risk patients should be turned in bed. Every-2-hour turns are historically based and rarely achieved. Frequency should be judged individually. Use of modern mattresses may decrease frequency but doesn't remove the need for turns. Avoid friction and sheer by using correct manual handling devices and sufficient bedside staffing. Consider limiting sitting in a "geriatric" chair to 2 hours.

For pressure-relieving devices consider both beds and chairs. Most hospitals have access to these to reduce pressure injury risk and personnel cost. Whether use of these devices is more cost-effective than adequate bedside nursing is unknown. They include the following:

- High-specification foam mattresses
- Alternating-pressure mattresses (air pockets intermittently inflate and deflate), e.g., Nimbus
- Air fluidized (warm air is pumped through tiny spheres to produce a fluid-like cushion)

### Promote a healing environment

- Provide nutrition such as protein and calorie supplements. There is no evidence to support use of specific vitamins (e.g., vitamin C) or minerals (e.g., zinc), but they are unlikely to harm.
- Manage incontinence (one of the few times that a geriatrician might recommend a catheter).
- Maintain good glycemic control in diabetics.
- Correct anemia (normochromic, normocytic anemia is common).

### Debridement

Dead tissue should be removed with a scalpel. No anesthetic is required because dead tissue is insensate. Occasionally, topical collagenases are helpful. In some patients, surgery, e.g., debridement, skin grafting, or myocutaneous flaps, may be needed.

### Dressings

There is enormous choice available with little evidence to favor one type over another. Use gels to soften, hydrofiber/gels (often seaweed based) for cavities, then a secondary dressing over the top. The general principles in sorting out dressings are as follows:

1. Mesodermic (deep) wounds require hydrophilic dressing with or without microbicides.
2. In stagnant but clean wounds that are tunneled use a vacuum system.
3. To heal skin once a wound is filled in, use hydrophobic dressings and absorbent materials.
4. Collagen-based dressing may be used for wounds not responding to other methods, to stimulate granulation.

*Antimicrobial agents*

All ulcers are colonized (surface swabs positive 100%); only 1% at any given time have active infection causing illness. Look for systemic surrounding cellulitis and signs of infection, and check blood cultures.

## Further reading

Bergstrom N, Braden BA (1992). A prospective study of pressure sore risk among institutionalized elderly. *J Am Geriatr Soc* **40**:747–758.

Reddy M, Gill SS, Rochon PA (2006). Preventing pressure ulcers: a systematic review. *JAMA* **296**:974–984.

# Compression mononeuropathy

- Where nerves are compressed against bone they can be damaged (see Table 18.1).
- This is usually a demyelination injury (neuropraxia), which resolves spontaneously in 2–12 weeks.
- Alcohol, diabetes, and malnutrition increase susceptibility.
- Any patient who has had a period of immobility on a hard surface is at risk, especially if they were unconscious.
- Such injuries can be misdiagnosed as strokes but are lower motor neuron in one nerve territory only.
- Nerve conduction studies are rarely required to confirm diagnosis.
- Treatment is supportive—many such patients are acutely unwell—but recognition becomes more important during rehabilitation.

**Table 18.1** Effects of nerve damage

| Nerve damaged | Site/mechanism | Motor effects | Sensory effects |
|---|---|---|---|
| Radial | Upper arm—spiral groove on humerus | Wrist drop and finger extension weakness | Small area of numbness at base of thumb |
| Ulnar | Elbow—cubital groove | Little and ring finger flexors and finger abduction and adduction | Little and ring finger |
| Common peroneal | Knee—fibula head | Foot drop and failure of foot eversion and toe extension | Lateral calf and top of foot |
| Sciatic | Buttock or thigh | Knee flexors plus common peroneal as above | Posterior thigh plus common peroneal as above |

# Rhabdomyolysis

Following prolonged pressure (e.g., if patient cannot get up after a fall or stroke or after a period of unconsciousness), muscle necrosis can occur, which releases myoglobin. High levels are nephrotoxic, precipitating to cause tubule obstruction with acute renal failure, especially as these patients are usually dehydrated.

Remember to check creatinine kinase (CK) and electrolytes in all patients who have been found on the floor for a prolonged or indeterminate period.

Many frail older patients with bruises after a fall will have raised CK levels without developing renal problems, but ensuring good hydration (often with 24–48 hours of intravenous fluids) and repeating renal function in such patients is good practice.

Suspect the full rhabdomyolysis syndrome in any patient with

- Prolonged unconsciousness
- Signs of acute pressure sores of the skin, and
- CK levels at least five times normal.

Urine may be dark ("Coca-Cola" urine) and urinalysis is positive to hemoglobin but without red blood cells. Hyperkelamia and hypocalcemia can occur.

Treat with aggressive rehydration. Monitor urine output, electrolytes, and renal function closely. If renal failure occurs, consider temporary dialysis. Prognosis is good if the patient survives the initial few days.

Other causes of rhabdomyolysis include drugs (especially statins), compartment syndrome, acute myositis, severe exertion, e.g., seizures or rigors, heat stroke (p. 430), and neuroleptic malignant syndrome (p. 155).

# Genitourinary medicine

**Wilmer Roberts**
**Misop Han**

# The aging genitourinary system

### Changes in women

Estrogen levels fall following menopause (usually around age 50). This leads to vaginal epithelial atrophy, decreased vaginal lubrication, and acidification and greater vulnerability to vaginal and urinary infection. The uterus and ovaries atrophy and the vagina becomes smaller and less elastic.

Hormone replacement therapy (HRT) improves menopausal symptoms but has other serious adverse effects that severely limit its use.

### Changes in men

There are gradual changes in anatomy and function but no sudden change in fertility. Most older men remain fertile. Testicular mass and sperm production fall as does semen quality. The prostate gland enlarges—benign prostatic hyperplasia (BPH)—but the volume of ejaculate remains similar.

Erection becomes less sustained and less firm, and the refractory period between erections lengthens.

Testosterone levels remain stable or decrease slightly. In a minority of men more severe falls are seen and hypogonadism may become symptomatic, manifesting as fatigue, weakness, muscle atrophy, and impaired cognition. Male HRT may have symptomatic benefit but risks serious disease. There are no good-quality long-term trials of replacement therapy in men.

### Changes in both sexes

Cross-sectional studies show much reduced frequency of sexual behavior of all kinds in older people. However, longitudinal studies show much smaller changes, suggesting that many changes are due to cohort effects, e.g., changes in the prevailing social environment during early adulthood.

Other factors include physical and psychological illness (e.g., arthritis, depression), reduced potency, and social changes (e.g., lack of a partner due to bereavement). Most of these factors are modifiable.

# Benign prostatic hyperplasia: presentation

Benign prostatic hyperplasia (BPH) is characterized by nonmalignant enlargement of the prostate gland and an increase in prostatic smooth muscle tone. The resulting bladder outlet obstruction leads to lower urinary tract symptoms (LUTS; "prostatism").

LUTS affect 25%–50% of men over 65 years, although the histological changes of BPH are even more common—almost universal in those over 70. The natural history is variable; some deteriorate, some stay the same, and some improve, even without treatment.

The prostatic hyperplasia occurs mostly in the periurethral zone and theus may not result in palpable enlargement of the prostate.

## Assessment

### Symptoms

Lower urinary tract symptoms are variable and may be mostly either

- *Obstructive*, with weak stream, straining, hesitancy, post-void dribbling, nocturia, acute urinary retention, or chronic retention with overflow incontinence; or
- *Irritative*, with frequency, dysuria, urgency, and urge incontinence.

Other presentations include hematuria, urinary tract infection (UTI), and renal failure secondary to hydronephrosis. Obstructive symptoms may be worsened by drugs, e.g., sedating antihistamines. Tricyclic antidepressants may improve irritative symptoms but may cause worsening obstructive symptoms and/or urinary retention.

Scoring systems (see Box 19.1) can help determine symptom severity and track progression and response to treatment.

### Examination

This includes the genitals (phimosis or meatal stenosis), abdomen (palpable bladder), neurological system, and digital rectal examination (DRE). DRE should be performed in every male >40 years of age and any man presenting for urological evaluation.

In BPH, the prostate is usually smooth and enlarged. An irregular prostate (nodule or induration) can occur, particularly with the presence of calculi, infection, or cancer.

### Investigations

Tests may help confirm the diagnosis and exclude other pathology:

- **Urinary flow rate** (only accurate if voided volume >150 cc): low value suggests obstruction, but is rarely needed.
- **Blood glucose** to exclude diabetes and serum creatinine to exclude diabetic complications or renal failure
- **Urinalysis** to exclude infection, hematuria
- **Ultrasound of urinary tract** to exclude hydronephrosis and/or high post-void residual bladder volume
- **Serum PSA** level after a discussion of risks and benefits of further investigation and treatment
- **Cystoscopy** and upper urinary tract imaging to exclude bladder and renal pathology

**Box 19.1 International prostate symptom score (IPSS)**

This is a well-validated, widely used assessment tool that can be either self-administered or given as part of a structured assessment by a health professional. Aggregate scores from the seven questions to give a total score range of 0–35:

| 0–7 | Mildly symptomatic |
|---|---|
| 8–19 | Moderately symptomatic |
| 20–35 | Severely symptomatic |

|  | Not at all | Less than 1 time in 5 | Less than half the time | About half the time | More than half the time | Almost always |
|---|---|---|---|---|---|---|
| **Incomplete emptying.** Over the past month, how often have you had a sensation of not emptying your bladder completely after you finish urinating? | 0 | 1 | 2 | 3 | 4 | 5 |
| **Frequency.** Over the past month, how often have you had to urinate again less than 2 hours after you finished urinating? | 0 | 1 | 2 | 3 | 4 | 5 |
| **Intermittency.** Over the past month, how often have you found you stopped and started again several times when you urinated? | 0 | 1 | 2 | 3 | 4 | 5 |
| **Urgency.** Over the past month, how difficult have you found it to postpone urination? | 0 | 1 | 2 | 3 | 4 | 5 |
| **Weak stream.** Over the past month, how often have you had a weak urinary stream? | 0 | 1 | 2 | 3 | 4 | 5 |
| **Straining.** Over the past month, how often have you had to push or strain to begin urination? | 0 | 1 | 2 | 3 | 4 | 5 |

|  | None | 1 time | 2 times | 3 times | 4 times | 5 times or more |
|---|---|---|---|---|---|---|
| **Nocturia.** Over the past month, how many times did you most typically get up to urinate, from the time you went to bed until the time you got up in the morning? | 0 | 1 | 2 | 3 | 4 | 5 |

# Benign prostatic hyperplasia: treatment

The treatment choice is influenced by patient preference, severity of symptoms, potential complications, and fitness for surgery.

## Conservative measures

"Watchful waiting" is reasonable if symptoms are mild or moderate. Reassess clinically and check renal function at 6- to 12-month intervals. Advise reduction in evening fluid intake; stop unnecessary diuretics. The main risk is acute urinary retention (1%–2% per year).

## Herbal preparations

These are widely used by patients, purchased without prescription. The most widely used is saw palmetto (*Serenoa repens*) extract.

### Medications

#### Alpha-adrenergic blockers

Alpha-blockers include, e.g., doxazosin, terazosin, tamsulosin, alfuzosin. They relax prostatic smooth muscle, increasing urine flow rates and reducing symptoms in days. Side effects are common: the most important ones are hypotension (see Box 19.2), especially orthostatic hypotension, syncope, and retrograde ejaculation.

Use cautiously, starting with a low dose (e.g., doxazosin 1 mg daily, increased in 1-mg increments at 2-week intervals to 4 mg). Exercise great caution if prescribed with diuretics or other vasodilators, if there is a past history of syncope, and in frail men. Tamsulosin (400 mcg daily) may be more prostate-selective than other alpha-blockers and may have fewer circulatory side effects.

#### 5-alpha reductase inhibitors

These include finasteride, dutasteride. They inhibit prostatic testosterone metabolism, reducing prostatic size. Benefit occurs slowly (months) and is most likely if the prostate is large (>40 mL). Side effects are uncommon but include erectile dysfunction (<5%), gynecomastia, and loss of libido. Given the absence of cardiovascular side effects, 5-alpha reductase inhibitors may be a better option in the frail older person. Prostate-specific antigen (PSA) levels fall by >50%, so double the observed value to give an indication of prostate cancer risk.

#### Combination treatment: alpha-blocker and 5-alpha-reductase inhibitor

This combination is shown to be more effective than monotherapy with either agent alone.

## Box 19.2 Alpha-blockers, BPH, and hypertension

Many men have both lower urinary tract symptoms due to BPH and are hypertensive. Alpha-blockers can be an attractive option as the one drug may treat both. However, alpha-blockers in the treatment of hypertension are less effective than several other drug classes (e.g., ACE inhibitors). Assess the impact on each problem separately and consider prescribing the most appropriate treatment for each individual condition.

## Surgery

Surgery is more effective than medications or "watchful waiting," but potential side effects are more significant. It is indicated if:
- Symptoms are moderate or severe (with patient preference).
- There are complications (recurrent UTI or hematuria, urinary retention requiring catheterization, renal failure).
- A trial of medical treatment has failed.

### Transurethral resection of the prostate (TURP)

TURP is the gold-standard procedure. Success rates are >90%. Potential adverse effects include retrograde ejaculation (most), erectile dysfunction (5%–10%), incontinence (1%) and death (<1%). 10% need further surgery within a few years.

### Newer procedures

Several have been developed. They are generally less invasive and probably have fewer adverse effects, but long-term outcome data are lacking. Local availability may be limited. The following are examples.

*Transurethral incision of the prostate (TUIP)*

TUIP is effective in those with smaller prostate glands. It has a low incidence of side effects.

*Laser ablation of the prostate*

This provides effective ablation of tissue without the concomitant bleeding and risk of hyponatremia and altered mental status (TUR-syndrome) potentially associated with TURP.

*Transurethral microwave thermotherapy (TUMT) and transurethral needle ablation (TUNA)*

These newer systems are well tolerated and require only local anesthetic in an outpatient setting. However, some are time consuming and difficult to learn, long-term results are less well known, and availability varies locally.

*Open prostatectomy*

This is reserved for very large glands (>75 grams) and when other interventions are needed, e.g., removal of bladder stones. It is very effective, but potential comorbidity is higher.

### Urinary catheterization

Long-term urinary catheterization is an option in the following situations:
- Symptoms are severe, or significant complications have occurred.
- Surgical mortality and morbidity would be high.
- Medical treatment has not been tolerated or is unlikely to be effective.

The usual example is acute or chronic urinary retention for which other contributory causes (e.g., constipation) have been addressed but the patient remains in retention and has failed a trial (or trials) without a catheter.

# Prostate cancer: presentation

This is a very common cancer in men, much more so with age: median age at diagnosis is over 70. However:
• Many tumors do not progress, even without treatment.
• Most men with prostate cancer are asymptomatic or have only obstructive symptoms from concurrent BPH.

This leads to difficult management decisions, especially in older people, for whom life expectancy for other reasons may be low and expensive, unpleasant, or risky treatments may not be worthwhile. Thus, the U.S. Preventive Services Task Force recommends against prostate cancer screening in men age 75 years or older.

## Assessment

Predictors of an adverse disease course (recurrence after treatment, local progression, metastases and death) include more advanced stage (TNM classification) and histological grade (e.g., Gleason score, see p. 538).

### Localized cancer

This is usually detected when evaluating a man with an elevated serum PSA level, abnormal DRE, or incidentally, e.g., at TURP for BPH. Tumor remains within the gland capsule; the tumor focus may be very small and unlikely responsible for symptoms. Prognosis is generally excellent, especially if the grade is favorable. Cure, via radiotherapy or surgery, may be possible, although for more indolent tumors, potential risks of aggressive treatment may outweigh its benefits.

### Locally advanced cancer without metastases

This is usually detected in patients with urinary symptoms or at DRE performed for other reasons. This patient group is much larger now that PSA testing is more common. The tumor has broken through the capsule, and prognosis is more adverse.

### Metastatic cancer

Some newly diagnosed patients have metastatic disease. However, due to PSA-based screening, there has been a significant decrease in incidence of metastatic disease at presentation. Many cases are asymptomatic.

Features (decreasing frequency) include urinary symptoms, bone pain, constitutional symptoms (e.g., weight loss), renal failure, pathological fracture, and anemia due to bone marrow infiltration. A minority of men experience an indolent course and, with treatment, may survive many years.

## Gleason score

This histological grading system correlates well with outcome and helps guide treatment choice. A composite of two scores of Gleason pattern (each range 1–5) is reported as X+Y, with X, the predominant pattern observed, and Y, the second most prevalent pattern. Therefore, the range is 2–10:

| | |
|---|---|
| 2–4 | Well differentiated (rare in the modern era) |
| 5–7 | Moderately differentiated (most common) |
| 8–10 | Poorly differentiated |

## Screening

There is increased locoregional incidence and decreased metastatic incidence (clinical stage migration) due to PSA-based screening and associated improvement in survival.

Combined DRE and serum PSA testing is recommended. Digital rectal examination alone is insensitive; tumors detected in this way are often locally advanced. PSA alone has good sensitivity but not high specificity, resulting in unnecessary prostate biopsies.

## Tests

The following should be selected advisedly, after considering the patient's wishes, the implications of a negative or positive result, and any risks of the test.

* *PSA*: See Prostate-specific antigen section (next page).
* *BMP* shows evidence of postrenal renal failure.
* *Transrectal ultrasound and biopsy* provides tissue for histological diagnosis and grading. Risks are hemorrhage and infection.
* *Bone scan or X-rays* are used if there are symptoms or bone biochemistry is suggestive. Metastasis to bone is common; appearance is sclerotic much more commonly than lytic. They are recommended if PSA >10 ng/mL.
* *CT/MRI scan* is used for tumor staging when surgery is contemplated and if PSA >20 ng/mL.

## Further reading

U.S. Preventive Services Task Force (2008). Screening for prostate cancer: U.S. Preventive Services Task Force recommendation statement. *Ann Intern Med* **149**(3):185–191.

# Prostate-specific antigen

Prostate-specific antigen (PSA) is produced by both benign and malignant prostatic glands. There is no single useful cutoff point that separates those with cancer from those without:

- Two-thirds of men with a high PSA do not have prostate cancer.
- One-fifth of men with prostate cancer have a normal PSA.

The higher the PSA level, the more likely cancer exists, but cancer can be present even in men with lower PSA levels (<4 ng/mL). Specificity is even less in older people, as the benign causes of elevated PSA are more common.

PSA increases with age and with BPH, prostatitis, urinary tract infection, digital rectal examination, prostate biopsy, urethral catheterization and instrumentation, and ejaculation.

PSA has two definite useful roles:

- In early detection of localized prostate cancer when treatment may be curative
- In monitoring tumor recurrence or progression following definitive treatment

PSA levels may be reduced with medical treatment (e.g., 5-alpha-reductase inhibitors, herbal remedies such as saw palmetto [*Serenoa repens*]) and may therefore reduce the above thresholds for referral.

# Prostate cancer: treatment

### Localized cancer

There are several treatment options, including "watchful waiting," hormonal treatment, radiotherapy, or surgery.

#### "Watchful waiting"

This is usually reserved for those with modest life expectancy (<10 years) and lower-grade (Gleason score 2–6) localized tumors, where progression is rare within 10 years. Check the PSA/DRE every 4–6 months. Start treatment (usually hormonal) if symptoms or if PSA/DRE changes.

#### Expectant management

This is usually reserved for those between 65 and 75 years of age, lower-grade (Gleason score 2–6), localized, and low-volume (as assessed by percentage of biopsy cores) tumors where progression is rare within 10 years. Check the PSA/DRE every 4–6 months. Repeat prostate biopsy yearly. Definitive therapy may be offered if symptoms appear, the rate of change of PSA suggests tumor progression, or any high-grade disease (Gleason pattern 4) is observed on biopsy.

#### Hormone treatment (see Metastatic disease, below)

There is great doubt as to whether early hormone treatment improves overall survival.

#### Radiotherapy

This is the most usual choice for high-grade localized tumors. It is probably as effective as surgery, but better tolerated. Side effects include erectile dysfunction, irritative urinary symptoms, and radiation proctitis.

#### Surgery

Radical prostatectomy is a major procedure, usually indicated only for those with long (at least 10–15 years) life expectancy, with moderate- to high-grade tumors, and in good health. Major side effects are urinary incontinence, impotence, and hemorrhage.

### Locally advanced disease without metastases

Key treatments are radiotherapy (see above) and/or androgen deprivation (see below). The relative benefits are unclear. Surgery probably offers no benefit, other than TURP, to relieve outflow symptoms.

### Metastatic disease

Androgen deprivation ("hormone treatment") is the linchpin of treatment. This can be achieved by castration (bilateral orchiectomy), but is usually done chemically, largely for reasons of patient preference. Luteinizing hormone–releasing hormone (LHRH) agonists are used commonly and are usually effective for 12–18 months. Surgery offers no benefits.

*LHRH agonists*

These include, e.g., goserelin (Zoladex®) and luprolide (Lupron®). Given as injections or implants, these agents cause initial (2 weeks) stimulation and then sustained depression of testosterone release. The initial increase can cause tumor growth ("flare") with adverse effects, e.g., urinary outflow obstruction, spinal cord compression, or bone pain. If anticipated, a short-term anti-androgen may help. Continuous therapy is not needed: survival appears similar if therapy is stopped when PSA levels are normal and restarted when they rise.

*Antiandrogens*

These include, e.g., bicalutamide (Casodex®), flutamide (Eulexin®), and nilutamide (Anandron®). They are useful in inhibiting tumor flare after LHRH agonist initiation, in tumor refractory to LHRH agonists, if LHRH agonists are not tolerated or accepted (e.g., because of erectile dysfunction), or when oral drugs are preferred. There is no evidence that long-term combined antiandrogens and LHRH agonists are more helpful.

*Side effects*

Side effects of LHRH agonists and antiandrogens include hot flushes, erectile dysfunction, and gynecomastia.

## Late-stage prostate cancer

Eventually, prostate cancer may become resistant (refractory) to hormone treatment, manifesting as a rising PSA and/or worsening symptoms while on treatment. Other treatments (e.g., estrogens or docetaxel-based chemotherapy) may be tried, but are rarely very effective. Death follows, often in months. Common complications, usually in more advanced disease, include the following:

- *Bone pain* is a major cause of reduced quality of life. Optimize oral analgesia: combinations of acetaminophen, opiates, and NSAIDs are effective. Local pain is helped by radiotherapy. Bisphosphonates or steroids may also help.
- *Pathological bone fracture* usually requires surgical fixation.
- *Acute urinary retention:* Catheterize. Intensify anti-tumor treatment if appropriate (e.g., hormone treatment, radiotherapy). Consider TURP.
- *Postrenal renal failure:* Determine site of obstruction by imaging.
  - Prostatic obstruction: catheter, TURP, intensify anti-tumor treatment
  - Ureteric obstruction: ureteral stenting or percutaneous nephrostomy
- *Spinal cord compression* is an emergency, as early decompression improves neurological outcome. Confirm with CT or MRI. Steroids, radiotherapy, or surgery may help decompress the cord.

# Postmenopausal vaginal bleeding

This is defined as bleeding from the genital tract over 1 year after onset of menopausal amenorrhea. The time criterion reflects the fact that menstruation is often irregular and infrequent around menopause, and investigations for sinister pathology are not then worthwhile.

Most cases are secondary to benign pathology, but treatment of the few cases of cancer (mostly endometrial) is far more effective if identified early, so do not delay assessment. Malignancy is more likely if bleeding is significant and recurrent—investigate vigorously if no cause is apparent.

## Assessment

### History
Assess the amount and frequency of bleeding, if necessary by discussing it with the caregiver. Consider other possible sources of blood, e.g., urinary or rectal. Take an accurate drug history.

### Examine
Examine the genitalia, perineum, and rectum to exclude tumor, trauma, and bleeding from atrophic sites. Obesity or osteoarthritis may make examination difficult; the left or right lateral positions are usually more successful.

### Investigation
Obtain a CBC to exclude severe anemia. Urine dipstick for hematuria is unlikely to be specific to blood of urinary-tract origin, especially if bleeding is recurrent or ongoing. Further tests are usually guided by expert gynecological advice, but may include the following:
- Cervical smear
- Vaginal ultrasound to assess endometrial thickness (<5 mm effectively excludes cancer and may prevent the need for more tests)
- Sonohysterography and endometrial biopsy may be required to diagnose benign causes of endometrial bleeding.
- Hysteroscopy—can be done under local or general anesthetic
- Dilatation and curettage
- Consider investigation of the urinary and GI tracts (cystoscopy, sigmoidoscopy).

## Treatment
Treatment is directed at the underlying cause, for example:
- **Atrophic vaginitis:** Topical estrogens are used because of their systemic absorption. If abnormal bleeding persists, biopsy of the endometrium is indicated to exclude hyperplasia or cancer. Use HRT if topical estrogens fail.
- **HRT**: Review the balance of risks and benefits and consider stopping the drug. Consider change of preparation, e.g., reduction of estrogen dose, increase in progesterone dose.

- *Endometrial carcinoma:* Total abdominal hysterectomy and bilateral salpingo-oophorectomy and/or radiotherapy are the usual interventions. In those unfit for surgery, progestins (e.g., medroxyprogesterone) may control the tumor.

## Causes of postmenopausal vaginal bleeding

Causes in approximate order of frequency are as follows:
- *Atrophic vaginitis.* Inflammation results as the thinner, less cornified epithelium is exposed to a more alkaline vaginal environment (pH 6–7.5 compared to pH <4.5 in women of reproductive age) colonized by a broad microbial flora.
- *Endometrial hyperplasia* secondary to
  - Exogenous estrogen (e.g., HRT)
  - Unopposed endogenous estrogen (especially in older, obese women, in whom peripheral conversion of steroid hormones to estrogens by adipose cells is higher).
- *Benign tumor,* e.g., cervical or endometrial polyps
- *Vaginal prolapse* and ulceration
- *Vaginal infection*
- *Carcinoma*
  - Endometrial
  - Cervical
  - Vulval
  - Vaginal
  - Ovarian

Other relatively common causes of "vaginal" bleeding include hematuria and rectal bleeding.

After hysterectomy, bleeding is commonly due to atrophic vaginitis or overgrowth of postsurgical granulation tissue.

Drugs causing endometrial disease (hyperplasia, polyps, and cancer) include the following:
- *HRT*
  - Cyclical replacement: investigate if bleeding is at unexpected times.
  - Continuous estrogen and progesterone: investigate if irregular bleeding persists for >12 months after treatment initiation.
- *Tamoxifen* (via a paradoxical endometrial estrogen-like effect)

# Vaginal prolapse

A *prolapse* is a protrusion into the vagina by a pelvic organ (bladder, bowel, or uterus) caused by one of the following:
- Weakness of pelvic connective tissue and musculature due to cumulative effects of childbirth trauma, aging, and estrogen deficiency
- Increased abdominal pressure, e.g., constipation, obesity, and coughing.

Depending on which structures are weak, the following may be seen:
- *Cystocoele:* The bladder protrudes through the anterior vaginal wall.
- *Rectocoele:* The rectum protrudes through the posterior vaginal wall.
- *Enterocoele:* Herniation of peritoneum and small bowel (the pouch of Douglas) occurs through the posterior vaginal wall.
- *Uterine prolapse* is descent of the cervix and uterus down the vagina.
  - First degree: cervix lies within the vagina
  - Second degree: cervix protrudes from the vagina on standing or straining
  - Third degree (procidentia): cervix lies outside the vagina

## Assessment

Often vaginal prolapse is asymptomatic. Most commonly there is a sensation of heaviness, fullness, or bearing down; a palpable mass; or a dull pelvic aching or backache. Symptoms may be diminished by lying down.
- *Cystocoele* may cause stress or overflow urinary incontinence, urinary tract infection, or bladder outflow obstruction.
- *Rectocoele* may cause fecal incontinence or difficulty in defecation; manual evacuation or digital reduction of the prolapse may be needed.
- *Enterocoele* causes pelvic fullness and discomfort.
- *Third-degree uterine prolapse* may cause ulceration and bleeding and bladder symptoms, e.g., difficulty in urinating.

Perform a pelvic examination, using a speculum if available. Severe prolapse will be immediately apparent. Ask the patient to bear down; this may reveal smaller degrees of prolapse. Some prolapses (e.g., rectocoele) are detected only by bimanual examination of the rectum and vagina.

## Treatment

This is dictated by symptoms, prolapse severity, the organs involved, general fitness, and patient preference. Urodynamic testing and imaging may be needed prior to treatment.
- Mild symptoms: topical estrogen cream and pelvic floor exercises
- Moderate or severe symptoms: pessary or surgery

### Surgery

Surgery is now generally well tolerated and effective. Usually via a transvaginal approach, weakened structures of the pelvic floor are strengthened and fixed in place or supported by mesh. Hysterectomy is sometimes necessary.

*Pessaries*

Fitting of a pessary is indicated for reasons of patient preference, when the risks of surgery are unfavorable, and as a temporary measure prior to surgery. They come in many shapes and sizes, but the most commonly used is the ring pessary. Other shapes may be used, commonly for severe disease, but can be difficult to insert and remove.

## How to care for a vaginal pessary

Every 4–6 months:
- Remove and clean the pessary
- Examine the vagina for evidence of ulceration
- Replace a damaged pessary
- Reinsert if all is well.

*Complications*
- If vaginal ulceration occurs, the pessary should be removed for several weeks, until complete healing has occurred. Local estrogen creams assist healing and may prevent recurrent ulceration. Try a different shape or size of pessary.
- Pessaries can embed in inflamed vaginal mucosa and become stuck. Topical estrogens and treatment of infection (e.g., candida) may reduce inflammation and assist removal. If the pessary remains stuck, refer patient for specialist gynecological assessment.

# Vulval disorders

Most nonmalignant vulval disorders are worsened by local irritants (e.g., soap, deodorant, perfume) and improve if avoided. Good perineal hygiene also helps, e.g., wiping front-to-back after urination or defecation, keeping the area dry, and wearing loose-fitting, nonsynthetic clothing.

## Vulvitis

### Symptoms
Symptoms are itching, discharge, and burning discomfort.

### Causes
These include the following:
- Candida is the most common cause. Risk factors include diabetes, HIV, recent antibiotic use, and obesity. Vaginal infection almost always coexists.
- Local dermatitis is often exacerbated by soap and deodorants.
- Sexually transmitted pathogens occur uncommonly, e.g., chlamydia.

### Diagnosis
Wet mount preparation KOH. Culture may be indicated for persistent or recurrent infection or to dictate therapy for noncandidal genera.

### Treatment
Treat candida with antifungal cream to the vulva (e.g., clotrimazole 1% cream) and pessaries or cream inserted high into the vagina (e.g., clotrimazole 200 mg pessary daily for 3 days). Single-dose pessaries (e.g., clotrimazole 500 mg pessary once) are effective and may be better tolerated. Oral treatment is also effective, e.g., fluconazole 150 mg once. There is no need to treat the male partner as candida is not sexually transmitted.

Treat irritant dermatitis by removing the cause and applying topical steroid cream regularly (e.g., hydrocortisone 1%) for 7–14 days.

Recurrent candidal infection is common, especially in diabetics and in those receiving repeated antibiotics. Consider longer-term treatment, e.g., weekly clotrimazole (500 mg pessary) or fluconazole (100 mg PO for 6 months).

If vulval itch persists without obvious cause, consider the following:
- Systemic disease, e.g., iron deficiency, thyroid disorders
- Use emollients and low-potency topical steroid to break the itch-scratch-itch cycle. Antihistamines are not effective.

## Vulvodynia

This is a chronic pain syndrome manifesting as burning, pain, or tenderness of the vulva. There are often psychological contributors. Infection, dermatitis, and epithelial disorders (neoplastic and non-neoplastic) should be excluded. Refer patient for specialist assessment and consider treating depression and empirical treatment with topical steroids or estrogens.

## Non-neoplastic epithelial disorders

### Lichen sclerosus

This is common in middle-aged and older women. It is either asymptomatic or causes itching or soreness or dyspareunia. It may even cause dysuria or pain on defecation. It is seen as white or pink/purple macules or papules resembling thin parchment paper and often in a figure-of-eight distribution around the vulva. Conduct biopsy to exclude neoplasia.

Treat with potent topical steroids (clobetasol propionate for 2–3 months), tapering the potency and frequency as symptoms improve. Progression to squamous carcinoma can occur in 4%–5%. Long-term follow-up is indicated.

### Squamous hyperplasia

Raised white keratinized lesions may be localized. Biopsy may be needed to exclude malignancy. Treat with medium-potency topical steroids, tapering to a stop as symptoms improve.

### Other disorders

These include psoriasis and chronic dermatitis, which can usually be diagnosed clinically, but biopsy permits more confident management.

## Malignant epithelial disorders

### Vulval cancer

Vulval cancer is mostly squamous cell carcinoma. It is easily treated in its early stages and often preceded by a premalignant stage. Late presentation is more common with age. It is commonly asymptomatic and an incidental finding, but it may itch, discharge, bleed, or cause pain. Appearance is variable—it may be raised or ulcerated, or appear as white or colored macules. If there is in any doubt that a lesion may be malignant or premalignant refer the patient for biopsy.

Treatment depends on the size and invasiveness of the tumor, the presence or absence of metastases, and the condition of the patient. Options include topical cytotoxic creams, resection under local anesthetic, wide local excision, or radical vulvectomy. Extensive vulval surgery is relatively well tolerated in older people.

If any vulval lesion does not respond as expected to treatment, re-consider the possibility of malignancy.

# Sexual function

Studies show that most older people desire some sexual contact. However, the frequency of sexual intercourse, both penetrative and non-penetrative, falls with age. This decline is multifactorial:
- Lack of partner, e.g., death of spouse
- Physiological changes of aging, e.g., decreased vaginal secretions, less sustained penile erections
- Physical comorbidity and medication, e.g., circulatory disease, beta-blockers
- Psychological comorbidity, e.g., low self-esteem, depression
- Societal expectations and judgments
- Lack of privacy, especially in institutional care

The clinical response to a patient's report of sexual dysfunction involves addressing each of these factors in a supportive and understanding way.

## Erectile dysfunction

Erection requires intact neurological, circulatory, hormonal, and psychological processes. In older men, several factors more commonly contribute to erectile dysfunction (ED) or impotence. A solely psychological cause is uncommon. Common contributors are medication, vascular disease, and neurological disease (stroke, autonomic neuropathy, local surgery, e.g., prostatectomy).

### History

Assess onset and progression, circumstances, and associated psychological issues. ED is common, yet is rarely asked about. Older men may volunteer the symptom, but many will accept it as part of "normal aging." Do not assume that an older man is not sexually active, and always warn about impotence as a potential side effect of relevant medications.

### Drugs causing erectile dysfunction

Along with vascular disease, drugs are the most common cause in older people:
- Antihypertensives (especially beta-blockers and diuretics, ACE inhibitors less so)
- Alcohol
- Digoxin
- Antiandrogens, LHRH agonists, estrogens, progestins
- Antidepressants (all classes, except trazodone)
- Less commonly: cimetidine, spironolactone.

### Examination

Assess the patient's mental state (depression, anxiety), for presence of secondary sexual characteristics, and vascular disease, and conduct a genitourinary examination. Neurological examination should include perineal and perianal sensation.

*Investigation*

Exclude systemic illness with CBC, BMP, and glucose. Diagnostic tests to determine an underlying cause of ED do not often alter management and are rarely performed except in younger men with appropriate history such as trauma. Hypogonadism is an uncommon cause of ED, so checking testosterone level is not usually necessary.

If libido (rather than ED) is the problem, then exclude hypogonadism by checking testosterone. If the patient is hypogonadal, check LH, TSH, and prolactin.

*Treatment*

When possible, stop incriminated drugs. Treat underlying disease, including anxiety or depression. Recently developed drug treatments are highly effective.

*Phosphodiesterase type-5 inhibitors*

These include sildenafil (Viagra®), vardenafil (Levitra®), and tadalafil (Cialis®) and cause smooth muscle relaxation and increase blood flow. They are easily used (take PO before intercourse), effective, and relatively safe.

Contraindications include being on nitrates; exercise caution prescribing these agents for those with coronary or cerebrovascular disease. Side effects are blurred or blue vision, gastrointestinal (dyspepsia), and vascular (flushing, headache).

*Alprostadil (prostaglandin E1)*

This is usually given as an intraurethral pellet (MUSE®), is absorbed locally, and causes local smooth muscle relaxation, There is no significant systemic absorption, so systemic side effects are rare and vascular disease is not a contraindication.

*Other options*

These include intracavernosal injections (the most effective treatment, but may cause corporeal fibrosis or priapism) and non-drug options such as vacuum devices (effective, but often discontinued due to discomfort).

# Incontinence

**James Wright**

# Urinary incontinence: causes

Incontinence has a major adverse impact on quality of life and has significant associated morbidity (risk of falls is increased). Even long-standing cases may be reversible, so evaluation is always indicated.

Incontinence is very common (around 30% of older adults at home, 50% in nursing homes) and incidence increases with age. Most incontinence in the older adults is multifactorial with many of the following features.

## Age-related changes
- Diminished total bladder capacity but increased residual volume
- Diminished bladder contractile function
- Increased frequency of uninhibited bladder contractions
- Reduced ability to postpone voiding
- Reversal of diurnal urine output and increase in nocturnal volume
- Atrophy of vagina and urethra in females
- Loss of pelvic floor and urethral sphincter muscle tone
- Hypertrophy of the prostate in males

## Comorbidity
- Diminished mobility and manual dexterity
- Prescribed medications affect lower urinary tract or alertness
- Defecatory dysfunction with increased constipation
- Impaired cognition—confusion can cause inappropriate micturition or interfere with cortical control of normal continence reflex pathways.

Taking these factors into account, incontinence can be divided into three broad categories to direct evaluation and therapy.
1. **Stress incontinence** is due primarily to anatomic derangement of the urethral sphincter and/or bladder, leading to urine loss with increases in intra-abdominal pressure.
2. **Bladder overactivity** is spontaneous urine loss with or without the sensation of urgency due to neuromuscular derangement of reflex voiding mechanisms and/or local smooth muscle control.
3. **Mixed incontinence** has features of both stress and spontaneous urine loss.

In older adults, overactive bladder disorders are more common and often more difficult to remedy. A number of reversible factors may contribute to spontaneous incontinence and should be treated accordingly.

## Reversible factors
- Urinary tract infection (p. 654)
- Delirium
- Drugs—e.g., diuretics cause polyuria; anticholinergics such as tricyclics may cause retention; sedatives can reduce awareness or mobility.
- Constipation may cause voiding difficulty and increased residual volumes in both sexes (p. 564).

- Polyuria, e.g., poorly controlled diabetes, hypercalcemia, edema resorption at night can cause nocturnal polyuria, psychogenic polydipsia.
- Urethral irritability, e.g., atrophic vaginitis, candida infection
- Bladder stones and tumors, most commonly identified in the setting of microscopic or gross hematuria.

## Other treatable factors

- In males, prostatic hypertrophy or carcinoma can cause outflow obstruction, bladder hyperactivity, or "overflow" incontinence. Stress incontinence is rare and most commonly postsurgical (i.e., after prostatectomy) or secondary to neurological disease.
- In females, loss of pelvic organ support (pelvic organ prolapse) may contribute to urinary incontinence and urinary retention.
- Fistula (communication between the bladder and vagina) represents a smaller incidence of incontinence in older women and is most commonly seen in the setting of hysterectomy and therapy for gynecological malignancy (i.e., pelvic radiation).

# Urinary incontinence: assessment

Identification of specific incontinence symptoms is most helpful for diagnosis and therapy.

- **Bladder overactivity symptoms:** Frequent (>8 times/day) and/or precipitant voiding—inability to "hold" with spontaneous urine loss before reaching the toilet. Nocturia more than twice per night and nocturnal incontinence are common. A sensation of urgency to void may or may not be present prior to an incontinence episode.
- **Stress incontinence symptoms** include leakage during coughing, lifting, walking, or other exercise.
- **Obstructive symptoms** in men include decreased force of urinary stream, hesitancy, and intermittent flow.

Be aware that the different symptom complexes can overlap (i.e., mixed incontinence or outlet obstruction leading to urge incontinence or overflow in men).

A systematic approach to diagnosing incontinence includes the following:

- *History and symptom review*. A 24- to 72-hour diary of frequency and volume voided can help to assess symptom type and severity as well as provocative influences. See Table 20.1
- *Examination* Include vaginal, rectal, and neurological examination. Evaluate sphincter competence with moderately full bladder and valsalva maneuvers. Assess for pelvic organ prolapse.
- *Assess post-void residual volume* See Box 20.1.
- *Investigations* include urinalysis and culture, general screening blood tests, cytology, and cystoscopy if there is hematuria. Urodynamic testing can be helpful if incontinence cannot be explained, treatment is unsuccessful, neurological disease is present, or surgical intervention is contemplated.

**Box 20.1 Residual volume**

Normal young people have only a few milliliters of urine post-micturition, but normal elderly can have up to 100 mL.

Causes of increased residual volume include the following:
- Prostatic hypertrophy, carcinoma (rarely)
- Urethral stricture
- Bladder diverticulum
- Cystocele and other pelvic organ prolapse (females)
- Hypocontractile detrusor
- Neurological disease (including multiple sclerosis [MS], Parkinson's disease, spinal cord injury, herniated disc).

Acute retention is usually painful but can present atypically with delirium, renal failure, etc.

Chronic bladder distention is usually painless, presenting with infection, abdominal distension or mass, or incontinence (continuous dribbling due to overflow or urge incontinence due to detrusor instability).

Persistently elevated residual volume increases the risk of infection.

Elevated bladder pressure can cause dilation of the urinary tract with hydronephrosis and potential renal failure.

Residual volume can easily be estimated using a simple ultrasound bladder scan or a diagnostic (in/out) catheterization.

## Voiding diary assessment

It is helpful to have patients and/or caregivers construct a 24- to 72-hour diary of frequency and volume voided as part of the incontinence evaluation (see Table 20.1). Useful data points such as the 24-hour voided volume, number and severity of leakage episodes, diurnal urine output, and maximum and minimum voided volume are easily determined. Catheterized volumes and post-void residual (PVR) can also be assessed when necessary using this format.

**Table 20.1** Example of voiding diary

| Date | Time | Voided volume | Leakage episode and cause | Catheterized volume/PVR |
|------|------|---------------|---------------------------|-------------------------|
|      |      |               |                           |                         |
|      |      |               |                           |                         |
|      |      |               |                           |                         |

# Urinary incontinence: management

- Correct diagnosis is necessary for effective therapy.
- Incontinence is multifactorial in many older adults, so combining treatments may be necessary, e.g., a man with obstructive prostatic symptoms and detrusor hyperactivity may benefit from an alpha-blocker and an antimuscarinic agent.
- Balance effective management and curative strategies to maximize quality of life for patients and caregivers (see Table 20.2).

**Table 20.2** Managing urinary incontinence

| Treatment | Indication | Notes |
|-----------|-----------|-------|
| **Bladder retraining** (gradually increasing time between voiding) | Overactive bladder syndrome/detrusor over activity | May reset voiding threshold |
| **Timed voiding** (urinating every 2–4 hours) | Dementia<br>Overactive bladder syndrome | Decreases likelihood of incontinence episodes |
| **Pelvic floor exercises** | Stress incontinence and bladder overactivity | Variable patient ability and adherence |
| **Bladder-stabilizing drugs**<br>Tolterodine 2–4 mg daily<br>Solfenacin 5–10 mg daily<br>Darifenacin 7.5–15 mg daily<br>Trospium chloride 20 mg daily<br>Oxybutynin 10–30 mg daily | Overactive bladder syndrome/detrusor overactivity | May precipitate urinary retention—monitor carefully<br><br>Side effects of dry mouth, constipation, and mood disturbance may limit effectiveness.<br><br>Dose escalation possible. Assess over 2–6 weeks for maximal effect |
| *Surgery*<br>Female | For stress incontinence: pubovaginal sling, colposuspension, urethral bulking.<br><br>For refractory urge incontinence: sacral neuromodulation trial | Urodynamic testing prior to surgery |
| Male | For outlet obstruction: prostate ablation with radiofrequency, laser, transurethral resection<br><br>For stress incontinence: perineal sling, artificial urinary sphincter, urethral bulking | |

**Table 20.2** Managing urinary incontinence (*continued*)

| Treatment | Indication | Notes |
|---|---|---|
| **Anti-androgens** Finasteride 5 mg daily Deutasteride 0.5 mg daily | For prostatic hyperplasia Improves flow and obstructive symptoms | Slow onset of action Most effective in large prostates (>40 cc) |
| **Alpha-blockers** Doxazosin 1–4 mg qhs Tamsulosin 0.4 mg qhs Alfuzosin 10 mg qhs | Smooth muscle relaxant for BPH—improves flow and obstructive symptoms | Titrate dose slowly— watch for hypotension (especially postural) and syncope or falls |
| **Double voiding** (ask patient to repeat voiding) | Poor bladder contractility and increased PVR | May help reduce large residual volumes and UTI risk |
| **Intermittent catheterization** | Atonic/hypotonic bladder Can aid continence and reduce renal damage and infection risk | Safe and well tolerated if technique is feasible |
| **Synthetic vasopressin** either oral or intranasal | Nocturnal polyuria | Possible side effect is dilutional hyponatremia Caution in patients with comorbid conditions likely to be exacerbated |

# Catheters

*A catheter is indicated for the following:*
- Symptomatic urinary retention
- Obstructed outflow associated with deteriorating renal function or hydronephrosis
- Acute renal failure for accurate urine output monitoring
- Intensive care settings
- Sacral pressure sores with incontinence
- When other methods of bladder management cause undue distress to a frail older person

*A catheter is NOT usually indicated for the following:*
- Immobility—even from stroke
- Heart failure with concomitant diuretic therapy
- Monitoring fluid balance in a continent patient
- Convenience of nursing—at home or in the hospital (see How to manage urinary incontinence without a catheter)
- Asymptomatic chronic retention—refer to urology for assessment

---

### How to manage urinary incontinence without a catheter

In spite of correct diagnosis and attempts to treat reversible causes of incontinence, some patients will continue to have permanent or intermittent urine leakage. An indwelling catheter is not always the best solution, as it can increase morbidity (infection, stones, urethral erosion) and even mortality.

Suggesting that catheters be removed is one of a geriatrician's most important jobs in post-acute care. If in doubt, involve a specialist continence nurse or team.

Other options for continence management are as follows:
- *Environmental modifications:* Bedside urinals and commodes, easy-access clothing, etc. can minimize or prevent accidents.
- *Regular or individualized toileting programs* can be very successful for patients with cognitive impairment but are labor intensive.
- *Absorbent pads* can be very effective but are quite labor intensive for very immobile patients.
- *Condom catheter* for men is particularly useful for isolated nocturnal incontinence as it can be removed during the day. It is sometimes difficult to use in uncircumcised men.
- *Intermittent catheterization* is for those with obstruction or atonic bladders. Consider it in agile, cognitively intact patients.

## How to minimize and treat catheter complications

### General
- For long-term catheters consider silicone, silastic, or silver impregnated (expensive)—these result in fewer blockages and infections.
- Catheters should be changed at least every 3 months.
- Maintain adequate hydration.

### Blocked catheters
- Consider the possibility of stones, infection, or bladder tumor.
- Renew catheter, maintain good fluid intake.

### Leakage around catheter
- Catheters can irritate the bladder, causing contractions. The resulting leak of urine past the catheter can render them useless and occasionally causes very painful spasms.
- This is particularly common if detrusor overactivity was cause of incontinence.
- Leakage can be induced or aggravated by infection.
- First exclude catheter blockage (which presents with identical spasms and leaks).
- If there is no residual volume, try reducing the catheter diameter and balloon size.
- Antimuscarinic drugs can sometimes help.

### Catheter infections
- All catheters become colonized after a few days, all catheter urine will be dipstick positive, and all specimens will grow bacteria. *This alone is not an indication for antibiotics.*
- Foul-smelling, dark, or cloudy urine is more commonly due to dehydration and is not an indication for antibiotics per se.
- Only treat clinically significant infections (fever, malaise, delirium, pain, abnormal inflammatory markers, etc.) to avoid promoting bacterial resistance.
- If you believe a catheter is a source of significant infection:
  - Send a urine culture to guide antibiotic choice.
  - Remove the catheter when possible (even if only for 48 hours). If not, perhaps change the catheter.
  - Ensure adequate hydration.
  - Choose a narrow-spectrum antibiotic if sensitivities allow.
- For repeated significant infection consider if the catheter is really necessary.

# Fecal incontinence: causes

This is defined as the involuntary passage of feces in inappropriate circumstances. The importance of situational factors means there is potential for anyone to be incontinent in some circumstances.

- Incontinence of feces is always abnormal and nearly always curable.
- It is much less common than urinary incontinence but more distressing.
- There is gross underreferral for diagnosis and treatment.
- Prevalence is 10% of nursing home residents are incontinent at least once per week.

## Continence mechanisms

- **The sigmorectal "sphincter":** The rectum is usually empty. Passage of feces into the rectum initiates rectal contraction (and anal relaxation), normally temporarily inhibited. The acute angle in the pelvic loop of the sigmoid may be important in causing temporary holdup.
- **The anorectal angle:** The puborectalis sling maintains an acute angle between the rectum and anus, preventing passage of stool into the anal canal.
- **The anal sphincters:** The external sphincter (striated, voluntary muscle), the internal sphincter (smooth muscle), and the anal vascular cushions complete the seal.
- **Anorectal sensation:** Sensation in the anus and rectum is usually sufficiently accurate to distinguish gas from feces, permitting the passage of flatus without incontinence. Good sensation may be particularly important when diarrhea is present.

## Causes of fecal incontinence

- Disorders of the anal sphincter and lower rectum include sphincter laxity (from many causes), severe hemorrhoids, rectal prolapse, tumors, and constipation.
- Any cause of fecal urgency (occasionally associated with reduced mobility), constipation (with spurious diarrhea), and any cause of diarrhea (inflammatory bowel disease, drugs, etc.)
- Disorders of the neurological control of the anorectal muscle and sphincter: lower motor neuron lesions (neuropathic incontinence), spinal cord lesions, cognitive impairment (neurogenic incontinence)

Fecal impaction is the most common cause (>50%). This is important because 95% of cases are curable. Neurogenic incontinence the second most common cause, where the cure rate is still around 75%.

# Fecal incontinence: assessment

## History

- The duration of symptoms is not helpful: impaction is just as common in those who have been incontinent for more than 3 months as in those in whom the incontinence is recent.
- Daily bowel movement is usual in older patients with impaction.
- Complete constipation is unusual in impaction.
- A feeling of rectal fullness with constant seepage of semi-liquid feces is suggestive of impaction, but rectal carcinoma may also present in this way.
- The combination of urinary and fecal incontinence strongly suggests impaction as the cause of both.
- Soiling without patient awareness suggests neuropathy.

## Examination

- **Inspect the anus** and ask the patient to strain. Look for inflammation, deformities, large hemorrhoids (internal or external), and rectal prolapse (pronounced protrusion of rectal mucosa through anus).
- **Rectal examination.** Assess passive and active anal tone by asking the patient to tighten; feel for feces or mass. It is easy to miss even large internal hemorrhoids unless proctoscopy is performed.
- **Abdominal examination.** Feel for the descending colon. Work proximally to assess colonic fecal loading (this may be misleading, see Investigation, below).
- **Neurological examination.** Look for signs of peripheral neuropathy and other neurological damage. Check perianal sensation (sacral dermatomes). Include a mental status assessment if you think neurogenic incontinence is likely.

## Investigation

A plain abdominal radiograph may be necessary to detect proximal fecal loading of the colon. Investigation of the anal sphincter tone and neurological control of rectum and anus (rectal manometry) is in the province of the proctologist and may occasionally be needed for neuropathic incontinence.

# Fecal incontinence: management

### Treatment of constipation

Fecal impaction, fecal retention, and fecal loading are the most common causes of constipation in hospitalized older people. Assume that any incontinent patient is constipated until proven otherwise after an adequate therapeutic trial of enemas for high fecal impaction.

### Mechanism

Passage of feces from the sigmoid into the rectum (often soon after a meal—the gastrocolic reflex) produces a sensation of rectal fullness and a desire to defecate. If this is ignored, the sensation gradually habituates, and the rectum fills with progressively harder feces. Some leakage past the anal sphincter (incontinence) is almost inevitable.

Impaction of hard fecal material produces partial obstruction, stasis, irritation of the mucosa with excessive mucus production, and spurious diarrhea. Emptying the colon of feces has two main effects: it prevents spurious diarrhea and, therefore, urgency, and it permits normal colonic motility and habit to be restored.

### Treatment of neurogenic fecal incontinence

Loss of control of the intrinsic rectal contraction caused by passage of normal fecal material from the sigmoid into the rectum results in the involuntary passage of a normal, formed stool at infrequent intervals, and usually at a timing characteristic of that patient (typically after breakfast).

It is a syndrome analogous to the uninhibited neurogenic bladder and usually only occurs in the context of severe dementia. However, note that incontinence in demented patients is commonly due to constipation. The diagnosis is thus usually made in a severely demented patient with a characteristic history after excluding the other common causes.

Since the diagnosis is usually one of exclusion, it is reasonable to treat most patients as though they have impaction, particularly if you cannot exclude high impaction by radiology. Once impaction has been excluded, there are three strategies:

- In patients with a regular habit, toileting at the appropriate time (perhaps with the aid of a suppository) may be successful. This requires an aide who knows the patient well.
- Arrange for a planned evacuation to suit caregivers, by administering a constipating agent (e.g., loperamide 2 mg every other day) combined with a phosphate enema two or three times weekly.
- If the patient has no regular habit and refuses enemas, the situation may have to be accepted and suitable protective clothing provided.

## How to treat "overflow" fecal incontinence

- Rehydration (possibly intravenous), regular meals, and help with toileting are important.
- **Enemas,** e.g., phosphate enema (120 mL sodium phosphate [27%]) given once or (occasionally) twice daily. Continue until there is no result, the rectum is found to be empty on digital examination, and the colon is impalpable abdominally. This may take a week or more.
- **Complete colonic washout,** e.g., using bowel prep such as GoLytely®. This is a rather extreme method but is sometimes required. Ensure the patient is well hydrated before you start.
- **Manual evacuation of feces** can cause further damage to the anal sphincters and is rarely necessary.
- **Laxatives** are generally less effective than enemas but can be used for milder cases and in the very frail. If the stool is hard, use a stool-softening laxative such as lactulose (20 mL/day)—stimulant laxatives (e.g., senna) may produce severe pain. Stimulant laxatives or suppositories may be appropriate for those with soft fecal overloading. A combination of stool softener and stimulant are sometimes used. While extra fiber is useful in prophylaxis, stool-bulking agents such as methylcellulose are of limited value in treating constipation as they increase the volume of stool being passed.
- After treatment, think prevention.

If, despite the above measures, a patient becomes impacted for a second time (without an obvious and removable cause), then regular (say once or twice weekly) enemas should be prescribed. Progress can only be satisfactorily monitored by examining the patient abdominally and rectally.

# Ears

**Ben Crane**

# Age-related hearing loss

Hearing loss is a common, often debilitating condition that increases with age. The prevalence of hearing loss—great enough to impede communication—is 10% in the general population and increases to 40% in the population older than 65 years. Hearing loss should not be ignored and dismissed by the physician as "part of getting older." It is a major contributor to decrease in quality of life through social isolation, anxiety, depression, and functional decline.

Hearing aids can be beneficial for improving the quality of life in the elderly. Despite the advantages, many older adults who could benefit from a hearing aid do not have one. Barriers to using one include cost (most insurance does not cover it), perception of social stigma, and a false belief that a hearing aid is not needed. As a result, only about 20% of people who would benefit from a hearing aid actually have one.

Cochlear implants are an option for any individual with bilateral profound hearing loss that cannot be significantly improved with hearing aids. Older adults are often excellent candidates because of their developed language skills.

One of the most effective screening tools is simply to ask patients, "Do you have a hearing problem?" Patients who respond affirmatively and want evaluation and treatment should be referred to an audiologist or otolaryngologist.

## Normal aging

### Presbycusis

- Presbycusis is a general term that describes hearing loss of multiple causes in older adults.
- Both the sensory peripheral (cochlea) and central (neural) components of the auditory system are affected, with peripheral degeneration accounting for at least two-thirds of the clinical features of presbycusis.
- Aging and noise exposure are the main contributing factors. Previous exposure to ototoxic agents such as some chemotherapy drugs and aminoglycoside antibiotics (often gentamicin) may also contribute to hearing loss.
- The high frequencies are lost first, usually noticed when high-pitched female voices become hard to hear. Because consonants are high frequency, the patient can often hear noise but not understand it, feeling that everyone is "mumbling" (loss of discrimination).
- "Recruitment" is a common problem, where the thresholds for hearing and discomfort are very close ("Speak slowly and clearly… don't shout").
- Busy and noisy environments make hearing harder; as a result, patients may avoid social situations.
- There is no treatment to reverse progression, but hearing aids often provide symptomatic improvement.
- Prevalence of presbycusis is 25% of 65- to 75-year-olds, and 40%–50% of those older than 75.

*Other ear changes with age*
- Thinner walls to the external auditory canal, with fewer glands, making cerumen drier, causing itching
- Drier cerumen due to decreased sweat gland activity, making accumulation (a cause of reversible hearing impairment) more common
- Increased hair growth in the external auditory canal, which further exacerbates cerumen accumulation
- Degenerative changes of the inner ear and vestibular system contributing to increase in deafness, vertigo, and tinnitus

## Classifying deafness

### Conductive
This is a disturbance in the mechanical attenuation of sound waves, preventing sound energy from reaching the cochlea.
- It can be caused by outer ear obstruction (e.g., wax, foreign body, otitis externa), tympanic membrane perforation, tympanosclerosis (scaring of the tympanic membrane), middle ear effusions, or ossicular mobility problems such as otosclerosis, ossicular discontinuity, or erosion.
- Conductive hearing loss is often surgically treatable, thus these patients should consult an otolaryngologist prior to being fitted with a hearing aid.
- Superior canal dehiscence syndrome is an unusual cause of conductive hearing loss that arises from loss of bone coverage over the labyrinth in the middle cranial fossa.

### Sensorineural
This type of hearing loss constitutes a problem with the cochlea or auditory nerve, so impulses are not transmitted to the auditory cortex.
- 95% of hearing loss falls into this category.
- It often has a genetic component, usually irreversible.
- In adults it may be traumatic, infective (viral, chronic otitis media, meningitis, syphilis), noise induced, degenerative (presbycusis), ototoxic (e.g., aminoglycosides, cytotoxics), neoplastic (acoustic neuroma), or have other causes such as Meniere's disease.
- The appropriate hearing aid can be helpful.
- In cases of unilateral or asymmetric sensorineural hearing loss, an MRI of the internal auditory canals with gadolinium should ordered to rule out cerebellopontine-angle tumors, such as acoustic neuroma.

## How to assess hearing

### General

Asking the patient if he or she has a hearing problem and observing performance in conversation is a good screening tool. If family members are present at the visit they often can provide a history of hearing loss that the patient may not be aware of or may deny.

### History

- Rate of onset and progression
- Unilateral or bilateral
- History of trauma, noise exposure, or ear surgery
- Family history of hearing problems or hearing aid use
- Drug history of ototoxic drugs, e.g., aminoglycoside antibiotics (gentamicin, streptomycin, etc.) and high-dose furosemide. Patients frequently do not know what drugs they were given during hospitalizations so ask about hospital stays and serious infections.
- Associated symptoms (pain, discharge, tinnitus, vertigo, and balance problems)

### Examination

- External ear and canal (looking for wax, inflammation, discharge, blood, abnormal growths, etc.)
- Drum (perforations, myringitis, retraction, bulging of drum, etc.)
- The Whispered Voice Test has excellent sensitivity and specificity. The examiner stands 2 feet behind the patient and occludes the non-tested ear with a finger while creating a masking noise by rubbing 2 fingers together. Three letters or numbers are whispered very softly. Misidentifying 50% or more of the items is abnormal.
- Tuning fork tests (with a 512 kHz fork) may be helpful. Both the Rinne and Weber tests are based on the principle of improved bone conduction perception with a conductive hearing loss.

#### Rinne test

This test compares air and bone conduction and is a sensitive and specific test of conductive hearing loss. Hold the tuning fork in front of the ear, then place it on the mastoid to compare air and bone conduction. Air > bone is normal (Rinne positive). Bone > air (Rinne negative) implies defective middle and outer ear function.

#### Weber test

Hold the tuning fork at vertex of the head and ask which ear hears the sound loudest. With conductive hearing loss, it is heard louder in the worse-hearing ear; with sensorineural hearing loss it is heard louder in the normal ear. It is less accurate than the Rinne test and is only moderately specific for sensorineural hearing loss.

### Who to refer?

Patients with any of following conditionsshould be referred to an otolaryngologist:

- Recent or abrupt hearing loss
- Any unilateral hearing loss or tinnitus (consider MRI)

## How to assess hearing (cont'd.)

- Hearing loss with a conductive component
- Hearing loss with associated symptoms, e.g., otalgia (ear pain), imbalance, vertigo, or autophony (unusual or disturbing sound of one's own voice), or otorrhea (drainage).

Sudden-onset hearing loss is an emergency and requires urgent ENT referral. If the hearing loss cannot be explained by infection or trauma, the patient should be started on steroids as soon as possible to have the best chance of regaining hearing. If a patient has a contraindication to systemic steroids, such as diabetes, an intratympanic steroid injection should be considered.

## Further reading

McGee S (2007). *Hearing in Evidence-Based Physical Diagnosis*. Second Edition, Chapter 21. Philadelphia: Saunders Elsevier.

# Audiology

Most patients with hearing impairment are managed by audiologists. They conduct hearing tests, fit patients for hearing aids, and offer hearing-related advice and rehabilitation.

## Specialized hearing tests

*Audiometry* quantifies the degree and pattern of loss, which may be of "pure tone" (using tones at varying frequencies and intensities) or "speech" (discriminating spoken words at differing intensities). The hearing thresholds are charted on an audiogram and interpreted by the audiologist (indicates conduction or sensorineural deafness, which frequency and which ear). Both air conduction and bone conduction should be measured.

*Tympanometry* indirectly measures the compliance of the middle ear, identifying infection and effusion in the middle ear and eustachian tube dysfunction.

*Evoked-response audiometry* measures action potentials produced by sound. No conscious response is required by the patient, thus tests are less open to bias.

## Recommending and fitting hearing aids

Audiologists help patients sort through the large variety of hearing aids available and choose a type appropriate for the patient's needs. They also help patients to have realistic expectations about their hearing aids (none yield "normal" hearing) and train them in how to use their hearing aids optimally (e.g., by minimizing background noise).

## Practical advice

Audiologists give information on assistive listening devices:
- **Alternative signals:** buzzers and flashing lights instead of doorbell or telephone ring; vibrating devices that attach to the wrist and alert the wearer to environmental noises
- **Television:** subtitles, or devices that connect to the hearing aid, allowing the television signal to be amplified.
- **Telephones** with high- and low-volume control and "T" settings that amplify the telephone noise without the background noise
- **Transmitter and receiver devices** (infrared or FM radio wave) for use in theaters, etc., with transmission from the sound source. The listener can adjust the volume in their receiver.

They can also offer advice on developing better communication skills.

## Aural rehabilitation programs

Age-matched group sessions can help patients with adjustment to the sudden reintroduction of noise with a hearing aid (after what is usually a gradual hearing loss). Here the audiologist can teach skills (e.g., blocking out background noise, lip reading) and facilitate the sharing of practical tips (e.g., eating in a booth at a restaurant to limit background noise).

## How to communicate with the hearing impaired

- Speak loudly and clearly, but do not shout.
- Use sentences, not one word answers—this gives contextual cues to lip readers.
- Minimize background noise.
- Maximize face-to-face visual contact.
- Use visual cues when talking (e.g., hand gestures).
- Be patient—repeat or rephrase things if needed.
- If confusion arises, write things down. Using a computer with increased font size may be useful.

## How to use a hearing aid

### Turning it on

Most hearing aids have three settings: O = off; M = microphone (use this setting for normal conversation); T = telecoil (use this setting with listening equipment, such as loop devices. These transfer sound directly to the hearing aid and cut out background noise).

In addition, there will often be a volume wheel, which can be adjusted as needed.

### What to do if there is no sound

- Check the hearing aid is not switched to O or T.
- Check that the batteries are not dead or put in upside down.
- Turn the volume up.
- Check that the mold is not clogged with wax.
- Check that the tubing is not wet (dry with hairdryer) or twisted.
- A working hearing aid will usually whistle when not in the ear.

### What to do if there is a whistling or squealing noise (feedback)

- This occurs when the ear mold is not snug, allowing sound to escape into the microphone.
- It is worse at high volumes.
- Check that the ear mold is a good fit (return to audiologist if not), and is inserted correctly.
- Ensure that there is not excess earwax impeding fit.

### Try turning the volume down.

- Maintaining the hearing aid
- Handle carefully.
- Keep the hearing aid dry, away from strong heat or light.
- Use a clean, dry tissue to clean it, never a damp cloth.
- Use wax remover on a regular basis.

# Hearing aids

The past decade has seen many advances in hearing aid technology and performance. Modern hearing aids offer improved fidelity, greater amplification, and frequency-specific amplification. Patients who tried hearing aids in the past and did not find them beneficial should be encouraged to try them again. Most states mandate that hearing aids can be returned for a refund within a 30-day trial period.

## What do hearing aids do?

All consist of a microphone, an amplifier that increases the volume, and a receiver that transmits the sound to the ear. Most hearing aids also include circuitry that filters and processes sound prior to amplification.

## Hearing aid evaluation

Finding a proper hearing aid for the patient is key to the success of the fitting. The following decisions need to be made:

- Monaural vs. binaural hearing aids. Binaural hearing aids yield a subjective improvement in sound clarity. Monaural can be considered for unilateral loss or when cost is a concern.
- Size and style depend on the shape of the external canal, the degree of hearing loss, the patient's dexterity, and cosmetic concerns.
- Circuitry and options appropriate for the patient. Conductive hearing loss is the easiest to aid because often only simple amplification is needed. What are the different types?

### Sizes from largest to smallest

- Behind the ear (BTE): Most amplification, easiest to handle, longer battery life
- In the ear (ITE)
- In the canal (ITC)
- Completely in the canal (CIC): cosmetically most appealing. Best for mild to moderate hearing loss, makes use of natural amplification provided by the pinna

### Signal processing

In the past, hearing aids were divided into analog, digitally programmable, and fully digital. Digital signal processing has become cheaper to manufacture in recent years and now comprises the vast majority of hearing aids dispensed.

### Open-fit hearing aids

A vented mold is used to allow low-frequency sound to enter the ear canal and avoid the occlusion effect of tight-fitting molds that makes the wearer's own voice sound unusual. The greatest benefit is for those with high-frequency sensorineural hearing loss, which is the case in 90% of elderly patient with hearing loss.

## Further reading

Kim HH, Barrs DM (2006). Hearing aids: a review of what's new. *Otolaryngol Head Neck Surg* **134**(6):1043–1050.

# Tinnitus

*Tinnitus* is the perception of a sound in one or both ears, without an external stimulus. It may be intermittent or continuous. Varying kinds of noises (ringing, humming, buzzing, occasionally, other noises) and at varying pitches are described. A third of people experience tinnitus at some point in their life; about 15% will seek medical treatment. The incidence increases with age. For most individuals tinnitus is a minor annoyance, but a small fraction of patients find it significantly disabling.

Tinnitus can be divided into two types:
- **Objective (or conductive):** Sound is transmitted to the cochlea by other tissue or fluid, such as vascular tumors or aneurysms. Patients can often hear their own pulse. Rarely, objective tinnitus is due to muscle spasms in the middle ear (stapedius or tensor tympani).
- **Subjective (or sensorineural):** Tinnitus is not associated with physical sound but has its origin in abnormal neural activity in the inner ear, auditory nerve, or central nervous system.

The following factors are associated with tinnitus:
- **Hearing loss** is a very common cause in older people. The mechanism is unclear—it may be akin to phantom limb pain. Note that tinnitus may precede hearing loss. It may be associated with conductive (e.g., wax accumulation) or more commonly sensorineural hearing loss (including presbycusis). Treatment of hearing loss (with hearing aid or occasionally cochlear implant) often results in improvement of tinnitus.
- **Drugs:** Many commonly prescribed drugs can either cause or exacerbate tinnitus (see Box 21.1).
- **Vascular disease:** microvascular damage to the auditory system, or a stroke affecting the auditory cortex
- **Infection:** e.g., chronic otitis media. Treat the cause, but the patient may have residual problems.
- **Other:** Meniere's disease, diabetes, thyroid disease, Paget's disease, brain tumor (intracanalicular and cerebellopontine), trauma and autoimmune disease. Treat the underlying cause.

## History
- Obtain a description of tinnitus. This may indicate the cause, e.g., pulsatile, often vascular; clicking, often due to palatal muscle spasms; high-pitched continuous noise is usually due to sensorineural hearing loss; low-pitched continuous noise is more commonly seen with (but not exclusive to) Meniere's disease.
- Screen for possible causes (drug history, ear disease, noise exposure, injury etc.).

## Examination
This should include a full head and neck examination, cranial nerve examination, auscultation for bruits, and inspection of the auditory canal.

## Investigation
- Audiogram; also consider CBC, glucose and thyroid function
- Imaging if unilateral (MRI of brain with gadolinium)

## Treatment

Treatment is difficult and frustrating—often the tinnitus will not resolve regardless of treatment.

- Stop any ototoxic medication and avoid its use in the future.
- Assess whether caffeine, aspartame sweetener, alcohol, nicotine, and marijuana worsen tinnitus and if so, avoid their use.
- Treat the cause (i.e., hearing loss) whenever possible.
- There is a strong association with insomnia and depression, both of which worsen the suffering and should be treated. There is some inconclusive evidence to suggest that antidepressants (SSRIs) may help even when there is no overt depression.
- Many other treatments have been tried (e.g., lignocaine, magnetic and ultrasonic stimulation, melatonin, Ginkgo biloba, niacin, zinc) but there is limited evidence that they work and adverse effects are common.
- Hearing aids are useful for hearing loss—the increased awareness of the background sound tends to make the noise less apparent.
- Masking techniques involve using a white-noise generator that aims to distract the patient from the tinnitus by reducing the contrast between the tinnitus signal and background noise. This technique works well at night when the tinnitus is often most bothersome.
- The mainstay of treatment is aimed at adjusting patients' perception of the tinnitus, trying to habituate them to the noise, and limiting the negative emotions it generates. This includes tinnitus retraining therapy, biofeedback, stress reduction techniques, and cognitive and behavioral therapy.
- Tinnitus support groups can be helpful.

---

### Box 21.1 Drugs causing or exacerbating tinnitus

- Aspirin (high dose)
- Other non-teroidal anti-inflammatory drugs (NSAIDs)
- Loop diuretics
- ACE inhibitors
- Calcium channel-blockers
- Doxazosin
- Aminoglycoside antibiotics
- Clarithromycin
- Quinine and chloroquine
- Carbamazepine
- Tricyclic antidepressants
- Benzodiazepines
- Proton pump inhibitors
- Some chemotherapy agents

---

### Further reading

Heller AJ (2003). Classification and epidemiology of tinnitus. *Otolaryngol Clin North Am* **36**(2):239–248.

# Vertigo

## Definition

*Vertigo* is the illusion of motion either relative to the environment (subjective) or the environment relative to the patient (objective). The key element is a feeling of motion, without which a clinical diagnosis of vertigo should not be made. Dizziness, light-headedness, nausea, and unsteadiness (which are often multifactorial in older adults) are often confused with vertigo.

## Physiology

The peripheral vestibular system is composed of the semicircular canals, the saccule, and the utricle. These organs sense motion, which is processed in the brain stem and cerebellum. Normally, there is a constant input from both ears updating the central structures on head position. In the brain stem they are integrated with other sensory information to control motor functions such as posture, ambulation, and eye movement.

The vestibular system controls eye movement via the vestibulo-ocular reflex (VOR). When this system ceases to function, patients notice the visual image moving (oscillopsia) when the head is in motion, such as during ambulation. An acute change of the signal from the vestibular end organs causes a disruption of the VOR, which is evident as a nystagmus. Over time, however, almost all patients can adapt to this disruption, yielding a normalization of function. Because of this adaptation:

- Vertigo is not a chronic condition. Multiple recurrences may occur, but a complaint of long-standing, continuous dizziness is not vertigo and is almost certainly of central origin.
- Vertigo rarely occurs with slowly progressive conditions (e.g., acoustic neuroma) as adaptation has time to occur.
- Vertigo is made worse by head movement.
- The use of vestibular sedatives such as meclizine should be limited to the acute phase for symptom relief only—prolonged use will delay adaptation and fail to relieve symptoms.

## Clinical relevance (see Table 21.1)

- Around half of all patients complaining of dizziness will have vertigo.
- In 80% of individuals vertigo results in a physician visit, sick leave, or interruption of daily activities.
- Of patients who present to emergency rooms with falls of unknown cause, 80% have vestibular impairment, and 40% complain of vertigo.
- Benign paroxysmal positional vertigo (BPPV) is the most common cause of peripheral vertigo, representing up to 40% of peripheral vestibular disease, with the incidence increasing with age.
- Chronic dizziness symptoms are frequently caused by vestibular migraine. This diagnosis is very common in older adults and should especially be considered if the patient has frequent headaches, motion sickness, or dietary triggers.
- Stroke should be considered in older patients with vertigo symptoms when other neurological deficits are present.

Table 21.1 Common causes of vertigo

| Condition | Features | Cause | Treatment |
|---|---|---|---|
| Benign paroxysmal positional vertigo (BPPV) | Episodes last less than a minute often with rolling over in bed, recurring frequently over weeks to months | Calcium debris in semicircular canal Usually idiopathic, associated with migraine and head trauma | Resolves spontaneously but may recur Epley maneuver may help |
| Acute labyrinthitis | Acute onset of severe vertigo, lasting hours to days Associated nausea, vomiting, and postural instability Patient in bed, refuses to move head | Unclear, possible ischemia of vestibular apparatus, often preceded by viral respiratory tract infection | High-dose steroids acutely may speed recovery Treat with vestibular sedatives only while vomiting, then allow adaptation to occur May have recurrent (milder) episodes or BPPV |
| Meniere's disease | Recurrent episodes of severe vertigo, vomiting, tinnitus, ear fullness (lasting hours), and fluctuating predominantly low-frequency hearing loss | Dilation of endolymphatic space in the canals seen—primary cause still unknown | Symptomatic treatment of acute attacks, low-sodium diet, diuretics may be of benefit; surgical options include intratypanic dexamethason or gentamicin and vestibular nerve sectioning |
| Vestibular migraine | Often a history of migraine headache, or headache in childhood. Frequent motion sickness, intolerance of perceived motion. Female predominance, often family history | Often triggered by dietary factors such as caffeine, chocolate, yeast, and red wine. May also be triggered by stress, fatigue, or hormonal factors | Lifestyle changes (i.e., avoid diet triggers, get regular sleep, eliminate stress). Prophylactic medications include beta-blockers, tricyclic antidepressants such as nortriptyline, and serotonin reuptake inhibitors. |
| Vertebrobasilar stroke | Stroke will cause abrupt-onset symptoms. Vertigo is usually associated with other neurological symptoms (e.g, ataxia, diplopia, visual loss, slurred speech, motor or sensory impairment) | Age, hypertension, coagulopathy, atherosclerosis | After stroke, slow improvement is normal, but often with residual defects. Modify vascular risk factors to prevent recurrence. |

# Vertigo: assessment

## History

This is the most important diagnostic tool in vertigo and should consist of open questions with clarification.

- Have the patient describe the symptom—is it a sensation of movement of self or the room (vertigo), nausea, disequilibrium, or a light-headed feeling? One should try to get the patients to describe their symptoms as specifically as possible, terms such as *dizziness* can include a wide range of symptoms.
- The duration of the attack is important. Duration of a few seconds suggests BPPV; hours suggests Meniere's disease or migraine, and days suggests labyrinthitis.
- Ask about onset, severity, duration, progression, associated symptoms, and recurrence to narrow down cause (see Table 21.1).
- Ask about provoking factors—it may be spontaneous or brought on by changes in middle ear pressure (sneezing, coughing) or head and neck position (question carefully to distinguish this from orthostatic symptoms). Brief vertigo occurring when rolling over in bed is almost always BPPV; orthostatic hypotension causes light-headedness after rising from a seated position.
- Ask about associated symptoms. Tinnitus and hearing loss (often worse during an attack) may suggest Meniere's disease. Headache may suggest a migraine etiology.
- Ask about predisposing factors, e.g., vascular risk factors, recent infections, headache, ototoxic drugs (gentamicin, chemotherapy), ear discharge, hearing loss, tinnitus, etc.

## Examination

- General examination with careful attention to the vital signs, and cardiovascular and neurologic systems
- Use otoscopy to examine the external auditory canals and tympanic membranes.
- Postural blood pressure measurements if patient has symptoms related to changes in position
- Examine eye movements for pursuit and saccades. Abnormalities in a patient with balance complaints suggest a cerebellar origin.
- Gait assessment
- Weber and Rinne tests using 512 Hz tuning fork. Audiogram if available.
- Vestibular assessment (see How to examine the vestibular system).

## How to examine the vestibular system

This is hard to do directly—it relies largely on testing the integrity of the vestibulo-ocular reflex (VOR).

- Test eye movements with the head still, looking for nystagmus (the eyes drift slowly *toward* the bad side, and the rapid correction phase is toward the good side). Visual fixation will suppress a peripheral nystagmus, but not a central one. Examination of the eyes under Frenzel lenses can bring out nystagmus that would otherwise be suppressed by visual fixation.
- Ask the patient to fix the gaze on the examiner's nose, while the examiner turns the head rapidly to one side or the other. The patient should be able to keep gaze fixed. If there is a peripheral vestibular hypofunction the gaze may drift during rotation toward that side, which is manifest by a catch-up saccade back to the point of fixation. When done properly, the test has better than 80% sensitivity and specificity for vestibular hypofunction.
- Ask the patient to shake their head, and then check for nystagmus—if it is present, this implies unilateral impairment.
- Nystagmus after 30 seconds of hyperventilation can be an indicator of a vestibular schwannoma.
- Eye movement in response to loud sound, valsalva, or pressure in the external auditory canal may indicate superior canal dehiscence syndrome.

## Dix–Hallpike maneuver

This is used to test for BPPV.

- Sit the patient up and stand behind the patient.
- Hold their head turned 45 degrees to one side.
- Keep holding the head at this angle and rapidly lay the patient down so that the head is hanging backward as much as possible (steps 1 and 2 of Epley's maneuver).
- Ask about symptoms while watching for nystagmus (nystagmus in a vertical torsional direction indicates posterior-canal BPPV).
- BPPV can be diagnosed confidently when the nystagmus is **latent** (occurs after a few seconds) and **transient** (stops after <60 seconds).
- After nystagmus stops, one can go directly to the Epley maneuver by rotating the head 270° so that the patient is facing the floor. Then have the patient sit up. This should move the calcium carbonate crystals to an area where they do not cause symptoms.
- Repeat procedure to see if symptoms have resolved.
- Repeat procedure with the head turned in the other direction.

# Vertigo: management

There are some specific treatments, depending on the cause (see Table 21.1). Symptomatic relief in the short term can be done with vestibular sedatives:

- Meclizine (12.5 or 25 mg up to every 8 hours)
- Clonazepam (0.5 mg up to every 6 hours)
- Promethazine (12.5 mg or 25 mg oral or suppository, also available IV). Sedating but works when for acute peripheral vertigo

These drugs are **not for long-term use** as they will impair adaptation and are rarely beneficial in BPPV because attacks are so short. Most vertigo will resolve with vestibular adaptation, leaving only brief feelings of imbalance on rapid head turns.

Some patients, however, will develop chronic dysfunction, in which case management is directed toward facilitating adaptation and development of coping strategies through vestibular rehabilitation. This is done by physiotherapists or otolaryngology specialist nurses and through a holistic approach. It involves a series of habituating exercises performed regularly to enable adaptation via compensation to occur. In addition to vestibular rehabilitation, consider exercise to improve muscle strength and a walking stick to aid peripheral balance.

Specific maneuvers (Epley's maneuver—see Figs. 21.1–21.6) and exercises are used for BPPV.

## How to perform the Epley maneuver

- Aims to clear debris from the posterior semicircular canal
- Requires the patient to have a reasonable range of neck motion
- Premedication with a vestibular sedative can be considered in severely affected patients.
- Stand behind the patient, firmly holding the head between your hands.
- Make movements quickly and smoothly, holding each position for at least 30 seconds or long enough for the vertigo and nystagmus to resolve before moving to the next position.
- The procedure may take as long as 3–5 minutes.
- See Figs. 21.1–21.6 on pp. 583–585 for illustration of technique.

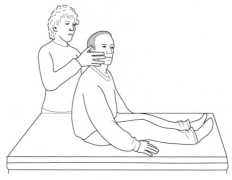

**Fig. 21.1** With the patient upright, turn the head 45 degrees to the affected side.

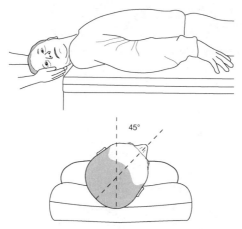

**Fig. 21.2** Lay the patient down, with the head still turned until the patient is reclined beyond the horizontal (as in the Hallpike maneuver).

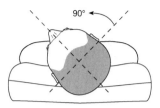

**Fig. 21.3** With the patient still reclined beyond horizontal, rotate the head through 90 degrees, with the face upward.

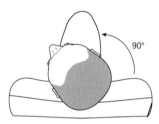

**Fig. 21.4** Keeping the head still, ask the patient to roll onto their side.

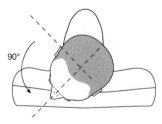

**Fig. 21.5** Rotate the head so the patient is facing downward.

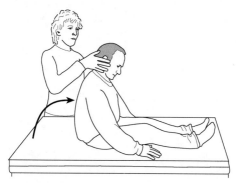

**Fig. 21.6** Keep the head at this angle and raise the patient to sitting position. Finally, rotate the head so it faces the midline with the neck flexed (facing forward, looking downward).

# Eyes

### Robert Weinberg

# The aging eye

Vision is a complex activity that involves eye function, cognition, reasoning, and memory.

With increasing age, the chance of visual impairment increases because of the following:

- Changes due to senescence
- Changes in associated functions (cognition, hearing, etc.)
- Increasing incidence of many eye diseases

Visual impairment is not inevitable—there is considerable diversity in both visual decline and compensatory adaptations.

There is a tendency for patients to blame failing vision on age and thus ignore it. Some changes may be age related, but there may be corrective action available or it may herald the onset of disease. Many eye disorders can be slowed or even stopped with prompt identification and treatment, and these actions may make all the difference between independence and dependence. Distinguishing what is "normal" and when to refer to a specialist is key.

## Changes in vision with age

### Visual acuity often decreases

- Multifactorial—changes in macula, lens, and cornea
- May be corrected (e.g., glasses or surgery)
- Consider eye disease if deterioration is rapid.

### Visual fields—peripheral vision is less sensitive

- Although formal field-testing is normal, consider cerebrovascular disease if there is a distinct homonymous field defect.
- Multifactorial—pupil smaller, lens cloudier, and peripheral retina less sensitive

### Near vision decreases

- Accommodative power diminishes due to increasingly rigid lens.
- Presbyopia is part of normal aging, beginning in middle age, and can be corrected with reading glasses or bifocals.

### Color vision

- Retinal receptors are unchanged.
- Alterations in color perception may relate to yellowing of the lens, altering the light reaching the retina.

### Light adaptation slower

- Rods and cones may be slower to react to changes in illumination, and the pupil may let in less light, requiring more light for good vision.
- This causes difficulty with night driving in particular.
- Glare may be a problem as the lens, cornea, and vitreous become less clear, and minute particles scatter light.

### Contrast sensitivity decreases
This is due to changes in the cornea, lens, and retina.

### Floaters
- Due to aggregation of collagen fibrils and liquefaction in the vitreous
- Usually normal, but if sudden onset, or large quantity, may indicate retinal detachment or vitreous hemorrhage.

# Visual impairment

Surveys indicate that 9.3% of the U.S. population has visual impairment (decreased vision not correctable by glasses or contact lenses) and 0.3% of the population is blind. The estimated incidence increases with age.

***Causes of visual impairment in people over age 75*** (from 2002 National Health Interview Survey):
- Cataract (53.4%)
- Glaucoma (10.3%)
- Diabetes (14.9%)
- Age-related macular degeneration (8.7%)

***Low-vision services*** may provide assistance with activities of daily living for those people with vision impairment that is not correctable by other means. Interventions include the following:
- Changing glasses prescription, using reading aids
- Explaining disease (it might *not* cause total blindness, e.g., with macular degeneration; improve patient's understanding of their future vision).
- Psychological support (often combined with hearing loss in older people—watch for social withdrawal. Acknowledge the problem and discuss the patient's fears).
- In some cases, consider a guide dog and the patient learning Braille.

Take specific history of certain activities and provide practical advice:
- **Reading**. What does the patient actually need to read? Advise about using good light, magnifiers, large-print books, photocopying recipes, etc., to a larger size.
- **Writing**. Use a black pen on white paper, consider Millard writing frame or bold-line paper, and discuss specific tasks such as writing checks.
- **Television**. Sit closer. Black and white sets may improve contrast; high-definition (HD) TV improves magnification and contrast.
- **Telling the time**. Use talking watches and clocks.
- **Cooking**. Improve lighting in the kitchen by removing dense-cloth curtains. Have tactile markers on oven and stove knobs, electronic fullness indicators on cups.
- **Telephoning**. Use large-button telephones.
- **Social interaction**. Sit with back to the window to improve light on visitors' faces. Discuss accessible holidays.

## How to optimize vision

*Bigger*
- Use magnifiers (glasses or contacts, hand magnifiers, stand magnifiers, illuminated magnifiers, reading telescopes). Consider portability, cosmetic aspects, and posture required to use them.
- Try larger print (large-print books; enlarge frequently used items with photocopier).

*Bolder*
- Contrasting colors, e.g., black on white
- Use highlighter to emphasize written word, reflective strips on door handles, stair edges, etc.
- Use white cups for dark drinks.
- Put contrasting strips round light fittings.

*Brighter*
- Use higher power bulbs (e.g., 150W rather than 60W).
- Use directable light sources (e.g., angle poise lamps).

# Blindness

### Definitions
- Blindness is partially sighted <20/200 in both eyes or reduced fields (e.g., homonymous hemianopia).
- Blindness need not mean total lack of vision. The statutory definition is that the person should be "so blind as to be unable to perform any work for which eyesight is essential." Pragmatically, it is vision <20/200, or very diminished fields.

### Benefits to individual
- Financial—personal income tax allowance, disability living allowance, eligibility for handicapped parking, easier access to help from social services.
- Loan from some libraries of cassette or CD player and CDs or tapes of talking books and newspapers

# Cataract

This term is used to describe any lens opacity. Cataract is the most ommon cause of treatable blindness worldwide. In the Unite States it is largely a disease of the older population, causing visual impairment in 9.3% of people aged 55–64, 31% of people aged 65–74, and 53% of people over 75. Everyone over 80 has some opacification. Causes of cataracts remain unknown.

## Possible causes

- Exposure to environmental agents (e.g., UV light, smoke, blood sugar)—more exposure with increasing age
- Ocular conditions (trauma, uveitis, previous intraocular surgery)
- Systemic conditions (e.g., diabetes, hypocalcemia, Down syndrome)
- Drugs (especially steroids—ocular and systemic)

## Symptoms

- Painless visual loss that varies depending on whether it is unilateral or bilateral and severity or position of the opacity.
- It commonly begins with difficulty in reading, recognizing faces, and watching television.
- It may be worse in bright light or be associated with glare around lights, affecting night driving.

## Signs

- Reduced visual acuity—usually gradual
- Diminished red reflex on ophthalmoscopy
- Change in appearance of the lens (appears cloudy brown or white when viewed with direct light)
- Beware of coexisting conditions: pupil responses are normal, and the patient should be able to point to the position of a light source.

## Management

New glasses prescription may delay the need for surgery.
- Optimizing visual conditions
- Surgical removal of opacified lens
- No effective medical treatment

## When to treat?

Treatment is individually tailored, depending on the visual requirements of the patient, severity of cataract, and presence of other ocular disease (which worsens outcome from surgery). Roughly speaking, <20/40 in both eyes is likely to benefit, but an older person who does not read much may be quite happy with this visual level. Conversely, someone who wishes to continue driving or needs precise vision for his or her life may want surgery much sooner.

**Previously, surgeons waited for the cataract to "ripen" to aid extraction; this is no longer the case. Surgery is generally performed on the poorer-seeing eye first and at some later time on the second eye. Timing for cataract surgery is not medically critical but is usually dictated by the patient's lifestyle and visual needs.**

**The surgeon should have a frank discussion about risks and benefits with each individual.**

## What the surgery involves

- It is usually done as an outpatient under local or topical anesthesia.
- Preoperative history and physical, and laboratory testing depending on those findings, are indicated.
- It is **not** necessary for patients to discontinue any systemic medications prior to cataract surgery. The procedure may be done safely even while a patient is taking an anticoagulant or aspirin.
- The patient must be able to lie reasonably flat and still and be able to communicate and cooperate with the surgeon. Hearing-impaired patients may need special hearing devices for surgery under local anesthesia, and demented patients may need sedation or general anesthetic (altering risk and benefit). Consider also history of heart failure, respiratory disease, and spinal deformity; can the patient lie flat or almost flat? If positioning is problematic, the surgeon must be able to adapt the procedure to ensure patient safety.
- The surgery is generally safe and a well-tolerated procedure.
- Phacoemulsification is most commonly used in the U.S. (a small incision in the eye to access the lens, which is then liquefied with an ultrasonic probe). A replacement lens is then folded into the empty lens capsule. Sutures are not usually needed, but dissolving or permanent sutures can be used to ensure a water-tight wound or increase wound stability in a patient with a chronic cough, as in COPD.
- Other methods (extracapsular and intracapsular extraction) are less commonly used.
- Conventional intraocular lenses, covered by insurance, can provide excellent vision without glasses for distance (the patient would need to wear glasses for reading) or for reading (the patient would need to wear glasses for distance). Many patients will choose to wear glasses (bifocal) to avoid having to put them on and take them off. Multifocal intraocular lenses that correct both distance and reading vision without glasses are available, but are not covered by insurance.
- Postoperatively the patient will wear an eye shield (usually at night) for a period and use steroid and antibiotic eyedrops.
- Surgery is done on one eye at a time. The second eye surgery may be done as soon as it has been determined that the first surgery is successful, or whenever the patient decides to undergo the procedure.

## Outcome

With no ocular comorbidity, >95% have a visual acuity of >20/50. Outcome is worse with other eye diseases, e.g., glaucoma, and in patients with diabetes and cerebrovascular disease.

New eyeglasses are usually prescribed a few weeks after surgery once postoperative inflammation has settled, unless the patient has selected a multifocal intraocular lens or is planning on having the second eye surgery done soon. In the latter case, eyeglasses are usually prescribed after recovery from the second surgery.

# Glaucoma

This is the third most common cause of blindness worldwide.

### Definition

Visual loss in glaucoma is due to increased optic nerve cupping resulting in visual field defect. It is usually associated with a rise in intraocular pressure sufficient to cause damage to the optic nerve fibers (either direct mechanical damage or by inducing ischemia). Specific mechanisms of optic nerve changes in glaucoma are still being investigated.

### Intraocular pressure

- Ciliary body (posterior) makes aqueous humor (fluid), which flows anteriorly through the pupil and drains via the trabecular network in the anterior chamber angle of the eye.
- Balance of production and drainage determines intraocular pressure.
- A wide range of pressures is seen in normal adults (detected with tonometry)—average, 15.5 mmHg; normal, <21 mmHg.
- It is individually determined at which pressure ocular damage ensues. There is a relationship between corneal thickness and safe intraocular pressure. Patients with thicker corneas can tolerate higher intraocular pressures without sustaining optic nerve damage.
- A person can develop glaucoma with "normal" pressure, called "normal-tension glaucoma" (may be high for that person, or other factors such as ischemia may be relevant). Fluctuating BP may be contributory.
- A person can have high pressures without having glaucoma; this is "ocular hypertension."
- Symptoms depend on the rate and degree of rise in pressure. Generally, increased pressure is asymptomatic unless advanced or acute.

### Primary ("chronic") open-angle glaucoma

- This is the most common form of glaucoma.
- Failure of outflow of aqueous humor causes a slow rise in pressure, allowing adaptation, so subtle or no symptoms occur until visual field defects progress.
- There is no pain, corneal cloudiness, or halos.
- A slow loss of visual field occurs, typically in an arc shape ("arcuate scotoma"), with preservation of central vision (macula has more nerve cells so is relatively protected). It may progress to tunnel vision and then blindness if left untreated.

Early detection can slow or halt progression of disease.

### Risk factors

- Age (1% in fifth decade, rising to 10% in ninth decade)
- African American origin (four times the risk)
- Blood relatives with glaucoma

*Screening*
- Target those at higher risk.
- Combination of ophthalmoscopy (looking for disc "cupping"), automated perimetry testing (for minor field defects), tonometry (for intraocular pressure), and measurement of corneal thickness (pachymetry)
- Encourage regular eye tests and include careful fundoscopy in physical examination.

*Treatment*
- *Topical treatments (eyedrops):* beta-blockers, e.g., timolol (decrease aqueous secretion; can cause systemic beta-blockade); prostaglandin analogs, e.g., latanoprost (improve drainage, may darken iris and cause eyelashes to grow longer); alpha-agonists (decrease aqueous production); carbonic anhydrase inhibitors, e.g., dorzolamide (decrease aqueous secretion); parasympathomimetics, e.g., pilocarpine (constrict pupil so will reduce visual field—not commonly used)
- *Oral treatments:* carbonic anhydrase inhibitors, e.g., acetazolamide (very powerful, with many side effects including electrolyte imbalance, decreased appetite, depression, and paresthesia of extremities)
- *Surgical treatment:* trabeculectomy—operation to improve aqueous outflow. Argon laser trabeculoplasty (laser energy applied to the trabecular meshwork) may be effective. Cyclodiode laser to the ciliary body (decreases production) is used in refractory cases.

## Acute-angle closure glaucoma
- Apposition of the lens to the back of the iris prevents outflow of aqueous fluid with a rapid rise in pressure.
- Causes red, painful eye with nausea and vomiting, blurred vision, and halos around lights (due to corneal edema).
- May be precipitated by pupil dilation, e.g., at dusk. Pupil constricts when asleep so episodes at night may be aborted by sleep.
- More common in older patients, women, and farsighted individuals— watch for it in the vomiting older woman with a red eye.
- On examination the cornea is usually cloudy and visual acuity is significantly reduced.

This is an emergency sight-threatening condition—it requires urgent referral and treatment.
- Treat with IV acetazolamide, topical glaucoma treatment, and laser iridotomy to restore flow. Treat the other eye prophylactically with laser iridotomy to prevent pupillary block.

# Age-related macular degeneration

Age-related macular degeneration (AMD) is an increasing cause of visual impairment in United States.

New treatments for early stages make detection crucial.

### Definition

As it sounds, age-related degenerative changes affect the macula (the central part of the retina responsible for clear central vision).

There are two types:
- 90% **dry** with gradual onset of symptoms (drusen and atrophy of the retinal pigment epithelium)
- 10% **wet**, where symptoms relate to leaking vessels causing distortion or sudden loss of central vision due to submacular hemorrhage (choroidal neovascularization—new vessels can leak, bleed, and scar, causing visual loss in a few months)

### Prevalence

- Increases with age
- 25–30 million worldwide
- Up to 30% of those over 75 may have early disease, and 7% have late disease.

### Risk factors

- The cause is unknown.
- Age, smoking, and family history are strongly associated.
- Female sex, Caucasian race, hypertension, blue eyes, other ocular conditions (lens opacities, aphakia), and low dietary antioxidants also possibly increase risk.

### Symptoms

- Asymptomatic in early stages, progressing to loss of central vision
- The patient may also have decreased contrast and color detection, flashing lights, and hallucinations.
- Distortion of straight lines is a feature of wet AMD.
- Peripheral vision is normal in the absence of other pathology.

### Detection

- Regular ocular examination with dilated fundus examination
- Use of Amsler grid in high-risk patients (see How to use an Amsler grid to detect macular pathology, p. 600).

### Prognosis

- The dry form progresses slowly and rarely causes blindness.
- The wet form may progress rapidly (blind in under 3 months). Sudden onset of distortion of central vision should prompt urgent referral.
- Bilateral disease occurs in 42% with wet AMD: first one eye will get it, and then the other will be affected within 5 years.

### Prevention

- Smoking is the most important modifiable risk factor.
- A diet rich in fruit and vegetables reduces the risk of development of AMD.
- A combination of beta-carotene, vitamins C and E, and zinc is effective in preventing severe visual loss in established moderate–severe AMD. In a multicentered study, antioxidant vitamins have been shown to halt progression of dry macular degeneration in approximately 30% of patients.

### Treatment

- Treatment is appropriate for a subset of wet AMD only. It halts progression, so early treatment is desirable. Several therapeutic approaches are now available and multiple additional therapeutic modalities are being investigated.
- Photodynamic therapy targets subfoveal neovascular areas (while preserving normal retina) by using a photosensitive drug (verteporfin) along with a nonthermal activating laser. Used in early disease, this therapy can slow or halt progression.
- Antiangeogenic (pegaptanib sodium) injections (FDA approved) into the vitreous cavity and repeated at 6-week intervals as needed can be effective in treating wet AMD.
- Ranibizumab, a recombinant humanized antibody fragment that inhibits angiogenesis (also FDA approved) is administered by intravitreal injection every month x3 then every 3 months as needed. After 1 year of treatment, 95% of patients with wet AMD treated with ranibizumab had no loss of vision, and approximately 1/3 of patients gained vision.
- Laser photocoagulation is sometimes used for extrafoveal lesions.

## How to use an Amsler grid to detect macular pathology

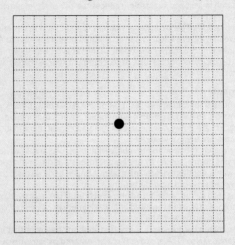

- Test one eye at a time.
- Usual reading glasses should be worn, and the grid held at acomfortable reading distance.
- Ask the patient to look at the central spot and not to look away.

Assess the following:
- Can all four corners of the grid be seen?
- Are any of the lines missing, wavy, blurred, or distorted?
- Do all of the boxes appear the same size and shape?

Any abnormalities may indicate macular pathology and should prompt referral to an ophthalmologist.

# The eye and systemic disease

Eye disease develops as a late complication of prolonged poor control of both diabetes and vascular disease. The important message is to strive to prevent these problems in the first place.

## Diabetes

Diabetes causes retinopathy, cataracts, and microvascular cranial nerve palsies.

### Retinopathy

- This is associated with increasing duration of diabetes—at 20 years, 80% of patients will have some retinopathy.
- All patients with diabetes require dilated annual screening (either photographic or by appropriately trained professional). Direct ophthalmoscopy alone is inadequate.
- Appearance includes microaneurysms, hemorrhages (background retinopathy) progressing to cotton-wool spots, blot hemorrhages and tortuous vessels (pre-proliferative retinopathy), then new vessels (proliferative retinopathy). Exudates and macular edema are indicators of maculopathy.
- Early detection of problems (especially when near the macula) should prompt referral to an ophthalmologist. Sight-threatening retinopathy requires laser photocoagulation to limit progression.

The benefits of intensive glucose control in older adults with type 2 diabetes mellitus to prevent retinopathy must be carefully weighed against the burden of care and risks to the individual. Benefit is more likely for robustly healthy older adults with greater than 10 years of average life expectancy or those with existing retinopathy. Meticulous control of hypertension has been shown to reduce all complications including retinopathy.

### Vascular disease

- This affects the eye directly with hypertensive retinopathy, and more indirectly when cerebrovascular disease affects vision. Vascular disease is associated with microvascular cranial nerve palsies.
- Early detection and control of risk factors for vascular disease will ameliorate this problem. Tight blood pressure control, smoking cessation, lipid lowering, diabetic control, and appropriate antiplatelet use should all be targeted at the older age group as aggressively as in younger patients.
- There is little in the way of treatment for the disease once it is established.
- Appearance includes silver wiring, arteriovenous crossing changes, arteriolar narrowing progressing to exudates, cotton-wool spots, hemorrhages, and papilledema.

## Giant cell arteritis

See Chapter 17, Temporal (giant cell) arteritis (p. 500).

# Visual hallucinations

Management varies with the cause.

## Organic brain disease

- Lewy body dementia (occurs in 50%–80%; hallucinations usually well formed, e.g., animals). Also occurs in other dementias such as Alzheimer's disease and dementia of Parkinson's disease. It can respond dramatically to cholinesterase inhibitors.
- Anoxia, migraine, and delirium—treat the underlying cause.
- Focal neurological disease (especially occipital and temporal lobe— ranges from unformed lines and lights, etc., to complex)
- Occipital lobe seizures—treat with anticonvulsants.

## Drugs

- Hallucinations are common with dopamine agonists and anticonvulsants (usually mild and unformed). They are also seen but less common with beta-blockers. Try reducing the dose, watching for rebound in symptoms.
- Overdose of anticholinergic drugs such as antihistamines or tricyclic antidepressants
- Use of amphetamines and LSD
- Alcohol withdrawal

## Psychiatric disease

Visual hallucinations occasionally occur with schizophrenia (auditory more common).

## Charles Bonnet's syndrome

- This is a diagnosis of exclusion.
- No other psychiatric symptoms or diseases are present.
- Hallucinations occur with bilateral visual loss (typically secondary to cataracts or glaucoma) as a "release phenomenon."
- These are usually well formed and vivid, occurring in clear consciousness.
- Insight is usually present.
- Duration is usually seconds to a minute or so.
- They may be simple (flashes, shapes) or complex (recognizable images).
- They are nonthreatening—the patient's reaction is often one of curiosity or amusement.
- The syndrome is probably underestimated, as patients are reluctant to tell doctors for fear of being labeled "crazy."
- This syndrome is not related to psychiatric problems.
- Reassurance is often all that is required, but symptoms may be improved by enhancing vision.

# Drugs and the eye

Many drugs frequently used in the older patient can cause ocular side effects. Older people are more vulnerable to developing side effects, but are least likely to report them (attributing them to getting older).

### Direct toxicity

- Chloroquine and hydroxychloroquine (used in treatment of rheumatoid arthritis and other connective tissue diseases as well as malaria), given in large, prolonged doses, can cause an irreversible toxic maculopathy causing permanent decrease in vision. Patients receiving these drugs should be monitored regularly for signs of maculopathy.
- Phenothiazines used for a long time (to treat psychosis) may cause retinal damage.
- Tamoxifen (for breast cancer treatment) may cause maculopathy.
- Amiodarone (for arrhythmias) deposits in the cornea in approximately 98% of patients and may cause glare. Less commonly, cataract can develop.
- Ethambutol (anti-tuberculous) can cause optic neuritis and red/green color blindness.

### Drugs altering accommodation

Drugs causing blurred vision include
- Antihistamines
- Some antihypertensives

### Drugs decreasing pupil size

Drugs causing less light accommodation include
- Opiates
- Miotic drops used for glaucoma

### Steroids

- Oral steroids over time can cause cataracts.
- Topical and oral steroids may raise the intraocular pressure.

### Drugs affecting tear production

The drugs listed below can cause changes in tear production, resulting in dry eye, burning, itching, and foreign-body sensation and may cause decreased vision. In addition, there is a decrease in tear production with age, causing similar symptoms.
- Antihistamines
- Beta blockers
- Diuretics

# Eyelid disorders

Eyelids provide physical protection to the eyes and ensure normal tear film and drainage. Disorders are common in older people, are often uncomfortable, and yet are underrecognized and undertreated.

### Entropion

This is in-turning of the (usually) lower lid. It occurs as the orbicularis muscle weakens with age (or with conjunctival scarring distorting the lid). Lashes irritate the eye and may abrade the cornea, causing red eye. Lubricants and taping of the eye may relieve symptoms. Surgery (under local anesthesia) provides definitive correction.

### Ectropion

This is eversion of the eyelid. It occurs with orbicularis weakness, scarring of the periorbital skin, or seventh nerve palsy. Distortion prevents correct drainage of tears and correct tear film, leading to watery eye with conjunctival dryness. Treat with ointment to protect conjunctiva. Surgery (local anesthesia) corrects this condition.

### Ptosis

*Ptosis* is drooping of the upper eyelid. When severe, it can cover the pupil and impair vision. Causes are aponeurotic (defects in levator aponeurosis), mechanical (lid lesion, lid edema), neurological (third nerve palsy—look for pupil and eye movement problems, Horner's syndrome), or myogenic (congenital levator dystrophy, muscular dystrophies, myasthenia gravis, chronic progressive external ophthalmoplegia).

Do not ignore ptosis in older people—it may not be long-standing. Look for signs of underlying disease.

### Dry eye

Dry eye is common in the elderly as tear secretion diminishes. The eye feels gritty but is not red. Diuretics may exacerbate it. The most common cause is blepharitis (inflamed lid margins with blocked meibomian gland orifices and crusting). This is usually worse in those with rosacea, eczema, and psoriasis.

Treat blepharitis with hot compresses (5 minutes bid), lid massage (upward toward lid margin lower lid, downward toward lid margin upper lid), eyelid cleaning that targets the base of the eyelashes at the lid margin (warm water ± baby shampoo on a cotton swab). Antibiotic ointment is not usually required unless staphylococcal infection is suspected.

Treat dry eye with artificial tears or ointment (this gives considerable relief).

### Eyelid tumors

The most common type (90%) is basal cell carcinoma. These are slow growing, nonmetastasizing but locally invasive. They are often ignored by the patient. They are more common in fairer skins after chronic sun exposure.

A waxy nodule with telangiectatic vessels on the surface and pearly rolled border (rodent ulcer) is the usual appearance. Treatment is with surgical excision (Mohs micrographic surgery preserves the most tissue and may be appropriate in some patients) or radiotherapy.

## Herpes zoster infection

This is facial shingles. Involvement of the ophthalmic division of the trigeminal nerve will cause vesicles and crusting periorbitally. Ocular involvement is common when vesicles appear on the nose (Hutchinson's sign).

## Parkinson's disease

Patients with Parkinson's disease have a decreased blink rate and may develop ocular problems related to tear dysfunction. These may include redness, foreign-body sensation, and blurring of vision. Supportive treatment with artificial tears used at least four or more times a day can be beneficial (see also Chapter 7, Parkinson's disease, p. 146).

# Skin

**Gerald Lazarus**
**Rachel Abuav**

# The aging skin

Skin changes with age are a result of intrinsic universal biological programs (intrinsic aging) (see Table 23.1) and sun exposure (photoaging).

**Table 23.1** Age-related skin changes

| Age-related change | Clinical implications |
|---|---|
| Epidermis thins, with flattening of dermo-epidermal junction, limiting transfer of nutrients and making separation of layers easier | Increased tendency to blistering |
| | Increased skin tearing |
| Slower cell turnover | Slower healing of wounds |
| Less melanocyte activity, with slower DNA repair | Increased photosensitivity, with increased tendency toward skin malignancy |
| Altered epidermal protein profile | Dry, rough, and flaky skin more common |
| | Abnormal skin barrier, so more prone to irritant contact dermatitis |
| Altered connective tissue structure and function | Reduced elasticity and strength of skin |
| Decreased blood flow through dermal vascular beds | Skin appears cooler and paler |
| | Thermoregulation is less efficient |
| | Hair and gland growth and function slow |
| Subcutaneous fat decreases in volume and is distributed differently (e.g., more abdominal fat) | Thermoregulation is less efficient |
| | Protection against pressure injury decreases |
| | Facial features appear more aged due to loss of facial fullness |
| Number of cutaneous nerve endings decreases | Cutaneous sensation blunts (e.g., fine touch, temperature, proprioception) |
| | Pain threshold increases |
| Fewer cutaneous glands | Thermoregulation is less efficient |
| Nail bed function decreases | Nails become thick, dry, brittle, and yellow, with longitudinal ridges |
| The immune functioning of the skin decreases | Increased risk of skin infections and malignancies |

# Photoaging

Photoaging is the most obvious manifestation of aging. Society's perception of aging is intricately tied to photoaging, which manifests as follows:

- Skin wrinkling (both coarse and fine), roughened texture, yellowed sallow complexion, and irregularities in pigmentation
- Solar (actinic) elastosis—thickened, yellow skin with rhomboid pattern on the posterior neck and comedones on the face and neck
- Actinic (or senile) purpura is a nonpalpable purpuric eruption often on the forearms due to red cell extravasation from sun-damaged vessels and minor trauma (the platelet count is normal).
- Lesions include brown macules (lentigines), multiple telangiectasia, actinic (solar) keratoses (scaly, rough hyperkeratotic areas on sun-exposed skin), and a tendency to develop skin tumors.
- Histologically, one sees a thickened dermis with tangled elastic fibers; the epidermis is variable in thickness with regions of both hypertrophy and atrophy.

Prevention is better than cure for these changes, but topical retinoids may reduce the appearance of wrinkles and pigment and certain plastic surgery techniques appear to have utility. Interventions include chemical peels, injections of fillers (i.e., hyaluronic acid or collagen), botulinum toxin, and laser resurfacing techniques.

## Sun protection

- Avoid unnecessary sun exposure.
- Stay out of the sun during the hottest time of the day (11 AM–3 PM).
- Sunscreens with sun protection factor (SPF) of at least 30 and broad-spectrum ingredients blocking both UVA and UVB are the most efficacious agents.
- Areas that are often forgotten include balding heads (wear a hat) and the tops of ears (apply sun screen).

# Skin cancers and pre-cancers

The following skin lesions are seen more frequently with aging, especially in patients with high cumulative sun exposure over their lifetimes. The lesions are most common on sun-exposed areas, especially the head and neck, are diagnosed by visual inspection, and confirmed by skin biopsy.

Any suspicious skin lesion should be biopsied when appropriate, or the practitioner should make a referral to a dermatologist for diagnosis and management. Particularly concerning areas for skin cancers are around the eyes, eyebrows, behind the ears, or in the malar creases, as tumors can infiltrate deeply and invade critical underlying anatomic structures.

## Actinic keratoses (AK)

- Rough, scaly patches on sun-exposed skin.
- Patients with lighter skin types are most commonly affected.
- Risk factors include sun exposure and arsenic exposure.
- Vary from skin colored to red, brown, yellow, and black (often patchy).
- Premalignant, with a small risk of becoming squamous cell carcinoma over years. Some resolve spontaneously.
- Treat established lesions. If a lesion does not respond or rapidly recurs after treatment, biopsy is recommended to rule out skin cancer (see Table 23.2).

**Table 23.2** Treating skin lesions

| Treatment option | Comments |
|---|---|
| Destruction with cryotherapy | Liquid nitrogen spray on a lesion for (15 seconds, 2 consecutive freeze–thaw cycles) <br> Blistering can occur, healing takes 5 days to 3 weeks, depending on site |
| Topical 5-fluorouracil cream or solution | Efudex®, Carac® 0.5%, 2%, or 5%—applied once to twice daily for 2–4 weeks <br> Causes erythema, burning, ulceration, and then healing |
| Topical 3% diclofenac sodium gel | Solaraze®: treat daily for 60–90 days <br> Therapeutic effect may occur up to 30 days after stopping <br> Usually less irritating than other methods |
| Topical 5% imiquimod cream | Aldara® applied 2 times per week x16 weeks <br> Can cause significant erythema, blistering |
| Photodynamic therapy | 20% 5-aminolevulinic acid solution (Levulan® is applied to AK <br> Skin is exposed to blue light (Blu-U®) |
| Tricholoracetic acid solution (20%–70%) | Applied to AK <br> Peeling of AK <br> Risk of scarring |
| CO$_2$ laser resurfacing | Excellent for treating the lip <br> Risk of scarring |

## Bowen's disease

- Intraepidermal carcinoma (squamous cell carcinoma in situ), with small risk of transformation into invasive squamous cell carcinoma of the skin
- Typically occurs on the lower leg of elderly women; head and neck of men and women equally
- Caused by sun exposure, arsenic exposure, or human papilloma virus (HPV) infection.
- Pink or reddish scaly plaques with well-defined edges.
- Histology should be confirmed; shave biopsy is appropriate.
- Surgical excision is generally the treatment of choice, Mohs micrographic surgery should be performed for large lesions or lesions in special sites (i.e., periungual).
- Topical treatments with lower cure rates include topical 5-fluorouracil (5-FU), imiquimod, cryosurgery, electrodessication and curettage, or radiation therapy.

## Basal cell carcinoma (see Plate 1)

- This is the most common skin tumor, accounting for 75% of all skin cancers.
- Risk factors include UV exposure, irradiation, arsenic ingestion, or chronic scarring.
- It is slow growing and usually only locally invasive (metastasis virtually unknown), but facial tumors left untreated can cause infiltration into and erosion of cartilage and bone with significant disfigurement.
- It begins as a pearly papule, which can then ulcerate. Lesions demonstrate a rolled border and surface telangiectasia.
- Less common morphologies include pigmented, which can mimic benign tumors; or sclerotic (morpheaform), which can look like a scar. These lack the classic features.
- Treatment depends on the location of the tumor and the size and histological pattern of the tumor (see Table 23.3)
- Recurrence is treatment dependent, 3%–20% at 5 years, so follow-up is required.

## Squamous cell carcinoma (SCC) (see Plate 2)

- This second most common skin cancer, accounting for 20% of non-melanoma skin cancers.
- Risk factors include sun exposure, irradiation, smoking, and exposure to industrial carcinogens. An important risk factor is chronic ulceration or scarring, (i.e., SCC may develop at the edge of a chronic leg ulcer).
- 5%–10% will metastasize if not treated, usually to local lymph nodes initially.
- It begins as an erythematous, indurated plaque that becomes elevated, scaly, and even wart-like. The plaque may then go on to ulceration.
- Excision with 4- to 60-mm margins or Mohs micrographic surgery is the standard therapeutic option for invasive SCC.
- Radiotherapy can be used for complicated cases in patients >60 years old, where excision is unreasonable (e.g., on the face of an elderly patient with significant comorbidities) or as an adjuvant to surgery (i.e., a recurrent tumor or when there is evidence of perineural invasion).

- Nonsurgical options for low-risk tumors include intralesional injection with interferon and topical immune-response modifiers (i.e., imiquimod), but cure rates are significantly lower.

**Table 23.3** Treatment options for basal cell carcinoma (BCC)

| Treatment | Indications |
| --- | --- |
| Mohs micrographic surgery | Tumors on face, genitals, fingers, and toes |
| | Tumors on trunk >2 cm in diameter, with indistinct borders, recurrent tumors, tumors in scars |
| | Aggressive histological findings |
| Excision (4 mm margin) | Well-defined tumors on the trunk |
| Electrodessication and Curettage | Superficial BCC |
| | Invasive BCC in non-hair-bearing areas, without aggressive histological features |
| Radiotherapy | For non-aggressive tumors in situations when excision will be disfiguring |
| | Elderly, frail patients who cannot endure surgery |
| | As an adjuvant to Mohs when there is perineural invasion |
| | Should be reserved for patients >60 years old |
| Topical immunomodulator (Imiquimod-Aldara®) | Superficial BCC when surgery not an option |
| | Cure rate may be lower |
| Photodynamic therapy (ALA-Blu U®) | Superficial BCC when surgery not an option |
| | Cure rate may be lower |

**Lentigo maligna (LM)** (melanoma—see Plate 3)
- Superficial melanoma, accounting for 5%–15% of all melanomas
- Frequently diagnosed in the seventh decade
- Occurs on chronically sun-damaged skin (nose and cheek)
- Slow-growing, irregularly pigmented reticulated patch that can be brown, black, red, or white
- Usually over 1 cm in size, occurring in areas of sun exposure
- Starts as an in situ lesion, lentigo maligna, where the radial growth phase is prolonged (10–40 years).
- 1%–2% become invasive with time, as demonstrated by a vertical growth phase; the lesion is called lentigo maligna melanoma.
- Excision is the standard of care (with a 5 mm margin, if in situ).
- If invasive (lentigo maligna melanoma), see section Malignant melanoma
- The best treatment of LM is being debated, and recommendations will likely be revised in the near future.

## Malignant melanoma (MM)

- Most lethal of skin tumors, commonly metastasizing when thick.
- 62,480 new diagnoses in the United States in 2008 (estimate); 8420 deaths in United States in 2008
- Risk factors: family history, prior melanoma, atypical moles, fair skin type (propensity to sunburn)

### Subtypes

- Superficial spreading melanoma (60%–70% of MM; plaque with irregular border and uneven pigmentation)
- Nodular melanoma (15%–30% of MM; dark pigmented nodule)
- Lentigo maligna melanoma (5%–15% of MM; see Lentigo maligna section)
- Acral lentiginous melanoma (5%–10% of MM; pigmented macule in nail beds, palms, and soles; most common type in patients with darker skin types)

Suspect MM if a pigmented lesion changes size or color, becomes irregular in shape, bleeds, itches, or looks inflamed.

- Early detection is key, as the thicker the lesion the worse the prognosis and once metastasized, the disease is frequently fatal.
- Removal is by surgical excision with wide margins (0.5 cm for in situ; 1 cm for tumors <1 mm in thickness; 1–2 cm for tumors up to 2 mm in thickness; 2 cm for tumors >2 mm in thickness).
- Sentinel lymph node biopsy should be done for intermediate-depth melanomas (provides staging and prognostic information).

Rigorous ongoing monitoring by a physician is essential and is the standard of care.

# Benign skin lesions

### Cherry angiomas (Campbell de Morgan spots)
- Small, bright red papules on the trunk
- Benign capillary proliferations
- Occur from middle age onward, almost universal by old age in Caucasians

### Skin tags and achrochordons
- Pedunculated, benign fibroepithelial polyps
- Occur more commonly in older patients; intertriginous areas often have multiple tags.
- Benign, usually multiple, cause unknown
- Removal for cosmetic reasons by snipping the stalk with scissors, cryotherapy (liquid nitrogen), or light electrodessication.

### Seborrheic keratoses (see Plate 4)
- Oval papules and plaques (1–6 cm diameter) occurring on the face and trunk of older patients. These can be seen in younger patients as well.
- Initially yellow, they become darker and more warty in appearance.
- They seem to be "stuck on," usually multiple.
- Removal can be done (usually for cosmetic reasons) by cryotherapy, curettage, or laser.
- Where concern exists about more serious pathology, skin biopsy should be performed or referral to a dermatologist made.

# Bacterial skin infections

## Cellulitis

Cellulitis constitutes red, edematous, circumscribed, sometimes painful plaque on the skin due to infection. The most common location in adults is the lower extremity. It is more common with increasing age, immunocompromise, and diabetes, and with a predisposing skin condition (leg ulcer, pressure sore, lymphedema, dermatophyte infection of the feet or toenails, traumatic wounds, etc.).

### Organisms

- Gram-positive cocci, including *Staphyloccocus aureus* and *Streptococcus* (group A, commonly *S. pyogenes*)
- At Johns Hopkins, 40% of the organisms are MRSA (methicillin-resistance *S. aureus*), 20% are MSSA (methicillin-sensitive *S. aureus*).
- Gram negatives and anaerobes cause a minority of cellulitis cases.
- With chronic leg ulcers, pressure sores, and lymphedema, colonization is broader so infecting organisms may be more diverse.

### Clinical features

- Warm, tender, raised area with circumscribed margins. Cellulitis is not always erythematous.
- Portal of entry for bacteria may be evident (e.g., trauma).
- Systemic signs and symptoms may follow (fever, malaise).
- Spread can cause lymphangitis with tender lymph nodes in the inguinal region.
- There is a risk of bacteremia.

### Investigations

- CBC: elevated white cell count in many patients
- Blood cultures will be positive in less than 5%.
- Local culture: e.g., wound swab, injection and aspiration of saline in the dermis (usually negative), skin biopsy (20–30% positive). This is rarely needed as empiric treatment for *Streptococcus* or *Staphylococcus* is often part of follow-up.

### Treatment

- Because community-acquired MRSA infection is so prevalent, empiric coverage is warranted, even if the cellulitis is minimal (see Table 23.4).
- Draw around the cellulitis with a water-resistant pen to allow accurate subsequent assessments and follow up at 24–48 hours for evidence of progression or clinical response to therapy.
- Elevate the limb—blistering due to excessive edema can lead to ulceration.
- If it is more extensive, with systemic symptoms and signs, lymphangitis, or worsening on oral therapy, then admit patient for rest, elevation, and parenteral therapy as needed (see Table 23.4).
- Total treatment should be for 7–10 days.
- If cellulitis complicates chronic ulcers, broader-spectrum antibiotics are needed at the outset; obtain cultures (aerobic and anaerobic) by vigorous rubbing of the advancing edge of an ulcer with a culturette.
- Look for and treat tinea pedis in all patients (with topical antifungals).

- Ensure that the patient has adequate analgesia.
- Older patients will often become dehydrated with bacteremia. Assess them clinically and biochemically, and give intravenous fluids in the acute phase if needed.
- Erysipelas is a more superficial infection, which obstructs lymphatic drainage; S. Pyogenes is pathogenic. It presents with fever and pain, on the face (bridge of nose and across cheeks), less commonly on limbs.

---

**Table 23.4** Therapeutic options for cellulitis and erysipelas

Trimethoprim/sulfamethoxazole DS (160 mg/800 mg) or clindamycin 300 mg PO tid x 7–10 days

- If condition is mild and the patient is well, oral therapy is appropriate.
- Presume MRSA and treat empirically.

Clindamycin 600 mg IV q8h or vancomycin 15 mg/kg IV q12h, or linezolid 600 mg IV q12h (for presumed MRSA infection) for 48 hours (or until the erythema starts to recede), then an oral course

- For patients with severe cellulitis, lymphangitis, worsening on oral therapy, or systemic signs

Penicillin V 500 mg PO qid x 10 days; amoxicillin 500 mg PO tid x 10 days; penicillin G benzathine 1.2 mil U IM x 1; cephalexin 500 mg PO qid x 10 days

- For erysipelas

Azithromycin 500 mg PO x 1 day, then 250 mg PO daily x 4 days; clarithromycin 250 mg PO bid x 7–10 days; clindamycin 300 mg PO tid x 7–10 days

- For erysipelas in penicillin-allergic patients

---

## Necrotizing fasciitis

- Rare and serious infection
- Affects soft tissues (usually arm and leg, abdominal wall, genital area (Fournier's gangrene, or perineum) and spreads rapidly along fascial planes
- Polymicrobial infection most frequently (e.g., *Staphylococcus, Pseudomonas, Bacteroides,* diphtheroids, coliforms), but *Streptococcus pyogenes* is common.
- Patient feels and looks ill with a high fever.
- Area of swelling, redness, and tenderness enlarges rapidly and becomes purple and discolored. Hemorrhagic bullae develop, followed by necrosis.
- Diagnosis requires incision of the area and culturing the pus, which wells up from below the fascial plane.
- Prompt parenteral antibiotics and early aggressive surgical debridement are essential.

The key to management is early recognition. Review a patient with cellulitis frequently if the patient is ill, and look for rapid spread beyond the drawn margin.

# Fungal skin infections

There are two main groups of fungi that cause infection in humans.

## Dermatophytes, e.g., *Tinea* species (ringworm)

- Infect the feet, groin, body, hands, nails, and scalp
- Suspect this if there is a distinct edge and scaling of an itchy lesion.
- Confirm diagnosis with skin scrapings, looking for septate hyphae under KOH examination or by fungal culture.

For localized uncomplicated lesions, topical therapy is adequate. Examples of available creams are as follows:

- Once-daily application x 2–4 weeks: terbinafine 1% (Lamisil) cream, naftifine 1% (Naftin) cream or gel, butenafine 1% (Mentax) cream
- Twice-daily application x 2–4 weeks: econazole 1% (Spectazole) cream, 2% (Nizoral) cream

Oral terbinafine will work for more resistant infection but should only be used if topical treatment fails and the diagnosis is confirmed.

## Yeasts, e.g., *Candida albicans* (thrush)

- Normal commensal organism of mouth and GI tract
- It produces infection in certain circumstances, e.g., moist skin folds, poor hygiene, diabetes, and use of broad-spectrum antibiotics—many of these commonly occur in older patients.
- Common sites include genital area (associated with catheter use), intertrigo (see p. 621), around the nail (chronic paronychia), and oral thrush (especially if dentures fit poorly).
- Topical imidazoles (e.g., clotrimazole) are effective for skin infection.
- Nystatin or miconazole lozenges, suspension, or gel can be used for oral infection.
- More widespread infection (e.g., esophageal candidiasis) or patients with severe immunodeficiency may require systemic therapy: fluconazole (IV or PO) 200 mg until symptoms improve, then 100 mg daily for 14–21 days.

## Seborrheic dermatitis

- Chronic inflammatory condition with erythematous scaly plaques
- Possibly due to a hypersensitivity to pityrosporum—a yeast skin commensal
- Classic distribution—face (eyebrows, eyelids, nasolabial folds, postauricular, beard area), scalp (dandruff), central chest, central back and in older patients only, flexural (axillae, groins, submammary)
- May cause otitis externa or blepharitis
- Exceedingly common in the elderly, exacerbated by poor skin hygiene
- Associated with Parkinsonism and HIV
- The scalp is treated with ketoconazole shampoo; improve efficacy by leaving it on for a few minutes before rinsing.
- Elsewhere, use ketoconazole shampoo as a wash and apply a number of low-potency topical steroids or topical antifungal, such as miconazole or ketoconazole creams.

- Blepharitis is treated with warm compresses, cleaning eyelids with Q-tips and diluted baby shampoo, and, if necessary, very low-potency steroid cream.
- It is difficult to treat—recurrence is common, and repeated treatments are often required. Aim for control, not cure.

## Intertrigo

- This a common complaint, often in older patients as well as the obese, when there is superficial inflammation of skin folds (e.g., flexures of limbs, groins, axillae, submammary).
- It is due to friction in a continually warm, moist environment.
- There may be underlying skin disease (e.g., seborrheic dermatitis, atopic dermatitis, irritant contact dermatitis [urine, feces], or psoriasis).
- Secondary infection with yeast is common.

### *Treatment*

- Improve hygiene.
- Wash carefully and always dry the skin thoroughly. Advise the patient to stop scrubbing.
- Use talcum powder or other drying powder (i.e., cornstarch) to keep areas dry.
- Apply topical antifungal (e.g., clotrimazole cream plus 1% hydrocortisone cream).
- Separate skin surfaces where possible.

# Leg ulcers

This is a common condition, afflicting 1%–2% of the adult population at any time. It is more common in older adults. Greater than 50% are venous ulcers, 10% are arterial, 25% are mixed venous and arterial, and the remainder due to other causes (diabetes, infection, malignancy, blood disorders, vasculitis, drug eruptions, etc.). It is important to distinguish the cause of an ulcer, as therapy is vastly different depending on the etiology.

## Clinical features of common ulcers

### Venous ulcers (see Plate 5)

- The medial malleolus is the most common site, though ulcers can be large and involve the lower extremity circumferentially.
- They are shallow and tender with irregular edges that are not undermined.
- The base is usually red, but may demonstrate a variety of surface features such as eschar or fibrinoid slough.

Look for associated skin features of chronic venous insufficiency (pitting edema, induration, hemosiderosis, varicosities, lipodermatosclerosis, atrophie blanche, and/or stasis dermatitis).

### Arterial ulcers (see Plate 6)

- These occur at sites of trauma or pressure—commonly the malleoli, toes, ball of foot, heel, and base of fifth metatarsal.
- They are round, with sharply demarcated, punched-out borders.
- Pain is significant and often worsened by leg elevation.

There are associated features of peripheral arterial disease (cool feet, loss of hair on surrounding skin, weak pedal pulses, and slow toe capillary refill on examination).

### Diabetic ulcers

- Occur at pressure points
- Painless (due to diabetic neuropathy)
- Often covered with a thick callus
- Often infected with undermined edges

### Pressure ulcers (see also p. 522)

- Propensity for skin overlying bony prominences (sacrum, hips, malleoli)
- Tissue compression exceeding the capillary filling pressure of 32 mmHg for longer than 2 hours causes local ischemia and necrosis.
- They begin with nonblanching erythema and progress to full-thickness skin loss.
- Patients who are immobilized or paralyzed are at highest risk.

### Vasculitis

- Palpable purpura is the earliest sign; dependent areas are most often affected.
- Ulcers then develop, especially if medium-sized blood vessels are affected by vasculitis.
- Exquisite pain is a universal feature.

- Ulcers are punched and round, and can be confused with arterial ulcers.
- Deep skin biopsy is needed to diagnosis vasculitis

### Pyoderma gangrenosum
- A noninfectious neutrophilic dermatosis causing recurrent painful ulcerations
- Pretibial areas are the most common location.
- Starts as a pustule, then ulcerates with violaceous undermined borders
- Associated with underlying disorders (inflammatory bowel disease, rheumatological disease, or hematological malignancy) in up to 70% of cases
- Trauma can precipitate a lesion (pathergy).

### Malignant ulcers
- Painless with a raised edge
- Be suspicious if an ulcer fails to heal or has an atypical appearance.

## A general approach to leg ulcers
- Examine the extremity to establish the cause; this is usually possible on clinical grounds. Look for markers of venous disease or arterial insufficiency (see Leg ulcers section).
- Use studies to confirm the clinical diagnosis: duplex ultrasonography to confirm the presence of venous insufficiency; ankle–brachial (ABI) or toe–brachial indices (TBI) to diagnose arterial insufficiency; 10-gram Weinstein filament exam to evaluate sensation (this will establish if the ulcer has a neuropathic component); skin biopsy (looking for malignancy or vasculitis, or for tissue culture if infection suspected), or blood tests (CBC, glucose, ESR, CRP, autoantibody screen, malignancy screen).
- Treat cause where possible, e.g., compression bandaging for venous disease (p. 626), revascularization for arterial disease (p. 622), or immunosuppression for vasculitis (p. 622).
- Ensure that there is adequate pain relief.
- Re-evaluate regularly. If the ulcer is not healing, then reassess the original diagnosis.
- Avoid antibiotics unless there is cellulitis or osteomyelitis. Colonization is inevitable, and surface swabs are usually unhelpful. Obtain deeper tissue for culture.
- Keep ulcer clean and avoid irritant topical applications. Many available products will cause a contact dermatitis (see p. 630).
- Consider patch testing a patient with a long-standing ulcer or worsening ulcer or surrounding inflammation to exclude an allergic contact dermatitis due to many topical agents used on ulcers.

# Chronic venous insufficiency

This is common, ranging from minor cosmetic problems to debilitating leg ulcers. It is more common after phlebitis or deep vein thrombosis (DVT) after leg injury, in obese patients, and with advancing age.

## Pathogenesis

Chronic venous insufficiency is due to failure of the venous pump in the legs. It is commonly caused by deep vein occlusion (although only half of patients will show signs of this on venography). Retrograde blood flow in the deep veins, valvular incompetence, and progressive pericapillary fibrin deposition also contribute to the process.

## Clinical changes

### Varicose veins
- Initially there may be no symptoms, just venous dilation (starts with submalleolar venous flares and progresses to dilated, tortuous, palpable varicose veins).
- Itch, ache, thrombophlebitis, or bleeding from varicosities
- Edema and a feeling of leg heaviness
- May initially be unilateral and wax and wane with position (classically occurring at the end of a day of standing).
- Thiazide diuretics may help, but watch for volume depletion.

### Skin changes
- Hemosiderin pigmentation due to red cell extravasation
- Telangiectasia
- Lacey white scars (atrophie blanche)
- Eczematous changes with itchy, weepy skin (stasis dermatitis)
- Lipodermatosclerosis occurs when fibrosis of the tissues leads to induration. It may become circumferential and girdle the lower leg, causing an inverted champagne-bottle appearance.

### Venous ulcers
Venous ulcers arise in the context of these skin changes, often precipitated by minor trauma (see pp. 648–9).

## Further reading

Bergan JJ, Schmid-Schnbein, Coleridge Smith PD, et al. (2006). Chronic venous disease. *N Engl J Med* **355**:488–498.

# Management of venous leg ulcers

Venous leg ulcers are a chronic and debilitating condition, with serious psychological and social implications. Median duration is 9 months, although 25% will still be present at 5 years. Correctly treated, 70% can be healed within 3 months, but 75% are recurrent.

### General measures

- Encourage mobility—this strengthens the muscle pump and helps prevent deep vein occlusion. If the patient is bed-bound, exercises such as toe and ankle wiggling and quadriceps movements can help.
- The patient should stop smoking.

### Limb elevation

- Raising the legs above the level of the heart improves venous return, reduces edema, and assists healing of venous ulcers. Unfortunately, this is rarely practical—many older patients cannot tolerate such a position owing to comorbidity (cardiac failure, COPD, arthritic hips, obesity, etc.) and even if they can, it is difficult to sustain.
- Balance benefits against risks of immobility and complications (thrombosis, deconditioning); limb elevation is usually only used for very resistant ulcers.
- Elevating the foot of the bed mattress at night is helpful (easiest with electronic hospital beds, otherwise use a wedge under the mattress).
- During the day, sitting with the feet on a stool is better than nothing, although it fails to raise the legs high enough.
- Elevation should *not* be used with peripheral arterial disease—check pedal pulses and ABI first.

### Compression

- Compression is first-line treatment for venous ulcers; it is superior to any other type of dressing.
- It relieves edema and stasis, and promotes healthier granulation tissue formation.
- Make sure of concomitant arterial insufficiency before applying compression: ABI or TBI of 0.9–1.2 is normal and can withstand compression; ABI <0.6, TBI <0.4, or either >1.2 (suggesting noncompressible vessels) indicates arterial insufficiency—compression must be avoided.
- When mixed-etiology ulcers are present, some compression is often required, but this has to be carefully moderated to compensate for the arterial insufficiency.
- Compression provides an active counterpressure to venous blood pressure and enhances function of the muscle pump.
- Use single-layer bandages, multilayer bandages, compression stockings, or a combination of stockings and bandages.
- Patients should be sent to an experienced surgical supply pharmacy for proper fitting of stockings.
- External pressure of 35–40 mmHg at the ankle is necessary to prevent capillary exudation.
- Unna boot is commonly used, but requires training to apply properly.

## Debridement

- Clean the ulcer by irrigation with saline.
- Debridement of dead tissue may improve healing by turning a chronic wound into an acute wound.
  - Scalpel (local EMLA cream may make this less uncomfortable)
  - Maggots (consume only dead tissue, leaving behind the healthy)
  - Autolytic debridement with moisture-donating dressing
  - Enzymatic debridement using topical proteases. No single wound dressing has been shown to improve healing.

## Wound dressings (see Table 23.5)

- An ideal dressing keeps the wound moist with exudates, but not macerated, at an ideal temperature and pH for healing without irritants, excessive slough, or infection.
- Simple, low-adherent and low-cost dressings are the mainstay.
- Impregnated dressings (e.g., with antiseptic, antibiotic, debriding enzymes, growth factors or silver sulfadiazine) can cause contact allergic or irritant dermatitis (up to 85% of patients), thus worsening the ulcer, so be aware of this.
- Occlusive or semi-occlusive dressings can aid with pain relief.
- Gel and hydrocolloid dressings can be useful to remove exudates and offer pain relief.

## Adjuncts to wound care

### Topical negative pressure devices
- Also known as vacuum-assisted closure devices
- May increase the healing rate of chronic wounds compared to that with saline gauze dressings.

### Growth factors
- Recombinant human platelet-derived growth factor isoform BB (rhPDGF-BB; Regranex®) is the only FDA-approved topical growth factor available.
- Promote wound repair mechanisms.
- Have been shown to be beneficial in some diabetic foot ulcers.

### Collagens
- Support wound healing by laying down a matrix that promotes new tissue deposition

### Pentoxifylline
- Has fibrinolytic and antithrombotic effects, and inhibits the production of proinflammatory cytokines
- Promotes healing of venous ulcers along with compression.

### Antimicrobials
- When bacterial colonization of chronic wounds exceeds $10^5$ organisms per gram of tissue, wound healing is impaired.
- Topical antimicrobials and antiseptics can be used to reduce wound bioburden.
- Mupirocin ointment and silver-releasing agents are examples.
- Be aware of potential allergic-contact dermatitis.

*Surgery*
- Skin grafts may be helpful. Pinch or punch skin grafts may stimulate healing.
- Surgical correction of deep vein incompetence is considered where bandaging has failed. This involves ligation of superficial veins and valvuloplasty.

**Table 23.5** Wound dressings

| Product | Advantages | Disadvantages | Indications | Examples |
|---------|-----------|---------------|-------------|----------|
| Gauzes | Inexpensive, accessible | Drying Poor barrier | Packing deep wounds | Curity gauze sponge or packing strip; Xeroform |
| Films | Moisture-retentive Transparent, semi-occlusive Protects wound from contamination | No absorption Fluid trapping, Skin stripping | Wounds with minimal exudate, Secondary dressing | Tegaderm HP; OpSite Flexigrid |
| Hydrogels | Moisture-retentive Nontraumatic removal Pain relief | May overhydrate | Dry wounds, painful wounds | Xcell cellulose dressing; Curagel |
| Hydrocolloids | Long wear-time Absorbent, occlusive Protects wound from contamination | Opaque Fluid trapping Skin Stripping Malodorous discharge | Wounds with light to moderate exudate | DuoDERM CGF; Tegasorb |
| Alginates and hydrofibers | Highly absorbent Hemostatic | Fibrous debris, Lateral wicking | Wounds with moderate to heavy exudate, mild hemostasis | Kaltostat; Aquacel Hydrofiber |
| Foams | Absorbent Thermal insulation Occlusive | Opaque, malodorous | Wounds with light to moderate exudate | 3M Adhesive Foam |

# Pruritus

Pruritis involves intense itching. Thirty percent of elderly suffer from persistent pruritus. The threshold for itch is affected by neurological and psychological factors, which are exacerbated by social isolation, sensory impairment (blind, deaf), and depression. This condition is often ignored, yet simple measures can make a big difference.

## Causes

### Medication

- The most common diagnosable cause for severe pruritus in the elderly is reaction to systemic medications.
- Often drug pruritus will disturb sleep. For the elderly this can be quite troublesome in a population that already has altered sleep patterns.
- The frequency of drug reactions is proportional to the number of medicines taken. Therefore, older patients with polypharmacy are prime candidates for drug-induced pruritus.

Note: a skin eruption need not be present. Drug-induced pruritus can take a month to cease once the offending drug is stopped.

### Xerosis cutis (dry skin)

- Xerosis is common with aging and frequently worse on lower legs, forearms, and hands.
- Skin is dry and scaly and may develop inflamed fissures when xerosis cutis is severe (asteatotic dermatitis).
- It is probably related to reduced levels of ceramides, leading to inability to efficiently retain moisture.

### Contact dermatitis

Contact dermatitis may show few skin changes if mild, yet cause troublesome itching. It is limited to areas exposed to allergen (e.g., under clothing if due to laundry detergent, fabric softeners, or dryer sheets).

### Systemic disease

- Liver failure (may be mild jaundice—itch caused by bile salts)
- Chronic renal failure
- Iron deficiency—even before anemia is apparent
- Hematological disorders (lymphoma, polycythemia—itch may be exacerbated by water)
- Infections (including fungal infection, scabies and lice infestations, GI parasite infections)
- Metabolic disorders (including thyroid disease, which affects 10% of hyperthyroid patients, and many hypothyroid patients because of dry skin; diabetes mellitus)
- Malignancy

## Assessment

- **History** should include a full review of systems, looking for underlying disease; a drug history; and specific inquiries about possible irritants (e.g., perfumes, cleansers). Ask if anyone else at home is itching.

- **Examination** should include inspection of all skin and thorough general examination (looking for, e.g., burrows or other signs of scabies, lymphadenopathy, hepatosplenomegaly, thyroid enlargement, etc.).
- **Investigations** should include CBC, iron and ferritin, ESR, renal and liver function, thyroid function, and blood glucose. Other tests may be included, guided by history, e.g., stool examination for ova, cysts, and parasites; abdominal ultrasound if there is organomegaly.

# Pruritus: treatment

- Treat the underlying cause whenever possible (i.e., iron supplements if stores are low, even if CBC is normal).
- Stop any drugs that may be causing or exacerbating the condition.
- Apply emollients—light preparations such as aqueous cream can help relieve itching, even if skin does not appear dry, and may be mixed with 0.25% menthol (Eucerin cream with 0.25% menthol and 0.125% camphor is a popular compound), which has a cooling and antiseptic action. Sarna Lotion® is also available, with the same ingredients.
- Greasier preparations (ointments) are useful when the dryness is more severe.
- Ammonium lactate preparations are available and are often useful for pruritus associated with xerosis (LacHydrin® and AmLactin® creams and lotions).
- Urea-containing emollients are used where the skin is scaly and are often useful in the elderly (Carmol® lotion)
- The patient should avoid excessive bathing and use preparations such as aqueous cream or emulsifying ointments instead of soap. Emollient bath additives can be added to the water (Aveeno Oatmeal Bath®).
- The patient should avoid exacerbating factors, such as heat (especially hot baths), alcohol, hot drinks, and vasodilating drugs.
- The patient should wear loose, cotton clothing.
- The patient should try to keep nails short to limit skin damage from scratching.
- Consider short-term bandaging where excoriation is severe to allow healing.
- Antihistamines may be useful, but caution should be exercised with the elderly population to avoid delirium and falls.
- Cholestyramine (4–8 g daily) is used to decrease itch associated with biliary disease.
- Light therapy (phototherapy) may help—either broad-band or narrow-band UVB therapy 2–3 times per week.

# Pruritic conditions

### Lichen simplex chronicus

- A local patch of pruritus, when scratched, leads to skin damage with thickening, discoloration, and excoriation.
- It is worse in times of emotional stress.
- Treat with steroids (topical or intralesional) and avoidance of scratching (bandaging may help). Capsaicin® cream may decrease itching by decreasing substance P in the skin.

### Pruritus ani

- This is a common complaint.
- It is occasionally due to infection (streptococci, candidiasis).
- Exclude allergic contact dermatitis, seborrheic dermatitis, or psoriasis.
- It is usually due to soiling of the perianal skin, which is worse with loose stool and difficulty in wiping effectively (e.g., with arthritis).
- The mainstay of treatment is improving hygiene after bowel movement (assist with wiping if physically difficult, consider wiping with a damp cloth).
- Use aqueous cream or Tucks® medicated pads (witch hazel) to cleanse.
- Avoid soap in the anal canal.
- Avoid toilet paper and fragranced toilet paper, which can cause irritation.
- Once developed, the itch may be self-perpetuating—break the cycle with steroids ± topical antifungals or antiseptics.
- Patch test to exclude allergy.

## How to recognize and manage scabies

Thinking of this diagnosis is the first step.

- Caused by *Sarcoptes scabiei* mite
- Spread by skin-to-skin contact
- Outbreaks can occur within institutions (e.g., nursing homes, hospital wards).
- Occasionally serious, even fatal

## Symptoms and signs

- Intense itch (worse at night)
- Widespread excoriation
- Examine the patient carefully for burrows and/or erythematous papules that are found
  - Between fingers and toes
  - On the wrist flexor surface
  - Around the nipples and umbilicus
  - In the axillae and groin.

## Treatment

- Isolate the patient (gloves, gowns).
- Apply topical pediculocide lotions or creams, e.g., permethrin 5%, lindane 1%, sulfur 5%.
- Apply to the whole body, including the scalp, neck, and face. Ensure that the interdigital webs are well covered.
- Treat all household members (or all others in close contact in an institution) simultaneously, including asymptomatic contacts.
- Wash clothes and bedding.
- Repeat treatment after a week.
- Prescribe 30–60 g cream and 100 mL lotion for each application.
- Antibiotics may be needed for secondary infection.
- Itch may persist for weeks after treatment has eradicated the mite, but should slowly diminish. Topical steroids and sedating antihistamines to aid sleep can be helpful.
- Persistent itch may indicate treatment failure.

**"Norwegian scabies"** occurs in immunosuppressed and frail older patients. A heavy load of mites produces hyperkeratotic lesions. It is highly contagious and may require additional oral treatment with ivermectin (250 mcg/kg) (off-label use).

# Blistering diseases

There are many disorders causing skin blistering in older people—see Table 23.6 for a differential. Common causes include blistering secondary to cellulitis or rapid-onset edema. Bullous pemphigoid is significant in that it occurs almost exclusively in the elderly population.

## Bullous pemphigoid

This is a chronic autoimmune bullous eruption.

### Clinical features

- The patient is systemically well.
- Skin becomes erythematous and itchy; often hive-like plaques are the initial presentation.
- Large, tense blisters then appear, usually on the limbs, trunk, and flexures (rarely mucous membranes).
- Blisters then heal without scarring.
- It may appear in normal-looking skin or at the site of previous skin damage (e.g., ulcer, trauma).
- This is a chronic and recurrent condition.
- This disease can present with generalized pruritus without characteristic skin lesions.

### Diagnosis

- It is confirmed by skin biopsy, which shows linear IgG deposited at the basement membrane.
- Circulating autoantibody (anti-BPAg1 and anti-BPAg2) is found in the serum of up to half of patients.

### Treatment

- It responds well to steroids.
- Mild, local disease can be treated with strong topical steroids.
- More widespread disease requires oral prednisolone (40–60 mg daily initially, with a gradual taper).
- Topical or intralesional steroids can be used for resistant lesions.
- Remember to monitor for and protect against steroid side effects (p. 130).
- Consider steroid-sparing agents for longer treatment courses (e.g., mycophenolate mofetil or azathioprine).

### Prognosis

- 50% of patients have self-limited disease.
- The majority will be off medication within 2 years.

## Further reading

Bolognia JL, Jorizzo JL, Rapini RP (2007). *Dermatology* (2nd ed.). Philadelphia: Mosby/Elsevier.
Fonder MA, Lazarus GS, Cowan DA, et al. (2008). Treating the chronic wound: a practical approach to the care of nonhealing wounds and wound care dressings. *J Am Acad Dermatol* **58**(2):185–205.

**Table 23.6** Causes of blistered skin

| Blistering disorder | Clinical features |
|---|---|
| Blisters secondary to cellulitis | Features of cellulitis present (see p. 618) |
| Blisters secondary to edema | Occurs when onset is rapid |
| Traumatic blisters | Due to friction, pressure, or trauma to skin |
| | Localized to site of insult, e.g., heel blister with ill-fitting shoes |
| Pressure blisters | Due to prolonged pressure that causes skin ischemia |
| | Can occur after 2 hours of immobility |
| | Risk factors include advancing age, immobility, dehydration, extremes of body size |
| | May progress to pressure sore (p. 522) |
| Fixed drug eruption | Itch, erythema, and blistering that appear and reappear at the same site after ingestion of a drug (e.g., furosemide) |
| | Reaction usually within 6 hours |
| Eczema | Blisters may occur in eczema, especially if there is secondary infection (e.g., eczema herpeticum, staphylococcal infection) |
| Infections | Herpes simplex—usually causes blisters on the face or genitals |
| | Herpes zoster—shingles is common in older patients (p. 752) |
| | Staphylococci and streptococci may cause primary infections (e.g., impetigo—facial blisters that rupture to leave a yellow crust; erysipelas—well defined area of redness and swelling that later blisters, usually on face or lower leg) or secondary infection of, e.g., a leg ulcer or wound. Either may result in blistering. |
| Bullous pemphigoid | See p. 636 |
| Pemphigus vulgaris | Serious autoimmune blistering disease |
| | A rare disorder, mainly affecting young or middle-aged patients |
| | Widespread flaccid, superficial blisters that rupture early |
| | The mouth is always involved initially. |
| | Patients are systemically unwell. |
| Dermatitis herpetiformis | Symmetrical extensor surface tense blisters, associated with celiac disease |
| | Rare, with peak incidence in the fourth decade |

# Infection and immunity

## Jonathan Zenilman

# The aging immune system

*The immune system ages in a complex manner*
- Some activities increase (e.g., production of memory T lymphocytes, immunoglobulin A [IgA], and autoantibodies).
- Other activities diminish (e.g., production of some interleukins, antibodies in response to foreign antigens, and macrophage clearance of antigens and complement during acute infection).
- Overall, immune responses become less efficient, less appropriate, and occasionally harmful with age.
- The immune system does not wear out—it becomes dysfunctional.
- This is an insidious process, often unnoticed until times of physiological stress (e.g., acute illness).
- It is more marked in older people with chronic disease, multiple comorbidities, and significant genetic and environmental factors.

*Immune dysfunction alters the response to infection in older people*
- Infectious disease is a more significant cause of morbidity and mortality in older people (up to 10 times more likely to be the cause of death).
- Impaired cellular immunity predisposes older people to reactivation of certain diseases, e.g.:
  - Shingles (p. 644)
  - Tuberculosis (p. 350).
- Altered antibody production increases fatality from pneumonia, influenza, bacterial endocarditis, and hospital-acquired infections.
- Decreased levels of lymphokines increase susceptibility to parasitic infections.
- Age-related immune dysfunction probably has a negative impact of the course of AIDS in older patients.

Investigations may not show characteristic changes associated with infection, or these changes may develop more slowly (e.g., rise in white cell count, CRP, and complement).

*Immune dysfunction also has other clinical consequences*
- Increased autoantibody production does not lead to an increase in autoimmune disease (this peaks in middle age) but may contribute to degenerative diseases.
- Response to vaccination may be less good.
- Falling immune surveillance may contribute to the rising incidence of cancer.
- T-lymphocyte dysfunction may contribute to the increasing incidence of monoclonal gammopathy with age (see p. 482).
- IgE-mediated hypersensitivity reactions are less frequent, so allergic symptoms tend to improve with age.

## Further reading
Evans JE, et al. (eds.) (2003). Immunity and ageing (section 4.3). In *Oxford Textbook of Geriatric Medicine*. Oxford: Oxford University Press.

# Overview of infection in older people

Infectious disease causes significant morbidity and mortality in older people. **Susceptibility** to infection is increased by
- Immune senescence (see p. 640)
- Altered skin and mucosal barriers

**Response** to established infection, which increases with use of a permanent prosthetic implant, might be compromised by the following:
- Decreased cardiac adaptation to stress
- Comorbid conditions and frailty
- Decreased lean body mass or even malnutrition
- Multiple previous hospital admissions or residence in long-term care facility
- Attenuated immune response

## Presentation
- Frequently atypical, e.g., global deterioration, nonspecific functional decline, delirium, falls, incontinence
- May initially give no clue to the site of sepsis, e.g., chest infections may present with falls, rather than cough
- Fever is often absent, reduced, delayed (due to senescent hypothalamic responses), or due to other medications.
- Often indolent with a slow deterioration over several days

By the time sepsis is obvious, the patient may be very sick. Infection of prosthetic devises is usually subclinical.

## Investigation
Obtaining samples can be difficult—e.g., the patient may be delirious and uncooperative, have urinary or fecal incontinence, or be unable to expectorate sputum. Misleading results are common:
- Positive urine dipstick does not necessarily indicate urine infection (see p. 654).
- Urine samples from a catheterized patient will often be heavily colonized, making dipsticks positive and culture results difficult to interpret.
- Ulcers will usually be colonized and swab results should be interpreted with caution (see p. 623).
- Abdominal ultrasound scan will often reveal gallstones in older patients—these are usually asymptomatic and do not necessarily imply biliary sepsis.
- Classic markers of infection (leukocytosis, elevated CRP, increased complement) may be absent or delayed in older patients.

## Treatment
Because of the difficulties in making an accurate diagnosis:
- Therapy is often empirical.
- Antibiotic failures are more common.
- Antibiotic resistance frequently develops.

Treatment may also be difficult to administer in delirious patients. Treatment options are often more limited for persons exposed to the health-care environment because of exposure to resistant organisms.

## How to accurately diagnose infection in an older patient

Making an accurate diagnosis with evidence to support it is important to allow tailored antibiotic therapy. Have a low threshold for considering sepsis as a cause for decline of any sort, but conversely, do not assume that all problems stem from infection.

### Investigations

- Full blood count: white cell count may be elevated, suppressed (poor prognostic indicator), or be unchanged.
- ESR, CRP often become elevated early on in infection, but this is very nonspecific and they may take 24–48 hours to rise or remain normal. Serial measurements advised.
- U, C + E: Septic older patients are prone to renal impairment.
- Blood and urine cultures should be sent **before** antibiotics are started.
- CXR: A patch of consolidation on an X-ray may be the first indicator that a global deterioration is due to pneumonia.
- Consider stool culture (if diarrhea) and sputum culture (if cough).
- Evaluate for presence of prosthetic devices—stents, vascular grafts, prosthetic joints or hardware, pacemakers, automatic implanatable cardiac defibrillators (AICDs), etc.

**If the source remains unclear**, repeat basic tests, then consider the following:

- **Skin:** Check carefully for cellulitis and/or ulceration (p. 618). Emphasize visualization of all pressure points.
- **Bones:** Osteomyelitis (particularly vertebral, after joint replacement or where there is chronic deep ulceration of skin) may present indolently. Check for boney tenderness and consider X-rays; MRI is the best choice. Check vertebrae for point tenderness, bone scans, or MRI (see p. 508).
- **Heart valves:** Bacterial endocarditis can be very hard to diagnose. Consider it in all patients with a murmur, and actively exclude it in those with prosthetic heart valves (see *Oxford Handbook of Clinical Medicine*, 6th ed. for more details).
- **Biliary tree:** Asymptomatic gallstones are common in older patients, but if an ultrasound also shows dilation of the gall bladder or biliary system with a thickened, edematous wall, then infection is likely. There is usually (but not always) abdominal pain. Send blood cultures. Endoscopic retrograde cholangiopancreatography (ERCP) may be needed to remove any obstruction.
- **Abdomen:** Diverticular disease is common, and abscesses may present atypically. Examine for masses and consider abdominal ultrasound or CT if there is a history of diverticulae or abdominal pain. Examine the genitourinary tract. Perform rectal exam to evaluate prosthetics.

**How to accurately diagnose infection in an older patient (cont'd.)**

- **Brain:** Meningitis, brain abscess, and encephalitis may present indolently in older patients, and the usual warning signs (confusion, drowsiness) may be misinterpreted. Headache and photophobia may be late or absent. Consider CT head followed by analysis of cerebrospinal fluid if a septic patient has focal neurology, headache, photophobia, or bizarre behavioral change.
- **Tuberculosis** may reactivate in older people and cause chronic infection. If there is known previous TB (clinical or CXR evidence), look very carefully for reactivation. Consider early-morning urines, sputum culture (induced if necessary), bronchoscopy, or biopsy of any abnormal tissue (e.g., enlarged lymph nodes).

Remember that fever and raised inflammatory markers can also be due to non-infectious conditions (e.g., malignancy, vasculitis, gout, etc.).

# Antibiotic use in older patients

Antibiotics are among the most frequently prescribed drugs, and their widespread use is promoting increasing antibiotic resistance. This is a particular problem in older patients where infections are more common, yet accurate diagnosis can be more difficult (see p. 643). Antibiotics are also associated with *Clostridium difficile* diarrhea.

## Antibiotic resistance

This occurs when a bacterium encounters an antibiotic and is not eradicated fully, the selection pressure being for antibiotic resistance. The resistant strain can then be transmitted to other patients. Resistance is encouraged by the following:

- "Blind" antibiotic therapy (where likely microbe and sensitivities are not known)
- Inappropriate antibiotic therapy (e.g., for viral respiratory tract infections)
- Inadequate treatment courses
- Poor adherence with therapy
- Transmission of resistant strains within health-care settings.

## Sensible antibiotic prescribing

This helps limit the problem. Sensible prescribing applies to all ages, but may be more of a challenge in older patients:

- Make a diagnosis—identify the source of sepsis (and thus possible pathogens), which will guide therapy before microbiological confirmation is obtained.
- Avoid using antibiotics for infections that are likely to be viral, e.g., pharyngitis, upper respiratory tract infection (URI).
- Always send samples for culture and sensitivity before initiating antibiotics.
- Local variations (e.g., diagnostic mix, local sensitivities) should be considered. Use guidelines from the local microbiological department.
- Choose the dose based on the patient (allergies, age, weight, renal function, etc.) and the severity of the infection. Inadequate doses promote resistance.
- Choose the route—aim for oral whenever possible, and convert IV therapy to oral as soon as feasible. IM antibiotic therapy can be useful in certain circumstances (e.g., demented patients who refuse oral medication because of added delirium) but are uncomfortable.
- Choose the duration based on the type of infection, e.g., simple urinary tract infection can be adequately treated in 3 days, whereas bacterial endocarditis can require many weeks of therapy. Unnecessarily long treatment courses will promote resistance, increase the risk of side effects, and increase cost.
- Empirical broad-spectrum antibiotics should be changed to narrow-spectrum alternatives as soon as sensitivities are known.

## Further reading

Johns Hopkins Antibiotic Guide: http://www.hopkins-abxguide.org/

# Methicillin-resistant *Staphylococcus aureus* (MRSA)

Methicillin was introduced in the 1960s to treat staphylococcal infections. It was used widely (including spraying solutions into the air on wards) and, initially, successfully. Methicillin has now been discontinued and replaced by flucloxacillin, but the term "methicillin-resistant *Staphylococcus aureus*" (MRSA) persists.

Resistance to methicillin gradually emerged, first in small numbers within hospitals, but the problem slowly increased and spread into the community until globally dispersed epidemic strains had emerged.

All staphylococci are easily transmissible and virulent (capacity to cause disease) and have the capacity to develop further antibiotic resistance.

## Contamination and transmission

- Anything coming into contact with an MRSA source can become contaminated, i.e., MRSA will exist for a short time on that surface.
- Transient carriage on the gloves or hands of health-care workers is likely to represent the main mode of transmission to other patients.
- Up to 35% of environmental surfaces in a room being used by an MRSA patient will culture positive (the role in transmission is unclear).
- Decontamination involves cleaning. Good hand hygiene and the use of alcohol hand gel after patient contact reduce transmission significantly.

## Colonization

- This is asymptomatic carriage of MRSA.
- Common sites are anterior nares, perineum, hands, axillae, wounds, ulcers, sputum, throat, urine, venous access sites, and catheters.
- Duration of colonization varies from days to years.
- Transmission from a colonized person is more likely if there is a heavy bacterial load with abnormal skin (e.g., ulcers, eczema), devices (e.g., catheters, cannulae), or sinusitis/respiratory tract infection.
- Health-care worker colonization is low.
- Eradication of MRSA in health-care workers and patients is sometimes accomplished during large outbreaks. This is done by applying topical mupirocin to the nose and using antimicrobial soap and oral antibiotics (e.g., trimethoprim/sulfa rifampicin).

# MRSA disease

Although MRSA does not cause a specific disease, the most common sites of infection are as follows:
- Wounds are the most common cause of postoperative wound infections.
- Intravenous lines often lead to bacteremia.
- Ulcers, including pressure, diabetic, and venous ulcers
- Deep abscesses—infection can seed to many sites, e.g., lungs, kidneys, bones, liver, and spleen.
- Bacteremia—there is compulsory reporting of this.

Hospital patients colonized with MRSA are at risk of developing infection. This is more likely if any of the following have occurred:
- Recent prior hospitalization
- Surgery or wound debridement
- Invasive procedures (including venipuncture and venous cannulation)

Infections due to MRSA cause increased morbidity and mortality, longer hospital stays, and increased cost compared to those due to a susceptible organism.

## Management

Infection-control measures to reduce the reservoir and lower the rate of transmission are crucial (see How to control MRSA, p. 649).

Antibiotic treatment is necessary when there is active infection—do not use it for colonization, as this will promote drug resistance. Responsibility to the patient (use the best drug available) and that to the community (do not promote antibiotic resistance) must be balanced. The choice of drug will depend on local resistance patterns and severity of the infection. When possible, wait for sensitivities from microbiology.

Options include the following:
- **Glycopeptide antibiotics** (e.g., vancomycin, daptomycin, teicoplanin) must be given intravenously; resistance is emerging.
- **Co-trimoxazole** is useful for susceptible skin, soft tissue and infections.
- **Fusidic acid, rifampicin, and doxycycline** can be effective, usually given in combination.
- **Clindamycin** is used for deeper infections, but most U.S. strains are resistant.
- **Fluoroquinolones**, e.g., ciprofloxacin. Resistance is rapidly emerging.
- **Linezolid** is a new oxazolidinone antibiotic with equivalent potency to vancomycin. It can be given orally or intravenously. Use it with caution because of the high cost and high incidence of side effects, including bone marrow suppression. It interacts with SSRIs.

## How to control MRSA

MRSA is endemic in most hospitals. The primary focus is reducing transmission rates in the hospital or health-care setting.

*Identify the reservoir*
- Commonly a patient with a heavily colonized or infected wound
- Health-care workers may also act as reservoirs.
- During an epidemic, it is usual to attempt to eradicate MRSA from likely reservoir sources (using nasal mupirocin, antimicrobial soap, and oral antibiotics).

*Reduce transmission rates*
Transmission usually occurs from patient to patient via a health-care worker, often when hands or gloves are transiently contaminated.
- **Hand hygiene** is the single most important factor in infection control. Good hand-washing technique and bedside alcohol-based hand gels should be used by staff, visitors, patients, therapists, volunteers, and service personnel after touching a patient.
- Known MRSA patients should be isolated where possible.
- **Gloves** should be worn on entering the room and removed before leaving.
- **Gowns and aprons** should be used if contact with the patient or environment is anticipated, or if the wound is open.
- **Masks** may reduce nasal acquisition by health-care workers.
- Patients should be **moved about the hospital as little as possible**. Radiological investigations should be done at the end of a list to allow cleaning after the test.
- Minimize the use of **foreign devices** (e.g., catheters, nasogastric tubes).
- Use **dedicated equipment** (e.g., stethoscopes, blood pressure cuffs, thermometers) or clean carefully after use.
- **Active surveillance** for MRSA colonization allows these procedures to be put in place earlier.

By following these guidelines, it is estimated that 70% of transmission can be prevented.

## Problems in geriatric care
- Isolation can cause problems with depression and lack of social stimulation.
- Patients may feel stigmatized or scared by the diagnosis.
- Rehabilitation may be restricted (e.g., if the patient is confined to a side room and cannot visit the rehabilitation unit or walk the floor).
- It may be difficult to enforce isolation of patients with dementia.
- Moving to nursing homes or community facilities may be delayed (e.g., while waiting for a side room).

# *Clostridium difficile*–associated diarrhea

*Clostridium difficile* (CD) is a gram-positive, spore-forming, anaerobic bacillus. It was rarely described before the late 1970s but is now a major cause of hospital-acquired infection on geriatric wards. *Clostridium difficile*–associated diarrhea (CDAD) is a major problem, causing a huge burden of morbidity, mortality, and cost.

## Pathogenesis
- Asymptomatic CD carriage occurs in less than 5% of the population. But it can be as high as 20% among nursing home patients.
- Spores persist for months to years in the environment and are resistant to many traditional cleaning fluids. Vegetative forms and spores can be transmitted from patient to patient.
- Gastrointestinal carriage is increased in the hospital population, with advancing age, other bowel disease, cytotoxic drug use, and debility (e.g., recent surgery, chronic renal impairment, cancer).
- Most antibiotics reduce the colonization resistance of the colon to CD.
- CDAD occurs when toxins (A and B) elaborated by CD bind to the colonic mucosa, causing inflammation. Broad-spectrum antibiotics such as quinolone and extended-spectrum cephalosporins confer increased risk.
- Rarely, outbreaks in the hospital can occur from cross-infection and can affect patients never exposed to antibiotics.

## Features
There is a wide range of manifestations, from asymptomatic carriage to fulminant colitis. The patient most commonly presents with the following:
- Foul-smelling watery diarrhea (mucous common but rarely blood)
- Abdominal pain and distension
- Fever

Severe cases can mimic an "acute abdomen." It occasionally causes chronic diarrhea.

Beware that acute decline in a patient's condition (e.g., fever, delirium, metabolic disturbance) can precede the diarrhea. Have a low threshold of suspicion for patients with multiple risk factors.

## Investigations
- Raised white cell count and inflammatory markers (following treatment of an infection; differential diagnosis includes relapse of original infection)
- CD toxin detection by enzyme-linked immunosorbent assay (ELISA) is both sensitive and specific for colitis. It can remain positive for weeks after resolution so is *not* useful in diagnosing recurrence.
- Stool culture may be positive in asymptomatic patients but is rarely done.

- Abdominal X-ray or CT may show distended, thick-walled large bowel.
- Sigmoidoscopy is often normal in mild disease or when colitis affects the proximal bowel. Characteristic colitis with pseudomembrane formation is present in more severe cases (also known as pseudomembranous colitis).
- The acute onset of diarrhea associated with leukocytosis and abdominal pain is strongly suggestive of CDAD.

## Complications

These rarely occur and include toxic megacolon, paralytic ileus, perforation, and bacteremia. Older patients requiring surgery have at least a 50% mortality rate.

## Relapse

Relapse is defined as a second event within 2 months, which occurs in around 20% of patients. It is rarely due to antibiotic resistance, but can be difficult to treat. Vancomycin, given orally, is an alternative to repeating the metronidazole course.

Patients with recurrence are more prone to further repeated infection. For repeated infection and recalcitrant CDAD, the following options are available:

- Further oral antibiotics, e.g., metronidazole, vancomycin, bacitracin.
- Patients with recurrent CDAD often require prolonged suppressive doses of antibiotics such as vancomycin.
- Probiotics such as yeast or lactobacillus have also been shown to help induce and maintain remission.
- Intravenous immunoglobulins and steroids have been used in severe recalcitrant colitis, but none have been shown definitely to work.

## How to manage *Clostridium difficile* infection

### Prevention
Use antibiotics wisely:
- Use only when there is good evidence of infection. Always try to obtain a microbiological diagnosis and treat only when you have diagnosed infection or if the patient is gravely ill and conservative management is judged unsafe.
- Use the smallest number of antibiotics with the narrowest spectrum possible. Some antibiotics are less likely to cause CD, e.g., ceftriaxone or ciprofloxacin are better than cefuroxime.
- Use the shortest course possible: 3 days for a simple urinary infection, 7 days for bronchitis, 10 days or longer only for septicemia, abscess, etc.

In the future, vaccines against CD might be available.

### Treatment
Have a high index of suspicion—if the patient is ill, commence treatment without waiting for confirmatory tests.
- Stop antibiotics unless there is very good evidence that they need a longer course.
- Use aggressive rehydration, as patients can become very hypovolemic even before they start to get diarrhea.
- Metronidazole 400 mg tid PO (for metronidazole intolerance, failure to respond, or recurrence use vancomycin 125 mcg qid PO). Both drugs must be enteral to obtain high intraluminal levels. If the patient is unable to swallow, consider a nasogastric tube or metronidazole PR 1 g bid. IV therapy may be added if septicemia is suspected. Vancomycin is recommended in clinically severe cases or WBC >20,000.
- Continue for 7–10 days or until there is a formed stool.
- A stool chart will indicate if diarrhea frequency is improving.
- Use of loperamide (2 mg with each loose stool) is controversial—it may mask response to treatment and increase chances of complications. However, proponents suggest that if the diagnosis is secure and treatment initiated it can reduce debilitating symptoms and speed recovery.
- Surgical complications may require colectomy.

### Infection control
- Have a nurse in the side room, where possible.
- Use gloves and aprons for all contact.
- Wash hands thoroughly with soap and water after each contact. Alcohol gels do not kill spores.
- Clean the environment thoroughly, especially after patient has left.

Patients are much less infectious once the diarrhea has resolved, so avoid moving the patient between wards until 48 hours after the last loose stool.

# Diagnosing urinary tract infection (UTI)

While urinary tract infection (UTI) is a common problem in older people, there is an even higher prevalence of asymptomatic bacteriuria and positive urinalysis without infection. In general, UTI is overdiagnosed.

It is important to know how to diagnose a UTI correctly and when to initiate treatment appropriately.

## Dipstick urine test

This quick, cheap test is commonly performed. It should only be done on urine collected, as described in How to sample urine for dipstick (p. 655).

### Urinary nitrite

- A positive result has a high predictive value for UTI.
- Many bacteria causing UTI convert urinary nitrate to nitrite, which is detected on the dipstick.
- False negatives occur with dilute urine.
- Certain bacteria (e.g., *Pseudomonas, Staphylococcus, Enterococcus*) may not convert urinary nitrate, so the dipstick will be negative.

### Leukocyte esterase

- A positive result has a high predictive value for UTI.
- Lysed white cells release esterase, which is detected on a dipstick.
- Corresponds to significant pyuria—may not detect low levels
- False-negative results also occur when there is glucose, albumin, ketones, or antibiotic in the urine.
- False positives ("sterile pyuria") occur with vaginal contamination, chronic interstitial nephritis, nephrolithiasis, and uroepithelial tumors. "Sterile" pyuria can indicate renal tuberculosis and sexually transmitted diseases (e.g., *Chlamydia*)—consider testing if history is suggestive.

### Blood

- A positive result for blood has a low predictive value for infection.
- Dipstick does not distinguish red cells from hemoglobin or myoglobin.
- Dipstick detects red blood cells (blood in the renal tract), hemoglobin (after hemolysis), and myoglobin (rhabdomyolysis).
- Causes of a positive blood dipstick are varied and may be prerenal (e.g., hemolysis), renal (e.g., tumors, glomerulonephritis), ureteric (e.g., stones), bladder (e.g., tumors, occasionally infection), urethral (e.g., trauma), or contamination (e.g., bleeding from the vaginal vault).
- Always repeat to ensure the hematuria has resolved with treatment.
- Management of persistent isolated dipstick hematuria without an apparent cause is difficult. In a fitter patient, referral for renal tract investigation by a urologist may be appropriate.

### Protein

- A positive result has a low predictive value for infection.
- Commercial dipsticks generally only detect albumin, and a positive result implies proteinuric renal disease.
- False positives occur in very concentrated or contaminated urine.

▶▶The combination of nitrites and leukocyte esterases on urine dipstick has the highest positive predictive value for infection. If these are negative and clinical suspicion is high, proceed to urinary microscopy and culture.

## How to sample urine for dipstick, microscopy, and culture

### Do not sample
- Urine that is not freshly collected
- Urine that has been contaminated with feces
- Urine from a catheter bag

### Mid-stream urine sample
- Ideal sampling method, but may be hard in confused or immobile patients
- The external genitalia should be cleaned, a small amount of urine voided, then the middle portion caught cleanly in a sterile container.
- Analysis should be performed while the urine is fresh.

### In–out catheter sample
- Carries a small risk of introducing infection (around 1%)
- Often well tolerated by older patients
- Discard the first urine, and sample the middle portion drained.

### Suprapubic sample
- Rarely done but may be necessary in a septic patient with outlet obstruction (usually men) when unable to pass a catheter
- Performed with ultrasound guidance

### Samples from catheterized patients
- These should only be sent if the patient is symptomatic, as the prevalence of positive dipstick is almost universal, and bacterial colonization of urine is common.
- Collect a fresh sample directly from the draining tube sampling port.
- Do not use urine that has collected in the bag.

# Asymptomatic bacteriuria

This is defined as a positive urine culture in the absence of symptoms of urinary tract disease.

- It becomes more common with increasing age (5% of community-dwelling females under the age of 60, rising to 30% over the age of 80).
- It is less common in men but again increases with age (<1% of those under 60, rising to 10% over the age of 80).
- Up to 50% of frail institutionalized patients and almost all catheterized patients will have bacteria in their urine (see p. 561).
- Other risk factors are as for urinary tract infection (see p. 658).
- Associated diseases include renal stones, diabetes, and chronic prostatitis in men.

## What does it mean?

- It probably represents urinary colonization rather than infection.
- There is no increase in mortality directly associated with asymptomatic bacteriuria.
- It seems to be transient in most—only 6% will grow the same organism over three sequential cultures; however, it is estimated that around 16% will go on to develop a symptomatic urinary tract infection.

## Treatment

No treatment is required for isolated bacteriuria. The use of antibiotics

- Does not affect morbidity and mortality.
- Does not improve continence.
- Promotes antibiotic resistance.
- Recurrence after antibiotic treatment is common.

Do not treat baceriuria unless the patient has symptoms.

# Urinary tract infection

UTI is a major cause of morbidity and mortality in the older population. UTIs account for a quarter of infections in healthy older patients and are the most common hospital-acquired infection. They are the most frequent cause of bacteremia in older patients. The annual incidence is up to 10% for older adults (but many cases are recurrent).

## Risk factors
- Advancing age
- Female sex (although the gap narrows with age)
- Atrophic vaginitis and urethritis in women
- Incomplete emptying (e.g., urethral strictures, prostatic hypertrophy or carcinoma, neuropathy)
- Abnormalities of the renal tract (e.g., tumors, fistulae, surgery)
- Foreign bodies (e.g., catheter, stones)
- Chronic infection (e.g., renal abscess, prostatitis)

## Organisms
- *Escherichia coli* is the most common organism, as in younger adults.
- Older patients are more prone to UTI caused by other pathogens, including other gram-negative organisms (e.g., *Proteus, Pseudomonas*) and some gram-positive organisms (e.g., group B *Streptococcus*, enterococcus, MRSA).
- Catheter-related UTI is often polymicrobial and antibiotic resistant.

## Presentation
The presence of symptoms is essential to make the diagnosis. Urinary frequency, dysuria (stinging or burning sensation on urinating), and new urinary incontinence are clear indications of urinary infection, but symptoms may be vague or atypical, including the following:
- Fever and general malaise
- Nausea and vomiting
- Confusion or delirium
- Deterioration in physical or functional ability

Infection may be
- Uncomplicated UTI (normal renal tract and function)
- Complicated UTI (abnormal renal tract, patient debility, virulent organism, development of complications such as impaired renal function, bacteremia, pyelonephritis, perinephric or prostatic abscess)
- Recurrent UTI (p. 662)
- Catheter-associated UTI (p. 561)

**Investigations**
- Urinalysis: Collect sample (p. 655), perform dipstick (p. 654), and send for microscopy and culture.
  - A negative dipstick does not exclude the diagnosis if the clinical suspicion is high. Always send for culture.
- If the patient is not well, consider checking blood tests, including renal function (risk of impairment), blood cultures (risk of bacteremia), full blood count, and inflammatory markers.

# Urinary tract infection: treatment

Treatment involves more than just antibiotics. Consider the following:
- Adequate hydration (oral hydration is often sufficient; sicker or more confused patients may require intravenous fluid)
- Medication review (consider suspending diuretics or drugs that are potentially nephrotoxic, such as nonsteroidals or ACE inhibitors)
- Management of any symptoms (e.g., confusion or decreased mobility may necessitate temporary increase in care at home, or even admission to hospital)
- Assessment for complications (e.g., pyelonephritis, bacteremia, abscess formation). Older patients are at high risk of dehydration and renal impairment. Consider admission for intravenous antibiotics and hydration if they are not well.
- Prevention of recurrence with measures such as ensuring good fluid intake and avoiding catheters if possible. Topical estrogens (vaginally) may be useful in postmenopausal women.

## Antibiotic choice

Choice of antibiotic is guided by local sensitivity patterns. The local microbiology department is likely to have guidelines for UTI management.
Uncomplicated UTI can be treated empirically as follows:
- Trimethoprim 200 mg twice a day (if local resistance is <20%) or
- Nitrofurantoin 50 mg daily or
- Co-amoxiclav 375 mg three times per day
- Ciprofloxacin 500 mg twice a day is effective, but because of concerns about emerging resistance, it should be reserved for resistant or complicated infection.
- In a patient with nosocomial UTI use intravenous therapy for resistant organisms.

## Duration of treatment

- Younger females with uncomplicated UTI can be successfully treated with a short course of antibiotics (3 days, or perhaps even single dose).
- There is limited evidence for the duration required in older patients, but it is likely that a longer course (5–10 days) is needed.

## Treatment failure

*Incorrect diagnosis*
- Delirium and a positive urine dipstick may be misleading.
- Is another etiology being missed?

*Resistant organisms*
- Review the results of the urine culture and pathogen sensitivities (ideally sent before empirical antibiotics were started).
- *E. coli* is resistant to ampicillin, resistance to sulfonamides is widespread, and trimethoprim resistance is increasing. Most are currently susceptible to nitrofurantoin and fluoroquinolones (e.g., ciprofloxacin), although fluoroquinolone resistance is increasing.
- Pathogens are more varied in older patients and these may not be susceptible to empirical treatment (e.g., nitrofurantoin is inactive against *Proteus* and *Klebsiella*).
- MRSA UTI may occur in older patients (especially with indwelling catheters), which may require intravenous therapy (e.g., vancomcin). However, when MRSA is found in urine, bacteremia needs to be considered.
- *Candida* may cause UTI in the frail, catheterized older patient (identified on microscopy). These cases are usually left untreated.
- If no culture result is available and the diagnosis is secure, try an empirical second-line agent such as co-amoxiclav or ciprofloxacin.

# Recurrent urinary tract infection

Recurrent UTI is defined as >3 symptomatic UTIs in a year, or >2 in 6 months. It may represent either a relapse (recurrent infection caused by original infecting organism) or a reinfection (infection with different species or strain). Urinary culture is indicated.

## Possible reasons for recurrent infection

- Ongoing source of infection (e.g., chronic prostatitis, renal abscess)
- Urological abnormality (e.g., stones, tumor, residual volume >50 mL, cystocoele)
- Catheterization.
- Poor hygiene (e.g., fecal soiling)
- Impaired immunity (e.g., diabetes, chronic disease)
- Genetic susceptibility

## Managing recurrent infection

- Repeat treatment with up to a week of antibiotics.
- Remove catheter, if possible.
- General measures include increasing fluid intake, treating constipation.
- Arrange renal tract ultrasound to look for residual volume and any urological abnormalities (lower threshold of investigation for males).
- Consider blood tests (e.g., glucose, renal function, full blood count, serum electrophoresis, PSA in men).
- Prophylactic antibiotics are rarely indicated (examples include multiple recurrences despite general measures or significant renal damage). Trimethoprim is well studied. Nitrofurantoin is effective but carries a risk of pulmonary fibrosis with prolonged use.
- Pre-emptive treatment can be useful in cognitively intact patients. A short course of antibiotics is held in reserve by the patient, to be taken when the UTI is symptomatic.

# Varicella zoster infection

Initial exposure usually occurs in childhood, causing chicken pox in suscep-tible individuals. The virus lies dormant in the sensory dorsal root ganglia of the spinal cord and can be reactivated later in life to cause shingles.

*Shingles* is a painful, self-limiting, unilateral eruption of vesicles in a dermatomal distribution. It occurs in 20% of the population at some time but is most common in older people (probably due to a decline in cell-mediated immunity with age).

## Clinical presentation

- A prodrome of fever, malaise, headache, and sensory symptoms (pain, tenderness or paraesthesia) occurs in the dermatome affected.
- Rash follows after a few days, initially with a cluster of vesicles that spread across the dermatome and then become pustular.
- 50% affect thoracic dermatomes (T5–T12), 16% lumbosacral, and 15%–20% have cranial nerve distribution.
- Usually affects single dermatome, but may involve several adjacent
- Acute herpetic pain is often a feature—it may precede the rash by days and is often described as sharp.
- Crusting occurs after about a week, then the patient is no longer infectious (prior to this, susceptible individuals may catch chickenpox).
- Healing generally occurs within a month but may leave scars.
- Recurrence is in around 5% of patients.

## Preventive

Vaccine for shingles is indicated in patients >60 years old, including those with previous episode of shingles.

## Treatment

- General measures include adequate oral fluid intake, simple analgesia (e.g., acetaminophen), and topical agents such as calamine lotion.
- **Antiviral therapy** (e.g., aciclovir 800 mg 5 times a day, famciclovir 250 mg tid, valaciclovir 1 g tid) should be given within 72 hours of rash onset to all patients over 50 years old, for a week, and has been shown to reduce severity of the attack, promote rash healing, and reduce the incidence of postherpetic neuralgia.
- **Prednisolone** (e.g., 40 mg tapering down over a week) can be given with antiviral therapy to reduce the severity of the attack, but has limited value and possible drawbacks (e.g., increasing bacterial superinfection, causing significant side effects) and should only be used when the infection is severe.
- **Analgesia** for neuralgia should be given early when indicated.

## Ophthalmic shingles

- More common in older patients
- Occurs when the ophthalmic division of the trigeminal nerve is involved, resulting in a rash on the forehead and around the eye

- Ocular involvement commonly occurs, causing a red, painful eye. Inflammation of the iris and cornea can cause vision loss, and topical steroid eyedrops are used to limit the inflammatory response.
- Prompt use of antivirals may limit the disease.

## Ramsay Hunt syndrome

- Shingles of several adjacent cranial nerves cause vesicles in the ear canal, ear pain, and a lower motor neuron facial droop.
- This may also cause vertigo, deafness, and disturbance of taste and lacrimation.

Always look in the ears for vesicles when a patient presents with a facial palsy.

- Facial paralysis is less likely to fully recover than in Bell's palsy.
- Treat with antivirals as described under Treatment (p. 664).

## Postherpetic neuralgia

- Occurs in up to 10% of cases.
- It is more common with older patients (up to a third of over 60s) who have sensory symptoms at prodrome and a more severe initial infection.
- Defined as sensory symptoms continuing >4 months beyond the onset of rash
- Subsides in most patients by a year; may become chronic and disabling
- Usually a deep, steady, burning sensation, sometimes exacerbated by movement or touch. Occasionally there is paroxysmal and stabbing.
- Can cause significant psychological symptoms (low mood, poor sleep, loss of appetite etc)
- Treatment is with tricyclic antidepressants (e.g., amitriptyline 10–150 mg every night), opioids (e.g., codeine 60 mg/day, tramadol 50–100 mg/day), or anticonvulsants (e.g., gabapentin, carbamazepine, phenytoin).
- Topical treatments with lidocaine or capsaicin are also effective.
- Other options can be used in specialist pain clinics, such as intravenous lidocaine, intrathecal steroids, or local nerve blocks.

## Other complications

The following complications are all more common in older patients:

- **Bacterial superinfection** (around 2%, can delay rash healing. Treat with topical antiseptic or antibiotic initially—more severe cases require systemic treatment.)
- **Motor neuropathy** (occurs when virus spreads to the anterior horn; symptoms depend on segment affected, e.g., C5/6 may cause diaphragmatic paralysis. Most patients will recover spontaneously.)
- **Meningeal irritation** (causes headache; occurs in up to 40%; the CSF shows reactive changes—lymphocytosis and elevated protein)
- **Meningitis and encephalitis** (rare; diagnosis enhanced by MRI imaging and CSF PCR. These usually occur with the rash, but may develop up to 6 months later.)
- **Transverse myelitis** (rare; occurs with thoracic shingles)
- **Stroke** (rare and serious; due to cerebral angiitis)

# Oncology

**Gary Shapiro**

# Malignancy in older people

Cancer is a disease of the older adult population, being relatively rare under age 35, and increasing in incidence with each decade. Currently, 60% of all cancers and 70% of all cancer deaths occur in people older than 65 years of age.

## Why is there more cancer in older people?

- Longevity: As more people avoid death from infection and vascular events, they remain alive to develop cancer.
- Environmental susceptibility: Increased longevity results in longer cumulative exposure to environmental carcinogens.
- Cellular alterations: Aging affects the process of cell replication, which increases the chance of malignant change. Senescence also contributes to diminished immune surveillance and other immunological abnormalities.

## Is cancer different in older people?

The stage-specific natural history of each cancer type usually determines outcome, but age can alter the expected behaviors of some cancers.

- *Non-Hodgkin's lymphoma:* Age is an independent negative risk factor and a key determinant of survival in the International Prognostic Index.
- *Acute myeloid leukemia:* The different biology of AML in older patients contributes to a relatively worse prognosis.
- *Breast cancer:* As women age, their breast tumors more frequently express hormone receptors, have lower rates of tumor cell proliferation, and have lower expression of Her-2/neu. Although these more favorable tumor characteristics suggest a more indolent course, the incidence of PR-negative tumors increases in the very old and their prognosis is often worse than that of their younger, postmenopausal, ER-positive, PR-positive counterparts.

Chronological age itself has limited influence over disease progression and prognosis. Biological and functional changes associated with aging are more reliable in estimating life expectancy, functional reserve, and risk of treatment complications. These include sarcopenia, body mass index (BMI), cytokine expression, glomerular filtration rate (GFR), and activities of daily living (ADL and IADL).

The impact of cancer may be different in an older person. Frail individuals have decreased reserve and resistance to stressors that cause vulnerability to adverse outcomes. Non-cancer deaths are common in frail older adults with malignancy.

Comorbidity is associated with mortality, both in general and specifically in cancer patients. This effect is independent of functional status and appears to have very little impact on behavior of the cancer itself. Studies do show that comorbidity has a major impact on toxicity and treatment outcome.

# An approach to malignancy

### Make the diagnosis

No matter how "typical" your patient's signs and symptoms, clinical impressions can be wrong. For example, the mass in the head of the pancreas seen on your patient's CT scan may be a treatable islet cell tumor, not an incurable adenocarcinoma.

Even if curative treatment is not possible, a diagnosis helps your patient and his or her family understand what to expect and how to prepare for the future. It allows you to target symptom control and minimize side effects by avoiding unnecessary nonspecific interventions. Many people find "not knowing" very hard, and are relieved when they receive an explanation for their symptoms.

Sometimes a frail patient is obviously dying, and diagnostic studies can be an additional burden. If knowing the diagnosis is unlikely to affect how you care for such a patient, it may be quite reasonable for you, your patient, and the family to decide that "blind" palliation of symptoms is the best course.

### Stage the disease

This allows accurate prognostication and gives the patient better information on which to base treatment decisions. Again, there are exceptions to this (e.g., the very frail who are likely to die from other causes), and each individual should be considered separately.

### Do not underestimate the patient's average life expectancy

Healthy older men and women often have an average life expectancy that exceeds median average life expectancy for others in their age cohort or life expectancy with untreated cancer. Functional status and presence or lack of comorbid illness is a better predictor of average life expectancy than age alone (see Fig. 32.1, Chapter 32, p. 750).

If a patient's life expectancy is so short due to comorbid illness that the cancer will not significantly affect it, anticancer treatment is not indicated. Anticancer treatment should be considered if the patient is likely to live long enough to experience cancer-related symptoms or premature cancer-related death.

### Understand the goals

*Goals of treatment*

- *Cure or palliation:* It is important to establish whether the goal of treatment is cure or palliation. It is also important to understand the probable duration of effects of the treatment.
- *Likelihood for achieving goals:* What is the likelihood of achieving these goals?

*Quality of life*
In addition to the traditional goals (e.g., tumor response, increased survival, and symptom control), the focus for older cancer patients is often maintaining independent function, making family events, staying out of the hospital, or even remaining economically stable.

## Balance benefits and harms

*Efficacy*
Fit older cancer patients respond to treatment similarly to their younger counterparts. However, a word of caution is in order. Until recently, few cancer clinical trials included older individuals, and it may not be appropriate to generalize these findings to the heterogeneous group of older cancer patients.

*Toxicity*
The toxic effects of cancer treatment are never less burdensome in older patients. In addition to the standard side effects of cancer treatment, there are significant age-related toxicities to consider. Though most are more a function of frailty than chronological age, even the fittest senior cannot avoid the physiological effects of aging. These include modifications of renal, hepatic, and gastrointestinal function, and changes in body fluid and muscle–fat composition.

These in turn affect the pharmacokinetic and pharmacodynamic properties of many drugs used in treating cancer. Also, drugs used for comorbid conditions increase potential for drug–drug interactions.

## Engage the patient

Health-care providers often underestimate the physical and mental abilities of older people and their willingness to face chronic and life-threatening conditions. Family members are no better at making these predictions.

Studies show that most older patients want detailed and comprehensible information about treatments and alternatives. Patients and families may consider cancer untreatable in the aged and not understand the possibilities offered by treatment.

While cognitively impaired patients pose a unique challenge, they are frequently capable of participating in goal setting and simple discussions about treatment side effects and logistics. Caring family members and friends are often able to share the patient's "life narrative story" so that health-care workers can work with them to make good substituted or best-interest judgments for those who are truly impaired.

# Treating malignancy in older people

### Use a specialist multidisciplinary approach

Cancer care changes rapidly and it is hard for the generalist to keep up to date, so specialist referral is needed. Cancer patients cared for in geriatric oncology programs benefit from multidisciplinary teams of oncologists, geriatricians, psychiatrists, pharmacists, physiatrists, social workers, nurses, and dieticians working together to identify and manage the stressors that can limit effective cancer treatment. These multidisciplinary teams use some form of the Comprehensive Geriatric Assessment (CGA; see p. 40) to assess functional status, comorbidities, socioeconomic issues, and nutritional status, and to determine the presence of polypharmacy or geriatric syndromes.

Decisions about cancer treatment should not be based on chronological age, rather on functional status and the presence of comorbid conditions.

The patient should be at the center of the decision-making process, as decisions are rarely clear-cut and require a balancing of the side effects of therapy against potential benefits. Frank discussion of what to expect should facilitate patient-led decisions, and there will be a wide variety of choices.

Some older people will wish to avoid any stress from treatment while others will accept a high level of discomfort for the chance of a few extra months of life. There is no substitute for having a thoughtful, unhurried discussion with the patient.

### Surgery

Surgical outcomes for non-frail older patients are not significantly different from those for their younger counterparts. Regardless of age, curative operations should always be considered. Even relatively frail patients may find palliative surgery the most effective and least toxic means for controlling symptoms related to, for example, bowel obstruction (pain, diarrhea, skin breakdown) or bleeding.

### Radiation therapy

Radiation therapy is well tolerated by fit seniors, and even frail patients may find the side effects acceptable if the benefits are sufficient. It is often the logistical details (such as daily travel to the hospital for a 6-week course of treatment) that are the hardest. These problems should be discussed with the patient, the family, and a social worker prior to starting radiation therapy.

### Hormonal therapy

Hormonal therapy is the mainstay of treatment for postmenopausal women with breast cancer and men with prostate cancer. In advanced disease, it usually provides very effective palliation, with acceptable side effects.

## Chemotherapy

Non-frail older cancer patients respond to chemotherapy similarly to their younger counterparts. Advances in supportive care (e.g., antiemetics, hematopoietic growth factors) have significantly decreased the side effects of chemotherapy and improved safety and the quality of life of older cancer patients. Nonetheless, they are at significant risk, especially if they are functionally impaired.

## Common treatment complications in older patients

### Bone marrow

Minimal stress will disrupt hematopoiesis in the older patient. Anemia and myelosuppression are common in older patients getting chemotherapy or radiation therapy. Primary prophylaxis with granulopoietic growth factors significantly decreases neutropenic infections and makes it possible for older patients to receive full doses of potentially curable chemotherapy.

### Mucositis, diarrhea, and dehydration

Older patients often have suboptimal fluid intake and are on diuretics. Since their gastrointestinal mucosa is particularly sensitive to damage from chemotherapy and radiation therapy, severe dehydration can occur when they develop diarrhea and mucositis from chemotherapy or radiation therapy.

### Neurotoxicity and cognitive effects

"Chemo-brain" can be profoundly debilitating in patients who are already cognitively impaired. Older patients with hearing loss or peripheral neuropathy (from, e.g., diabetes) have decreased reserve and are highly vulnerable to neurotoxic chemotherapy like the taxanes or platinum compound.

*Fatigue* is a near universal complaint of older cancer patients. It is particularly a problem for those who are socially isolated or dependent on others in ADLs or IADLs.

*Depression:* In contrast to younger patients who often respond to a cancer diagnosis with anxiety, depression is the more common disorder in older cancer patients.

*Cardiac problems* increase with age, and it is no surprise that older cancer patients have an increased risk of cardiac complications from anthracyclines, trastuzumab, and other potentially cardiotoxic anticancer agents.

*Osteoporosis* can be exacerbated by aromatase inhibitors, the mainmainstay of hormonal therapy in postmenopausal women with breast cancer. This, in turn, can result in fractures, falls, and progressive debility.

## Treatment timelines

When the goal of treatment is palliative, chemotherapy should never be administered without defined end points and timelines. It should be clear to everyone what "counts" as success, how it will be determined (a symptom controlled, a smaller mass on CT scan), and when. Patients and their families should understand what their options are at each step and how likely each is to meet the patients goals.

# Presentation of malignancy

Fit, cognitively intact older patients usually present with a fairly typical story—a breast lump, a thyroid nodule, altered bowel habits with iron deficiency anemia. By contrast, cancer in the frail older adult often presents in unusual ways. It may be found incidentally (e.g., a mass on a routine chest X-ray) or there may be a highly suggestive clinical scenario. Deciding how aggressive to purse a cancer diagnosis is a common challenge in geriatric practice.

## Common presenting scenarios

*Weight loss without apparent cause*
- Always check a dietary history, measure thyroid function, screen for depression, and assess cognitive state.
- Even subtle abnormalities should be investigated with the appropriate diagnostic studies.
- If a careful history and physical exam (H&P) finds no localizing signs or symptoms, consider selected appropriate screening diagnostic studies (see How to screen for malignancy when suspicion is high, p. 675).
- If the screening studies are normal, malignancy is unlikely. Dietary support with interval follow-up may be appropriate (see p. 371).

*Elevated inflammatory markers (ESR, CRP)*
- Without associated signs or symptoms of cancer, elevated inflammatory markers are usually not due to malignancy. They should not be used to screen for an occult cancer.
- Elevated inflammatory markers are usually due to infectious or rheumatologic disorders.
- The screening H&P should include a close look at the bones (osteomyelitis) and joints (gout, arthritis) and appropriate diagnostic investigations.
- Consider giving the patient a thermometer and temperature chart to fill in. A source of infection should be sought with cultures.
- Remember to check for diverticular and perirectal abscesses.
- Have a low threshold for endocarditis (see p. 643).
- Vasculitis (especially giant cell arteritis, see p. 500) should be considered. Temporal artery biopsy and a trial of steroids may be appropriate, even if the history is not classic, but remember to check response and rethink the diagnosis if the blood results do not normalize.

*Anemia*
- Iron deficiency anemia should always raise the possibility of gastrointestinal malignancy (see p. 471).
- Macrocytic anemia is probably due to a vitamin (folate or $B_{12}$) deficiency, alcohol, or medications, but it may also be the first sign of a myelodysplastic syndrome.
- Anemia is not uncommon in older people with chronic diseases or renal insufficiency, but confirmatory studies are almost always indicated. In addition to a good H&P, these usually include diagnostic blood, and, when appropriate, bone marrow studies.

# How to screen for malignancy when suspicion is high

*History*

History should include the following:

- Dietary history
- Mood assessment
- History of fevers and night sweats
- Travel history
- HIV risk factor assessment
- Full review of systems enquiry (especially meticulous inquiry into gastrointestinal symptoms and postmenopausal bleeding)

*Examination*

Full examination is required, including the following:

- Lymph nodes
- Skin nodules or rashes (check body surface fully)
- ENT/oral cavity examination
- Male external genitalia (testicular masses)
- Female breast and pelvic examination
- Rectal (and prostate) examination
- Thyroid examination

*Diagnostic studies*

- CBC with differential
- Electrolytes
- Blood sugar
- Creatinine and BUN
- Calcium
- Liver function tests and albumin
- Thyroid function tests
- Serum protein and protein electrophoresis (SPEP)
- Urinalysis (microscopic and dipstick)
- Chest X-ray (PA and lateral)
- Fecal occult blood tests
- PSA in men

Carcinoembryonic antigen (CEA) and most other tumor markers are nonspecific and should not be used to screen for occult malignancy.

## How to manage symptomatic hypercalcemia

Older patients often present with altered mental status or constipation. In patients with a known diagnosis of cancer, these symptoms may be mistakenly attributed to side effects of narcotic analgesics or anticancer treatment. Other symptoms iinclude dehydration, progressive weakness, anorexia, nausea, vomiting, thirst, polyuria, or dysrhythmias.

Look for symptoms and signs of malignancy, which almost always precede malignant hypercalcemia.

Hypoalbuminemia is common in older patients, and it can mask high calcium—always correct the calcium level or check the serum ionized calcium.

### Management

*1. Restore volume*

Infuse intravenous normal saline at an initial rate of 300–500 mL/hr, with frequent evaluations (and adjustments) for congestive heart failure. Decrease rate once the extracellular fluid volume deficit has been partially corrected. At least 3–4 liters of normal saline is typically needed in the first 24 hours.

*2. Saline diuresis*

Once the patient is rehydrated (a positive fluid balance of approximately 2 liters) a normal saline infusion rate of 100–200 mL/hr is usually sufficient to promote saline diuresis and calcium excretion.

*3. Monitor for CHF*

Because older patients may have difficulty handling large fluid loads, furosemide may also be needed. This diuretic increases urinary calcium and sodium excretion but should be given only if necessary, in appropriate doses, to prevent or treat fluid overload. Furosemide adds little to the effect of saline diuresis and may produce recurrent dehydration or hypotension. Thiazide diuretics impair calcium excretion and must be avoided.

*4. Monitor electrolytes*

Serum electrolytes, calcium, and magnesium should be measured every 6–12 hours. Adequate replacement of potassium and magnesium is essential.

*5. Intravenous bisphosphonates*

Bisphosphonates inhibit bone resorption and are usually quite effective in controlling hypercalcemia for 3–4 weeks. Pamidronate (IV over 2 hours, 60 mg or 90 mg) for severe hypercalcemia (>13.5) or zoledronic acid (4 mg IV over 15 minutes) is usually effective in 2 days. Treatment can be repeated after 7 days if the calcium level has not changed significantly. Bisphosphonates are adjuncts to volume restoration and saline diuretics and should not be used in place of them. They can cause nephrotoxicity and should be used with caution in patients with renal insufficiency and in combination with other nephrotoxic drugs.

## How to manage symptomatic hypercalcemia (cont'd.)

*6. Other acute treatments*
IV bisphosphonate therapy is much more efficacious and less toxic than older pharmacological agents (calcitonin, mithramycin, oral phosphates). With rare exception, they should no longer be used in the acute management of hypercalcemia of malignancy. Glucocorticoids may still have a limited role in treating selected patients with hypercalcemia due to multiple myeloma or other hematological malignancy. Rarely, hemodialysis is used to treat severe hypercalcemia unresponsive to other therapy.

*7. Long-term therapy*
Specific systemic anticancer therapy (chemotherapy, hormonal therapy, targeted therapy) is the best long-term treatment. Localized therapies (radiation, surgery) seldom influence serum calcium levels.

# Cancer with an unknown primary

Metastatic cancer from an unknown primary (CUP) makes up 5%–10% of all diagnosed cancers. They have a poor prognosis and, even after post-mortem examination, the primary tumor is only identified in about half of the patients. Though their peak incidence is in the sixth decade, they can pose a particularly vexing problem in the older patient.

Finding metastases during investigation for vague symptoms or when looking into more specific problems (such as bone pain, abnormal liver function tests, breathlessness, enlarged lymph nodes, etc.) is a commonly encountered problem in geriatric practice, and a structured approach to management is essential.

## Approach to investigation

When the primary cancer site cannot be identified, overall response to empirical treatment is only 20%–35%, with median survival times of 5–8 months. There are, however, several "don't miss" scenarios that have a relatively favorable prognosis, and it is incumbent upon the doctor to rule these out in all but the frailest older patient.

Every woman with an adenocarcinoma of unknown primary site should have bilateral mammograms and a pelvic examination. Although metastatic breast and ovarian cancer can't be cured, they can often be controlled for a number of years with reasonably good quality of life. An elevated CA-125 tumor marker may be sufficient circumstantial evidence to treat a CUP as if it were an ovarian primary, especially if the metastases have papillary characteristics and are in the peritoneal cavity. Even with a negative breast examination and breast imaging a woman with isolated adenocarcinoma metastases in the axilla should be treated as if she has breast cancer.

Men with CUP should have their prostate examined with a careful digital rectal examination and have their PSA checked. Germ cell tumors are also seen in older men, and it is important to investigate this possibility with a testicular examination.

Pathologists can often provide useful information regarding the likelihood of these treatable primary sites, especially when special immunohistochemical (IHC) stains are applied to the biopsy tissue. Lymphomas, germ cell tumors, and neuroendocrine tumors are not considered CUPs (which are usually defined as either adenocarcinoma or undifferentiated carcinoma), and it is useful for the pathologist to exclude these treatable malignancies from among the possible primaries.

Unknown metastatic squamous cell carcinomas in neck lymph nodes are generally regarded as arising from the head and neck region (even if they are not found by extensive ENT diagnostic studies), and they are treated accordingly.

Other than these, the evaluation follows the same diagnostic approach outlined in How to screen for malignancy when suspicion is high (p. 675). Endoscopic examinations are reserved for patients with (even the subtlest) signs or symptoms of GI or pulmonary pathology.

CT imaging studies are usually reserved for those with signs or symptoms, although there is a growing body of evidence supporting the use of PET scans, especially in those with limited sites of metastatic disease.

# Palliative care and end of life

## Grace Cordts

# Palliative care

*Palliative care* is interdisciplinary care aimed to relieve suffering and improve quality of life for patients with advanced disease and for their families. It involves a multidisciplinary team approach, with attention to relief of physical symptoms and provision of social, psychological, spiritual, and family support.

It is appropriate along the entire course of an illness, regardless of whether treatment is focused on cure or making someone comfortable at the end of life.

## General principles of palliative care

- Communication with the patient and family is important. Your presence is therapeutic.
- All symptoms should be evaluated and a diagnosis made on the basis of probability and pattern recognition.
- Explanation of the cause and treatment planned empowers the patient and keeps expectations realistic.
- Treatment involves correcting what can be corrected (e.g., treating oral candida infection contributing to odynophagia), counselling to help patients accept limitations imposed by the disease (e.g., a patient with COPD may not be able to walk in the garden, but supplying a wheelchair may allow them to go out), and drugs to control symptoms.
- Treatment is planned for each individual with attention to detail, its impact is monitored closely, and it is discontinued if ineffective.

# Hospice

*Hospice* is a specialized program of care and part of the palliative continuum. Medicare, Medicaid, and most third-party payers offer a hospice benefit. Patients are eligible for the Medicare benefit if (1) a licensed physician certifies that the patient has an estimated life expectancy of 6 months or less and (2) the patient or designated decision-maker agrees to the hospice care plan for management of the terminal illness.

## Medicare hospice benefits

The Medicare hospice benefit is divided into benefit periods:
- An initial 90-day period
- A subsequent 90-day period
- After the first two 90-day periods there is an unlimited number of 60-day periods.

The beneficiary must be recertified as terminally ill at the beginning of each benefit period.

The following covered hospice services are provided as necessary to give palliative treatment for conditions related to the terminal illness:
- Nursing care
- Services of a medical social worker, physician, counselor (including dietary, pastoral, and other), and home care aide and homemaker
- Short-term inpatient care (including both respite care and procedures necessary for pain control and acute and chronic system management)
- Medical appliances and supplies, including drugs and biologicals
- Physical and occupational therapies, and speech–language pathology services
- Bereavement service for the family is provided for up to 13 months after the patient's death.

# Breaking bad news

Physicians caring for older adults must be skilled in breaking bad news. No matter how old or frail the patient is, bad news can be devastating. Paradoxically, news that seems bad may be taken well—someone who has felt ill for some time may welcome an explanation, even if it means a terminal diagnosis. Sometimes the patient expects the worse ("I've had a stroke? Thank goodness it isn't cancer.").

Each case needs to be considered individually and carefully modified as reactions become apparent.

## Who should be told bad news?

Information about a patient's diagnosis and prognosis belongs to the patient, and that individual has a right to know. The paternalistic tendency to "protect" the patient or relatives from bad news is now largely obsolete, but some patients and relatives still believe this exists, and this attitude may need to be corrected.

It is important to remember, however, that some older people do not wish to know details about diagnosis and prognosis; this may be a cultural bias. They prefer to trust others to make decisions for them. It is inappropriate to force information on such patients.

Determination of the patient's preference to know may take the form of a direct question, such as, "If you turn out to have something serious, are you the sort of person who would like to know exactly what is wrong?", or a more subtle inquiry: "We have some test results back, and your daughter is keen to talk to me about them. Would you like to know about them too?" The response to this is usually informative, either "Yes, of course I want to know," or "Oh well, I'd rather let my daughter deal with all that."

Well-meaning relatives (usually children, who are used to challenging authority) may be more proactive in seeking information than the patient is, and then try to shield the patient from the truth, believing that their parent would not be able to cope. In such situations, avoid giving information to relatives first—explain that you cannot discuss it with them without the patient's permission.

Be sympathetic, as these wishes are usually born from genuine concern. Explore why they don't want the patient to hear bad news, and help them to understand the true level of awareness that most patients have about their health—they know that they are ill and must have had thoughts about what is wrong. Point out that it becomes impossible to hide a diagnosis from a patient in a deteriorating condition and that such an approach often sets up major conflict between family members and health-care providers.

Be open—tell the relative(s) that you are going to talk to the patient, and promise discretion (i.e., you will not force unwanted information). A joint meeting can be valuable if the patient agrees. Of course, the family may be right; the patient does not want to be told about their diagnosis. But establish this for yourself first. Remember, always get permission from the patient before disclosing details to anyone else.

## How to break bad news

1. Prepare for the discussion: be sure you know the medical facts of the case; anticipate questions that might arise about prognosis, referral, or treatment.
2. Ensure that there is a quiet environment. Allow for an appropriate amount of uninterrupted time.
3. Suggest that family members or friends come along to support.
4. Invite other members of the multidisciplinary team who are involved in the patient's care (e.g., nurse and social worker).
5. Begin with introductions and context ("I am Dr. Brown, the doctor in charge of your mother's care since she arrived in the hospital. I already know Mrs. Jones, but perhaps I could also know who everyone else is?").
6. Establish what is known ("A lot has happened here today—perhaps you could begin by telling me what you already know.", or in a non-acute setting: "When did you last speak to a doctor?").
7. Set the scene and give a "warning shot" ("Your mother has been unwell for some time now, and when she came in today she was much more seriously ill" or "I'm afraid I have some bad news.")
8. Use simple, jargon-free language to describe events, giving "bite-sized" chunks of information and gauging comprehension and response as you go.
9. Avoid euphemisms—say "dying" or "cancer" if that is what you mean.
10. Allow time for the news to sink in. Long silences may be necessary; try not to fill them because you are uncomfortable.
11. Allow time for emotional reactions. Using verbal and nonverbal communication, reassure the patient and family that this is an acceptable and normal response.
12. Encourage questions.
13. Don't be afraid to show your own emotions, while maintaining professionalism—strive for genuine empathy.
14. Summarize and clarify understanding, if possible. If you feel that the message has been lost or misinterpreted, ask them to summarize what they have been told, allowing reinforcement and correction.
15. Establish a plan for follow-up and how to get in touch for any further questions.
16. Document your meeting carefully in the medical notes.

# Bereavement

With bereavement, physicians deal primarily with patients grieving over the loss of a loved one, but they also deal with patients grieving over the anticipated and real loss of health, the future, physical abilities, roles, and relationships. Physicians grieve the loss of patients they have cared for.

There is a normal grieving process that people experience. Most will adapt, but a quarter will develop major depression or complicated grief reaction.

The grieving process is amenable to positive and negative influences, so awareness of those who are at risk can help to target care.

## Normal stages of grief

These are not linear. People often go back and forth between stages.

- **Shock/denial** lasts from minutes to days. It lasts longer for an unexpected death. It resolves as reality is accepted.
- **Pining/searching:** People feel sad, angry, guilty, and vulnerable. They have the urge to look back and search for the dead person. They are restless, irritable, and tearful. Loss of appetite and weight can occur, as can poor short-term memory and concentration. This stage is resolved by feeling pain and expressing sadness. It may be hampered by social or cultural pressures to behave in a certain way.
- **Disorganization/despair:** People feel as if life has no meaning. They tend to relive events and try to put it right. It is common to experience hallucinations of the deceased when falling asleep (reassure those grieving that this is normal). This stage resolves as the grieving person adjusts to the new reality without the deceased.
- **Reorganization:** People begin to look forward and explore a new life without the deceased. They find things to carry forward into the future from the past. They may feel guilt and need reassurance. This is a period of adjustment.
- **Recurrence:** Grief may recur on anniversaries, birthdays, etc.

## Abnormal grief reactions

Abnormal grief reactions include bereavement-related depression and a complicated grief reaction. It is important to identify a complicated grief reaction since it does not respond to interventions for major depression.

A complicated grief reaction is suggested when a patient presents with symptoms of 6 months' duration that include searching for the deceased, preoccupation with thoughts of the deceased, detachment from others, loneliness, distrust, and expressing similar somatic complaints of the deceased. Patients with complicated grief require referral to a specialist.

### Risk factors for complicated grief

- Sudden or unexpected loss
- Low self-esteem
- Little social support
- Prior mental illness (especially depression)
- Multiple prior bereavements
- Ambivalent or dependent relationship with the deceased
- Having cared for the deceased in their final illness for more than 6 months
- Having fewer opportunities for developing new interests and relationships after the death

Although older people are generally more accepting of death than younger people, they commonly have a number of these risk factors. For example, an 80-year-old man who has cared for his demented wife for 3 years prior to her death is likely to have experienced an ambivalent relationship by being a spouse as well as a caregiver. He may have limited social support and opportunity for alternative social contacts.

Older widowers have the highest rate of suicide among all groups of bereaved persons.

Older persons experiencing loss of functional status or who are in the midst of a terminal illness may grieve over future losses. Physicians should encourage patients and caregivers to discuss their feelings, fears, and hopes.

Physicians caring for aging patients and their families should be cognizant of their own emotional reactions when patients die, and attend to their own emotional needs. Saying goodbye to patients, sending condolence letters, and attending their patient's funeral is usually welcomed and helpful.

### How to promote a "healthy bereavement"

- Identify those at risk of abnormal grief (see Abnormal grief).
- Encourage seeing the body after death, if wished.
- Encourage involvement in funeral arrangements.
- Give permission for "time out" and reassurance that the bereaved are experiencing a normal reaction.
- As time goes on, set small goals for progressive change to structure recovery.
- Some grieving people may need short-term medication for relief of anxiety or insomnia. Note that prolonged use of benzodiazepine can interfere with the normal grief process.

For the **confused, older patient**, repeated explanations, supported involvement in the funeral, and visiting the grave have been shown to reduce repetitive questioning about the whereabouts of the deceased.

# Symptom control in the terminally ill

### General principles of symptom management

- Conduct a thorough history and physical exam.
- Identify and treat the underlying cause, if appropriate (if someone is imminently dying, workup may not be appropriate).
- Use nonpharmacological and pharmacological approaches.
- Liver and kidney function can be impaired, so medication needs to be adjusted.
- Medications in older adults can cause adverse effects; use cautiously, "start low, go slow, but give enough."

### Pain

- Successful pain management involves thoroughly assessing pain and matching treatment to the type of pain.
- Use a scale to quantify pain, and reassess regularly.
- Identify likely cause(s) and treat underlying cause with appropriate nonpharmacological and pharmacological interventions.
- Use the WHO analgesia ladder, starting with nonopioids (acetaminophen, NSAIDs). Next add weak opioids (codeine, tramadol), escalate the dose, then replace with strong opioids (e.g., morphine slow release [MST]). Give regularly and treat all side effects (nausea, constipation).
- Medication should be given around the clock.
- Use short-acting opioids to escalate doses and switch to long-acting opioids when the patient is on a stable dose and pain is controlled.
- If using narcotics, prescribe bowel regimen unless contraindicated. See below section on constipation.
- Methylnaltrexone is FDA approved for opioid-related constipation. This should be used after other treatments have failed.
- Aim to use the oral route if possible, but consider subcutaneous, transdermal, or rectal routes if necessary. Patient-centered analgesia (PCA) is an option in the hospitalized patient.
- Neuropathic pain is often opioid responsive, but antidepressants and anticonvulsants can be added.
- Treat muscle spasm with physiotherapy, heat, antispasmodics, and benzodiazepines and nerve compression pain with steroids.

### Nausea and vomiting

- Complex symptoms involving several areas in brain and GI tract
- Mediated through several neurotransmitters (serotonin, dopamine, acetylcholine, and histamine) which allow multiple agents to be effective (dopamine agonist, antihistamines, anticholinergics, serotonin antagonists, and prokinetic agents)
- Identify the cause—is it reversible (e.g., medication, hypercalcemia, bowel obstruction)?
- Use regular antiemetics, start with the most appropriate antiemetic and maximize the dose. If there is no relief, switch to another class of medication or add another class of antiemetic.

- Give small portions of palatable food, sips of liquid, and ginger, and avoid strong smells.

## Constipation

- A stimulant laxative (e.g., senna) is necessary if the patient is on opioids, but a stool softener might otherwise be enough.
- Opiates decrease peristalsis so a stimulant laxative is needed. See Pain (above) and Constipation section in Chapter 12 (p. 380).

## Anorexia

- This is normal in advanced cancer and other conditions as death approaches.
- Family concerns may be the main problem—they may feel their relative is giving up.
- Deal with this directly. Eating more will not alter the outlook and pressuring the patient can make them miserable.
- Decrease medications that cause nausea or anorexia (opiates, SSRIs).
- Give good mouth care.
- Help with feeding if the patient is weak.
- Offer frequent, small meals.
- Prokinetics (e.g., metoclopramide) or steroids (prednisolone, medroxyprogesterone) may help but they may also hasten death (medroxyprogesterone) (see also Box 26.1).

## Dyspnea

- Treat the cause (transfuse for anemia, drain effusion, etc.).
- This is a terrifying symptom for the patient and family. Plan an approach to dealing with an attack (for the patient and family).
- Oxygen can help if the patient is hypoxic; a fan can be helpful.
- Low-dose opioids in opioid-naïve patients are helpful. Increasing the dose for patients already on opioids can help. Relief of dyspnea from opioids has shorter duration than pain relief, thus requiring more frequent dosing.
- Bronchodilators can help with bronchospasms
- Anxiolytics are helpful only if anxiety is a diagnosis; otherwise, it can make dyspnea worse.
- The goal of treatment is subjective improvement, not decreased respiratory rate.

## Delirium

- Identify the cause (infection, drugs, withdrawal from alcohol, electrolyte imbalances).
- Keep the patient in a calm, well-lit environment. Relatives can often help with reorientation.
- Drugs (e.g., haloperidol) can be used as a last resort, but antipsychotics are associated with increased death rate (see How to prescribe medications for delirium, p. 208)

### Dehydration

- Dying patients drink less (due to weakness, nausea, decreased level of consciousness). When this is chronic, the body slowly adapts and thirst is not felt.
- Good mouth-care is all that is required when decreased intake is part of the dying process.
- Reassure relatives that it is the disease that is killing the patient, not the dehydration.

### "Death rattle"

- The patient is usually unaware. Reassure the family of this.
- If excess secretion is causing distress or discomfort to the patient or the family, use hycosamine, glycopyrrolate or a scopolamine patch.

---

**Box 26.1 The principle of double effect**

Treatments given to relieve symptoms at the end of life can worsen the underlying disease and even hasten death, e.g., opiates given to relieve pain cause respiratory depression.

The treatment can be given if four conditions are met:

- The act itself must be good or neutral (e.g., giving medication by injection).
- The good effect is not caused by the bad effect (e.g., pain is not relieved by suppressing respiration).
- The good effect is intended, not the bad effect (e.g., pain relief intended, not respiratory depression).
- The good effect outweighs the bad effect (e.g., pain relief is more beneficial than the harm of respiratory suppression).

Good communication with the family and other members of the team ensure that everyone understands the rationale behind a treatment plan.

## How to order patient-centered analgesia (PCA)

PCA requires four orders
- Demand dose (also known as patient initiated dose or bolus dose)
- Delay interval or lock-out time period between demand dose
- Continuous infusion rate, if used
- Hourly limit—the maximum amount of drug dispensed in 1 hour

Morphine, hydromorphone, fentanyl, and methadone can be used.

The route of administration is primarily intravenous or subcutaneously. Epidural, intrathecal, or intraventriculr routes are used but require specialists for line placement.

The dosage of medication is dependent on the medication and on whether or not the patient is opioid naïve.

*Opioid-naïve patient*
- Use a low or no basal rate until opioid requirements are known.
- The lock-out period is determined by time for the drug to reach maximum effect, usually 10–12 minutes.
  - Morphine: no basal rate, 1 mg dose every 10 minutes
  - Hydromorphone: no basal rate, 0.2 mg dose every 10 minutes
  - Fentanyl: no basal rate, 10–15 mcg every 10 minutes

*Opioid-tolerant patient*
- Use basal rate to cover prior analgesic requirements.
- Demand dose is generally 25%–50% of the hourly rate.
- The lock-out period is 10–12 minutes.

Titration of the PCA dose is done every 30–60 minutes until the patient is pain free. If the patient is not on a basal rate and is using demand doses, then a basal rate should be added. This is done by adding up the amount of medication given over a specific number of hours and dividing that by the number of hours. A new demand rate should be calculated.

If a patient cannot push the mechanism to initiate a demand dose then a PCA is not appropriate (e.g., a patient with dementia or severe arthritis of the hands).

If a patient is at the end of life and medication is needed for symptom management, a continuous infusion can be run and adjusted for symptom relief.

# Documentation after death

### Verification of death

This is the confirmation that death has occurred and may be performed by any doctor, trained nurse, or paramedic. It must be done before a body can be moved to the mortuary. It is recommended that you look for the following:

- Absence of response to pain or stimulation
- Fixed dilated pupils
- Absence of a pulse (check for at least 30 seconds)
- Absence of heart sounds (check for at least 30 seconds)
- Absence of respiratory movements (check for at least 30 seconds)
- Absence of breath sounds (check for at least 30 seconds)

Always record your findings in full, along with the time of death and the time of verification (if different).

### Death notification

- Do this in person, when possible.
- Respect ethnic, cultural, and religious traditions.
- Use simple language, such as "died" or "dead." Do not use euphemisms.
- Express your condolences.
- Answer questions and allow time for information to sink in.
- Respond to emotions.
- Offer to contact other family members or clergy.
- Allow time for information to be absorbed before asking for autopsy or organ donation.

If telephone notification is the only option, in addition to the above:

- When possible, try to let the person(s) know when the patient starts to deteriorate.
- Identify the most appropriate person to tell, i.e., health-care power of attorney, etc.
- Do not leave a message about the death; leave explicit contact information.
- Offer to meet in person.
- Ask them if they will come to see the person who died.
- If you are uncomfortable with this, ask for help.

### Certification of death

This is the act of writing a death certificate. It is an important duty and legal requirement of the doctor who has recently been looking after the patient. It allows the family to arrange a funeral and provides very important statistics for disease surveillance and public health.

Inexperienced doctors tend to record the mechanism of death rather than the underlying cause, which may lead to underrepresentation of the real pathology in national statistics. Patients die of dementia and stroke, although their complications, e.g., aspiration pneumonia, may be the last thing that was treated.

# Resources

- American Association of Hospice and Palliative Medicine: www.aahpm.
  com

Educational material, including one page, "Fast Facts," about different topics relating to the care of terminally ill patients.

- End of Life/Palliative Education Resource Center.
  www.eperc.mcw.edu

Web site with educational material.

- Caring Connections—A program of the National Hospice and Palliative
  Care Organization:
  www.caringinfo.org

Web site that gives professional and patient information.

- WHO analgesic ladder:
  http://www.who.int/cancer/palliative/painladder/en/

# Ethics

### Thomas E. Finucane

This chapter is intended to be purely descriptive. Common law, statutes, and nomenclature vary from state to state, and country to country. No one involved with this chapter is a lawyer, and this chapter does not provide legal advice.

# Competency and capacity

*Competency* has a fairly special meaning when used in law. *Capacity* does as well, although it is a bit less well defined. In medical writings, both refer to the ability of a patient to make informed, authentic, and meaningful decisions about treatment. The terms are used variably in medicine; *competency* is often, but not always, used to refer to a court decision about the patient's decisional ability, whereas, *capacity* may refer to the physicians' judgment on this matter.

A cornerstone principle of Western biomedical ethics is that every competent person has the right to say, "Keep your hands off me."

To certify that a person is incompetent is a very serious matter, because it will limit or eliminate that person's freedom. Many serious problems arise when decisions about life-sustaining treatment (LST) must be made on behalf of an incompetent patient.

Competence generally depends on the task in question. One could be competent to play bridge but not basketball, and vice versa. No standardized test can identify incompetence in a communicative patient.

Over 30 years ago, Roth et al.[1] said, "the search for a single test of competence is a search for the Holy Grail. Unless it is realized that there is no magical definition of competency to make decisions about treatment, the search for an acceptable test will never end.... [J]udgments (about competency) reflect social considerations and societal biases as much as they reflect matters of law and medicine."

## Assessing competence

See Table 27.1 and How to assess competence.

**1.** Roth LH, Meisel S, Lidz CW (1977). Tests of competency to consent treatment. *Am J Psychiatry* **134**:279–284.

**Table 27.1** Assessing competence

| | |
|---|---|
| • Competence is decision-specific. Questions that are more complex and/or more important demand a higher level of competence. | • Assess competence for each relevant question individually. Global tests, e.g., mental test scores, are not a substitute and can be misleading. |
| • Competence is assumed for adults. | • The burden of responsibility is with the assessor to demonstrate incompetence. |
| • Competency levels may fluctuate. Some types of dementia and delirium can cause transient reversible incompetence. | • Ensure the patient is functioning at their best before assessing competence. If in doubt, repeat the assessment later. |
| • Ignorance is not the same as incompetence. | • Patients should be educated about a subject before being asked to make a decision (just as you would expect a surgeon to explain an operation before asking you to sign a consent form). |
| • A competent patient may make an unwise or unconventional decision. | • Competent patients can make decisions that lead to illness, discomfort, danger, or even death. Caregivers and relatives often need education and support when the patient chooses an unwise option. |

## How to assess competence

- *Trigger:* Doctors should be alert to the possibility of incompetence, but it is often people closer to the patient (relatives/caregivers) who highlight a problem. In real life, a competency assessment is usually only used when there is conflict or where an important step (such as a medical decision, will, or enduring power of attorney) is being attempted. Previous assessments of competency for other decisions or at other times are not a substitute for the latest assessment.
- *Education:* The patient should be given ample time to absorb and discuss the facts and advice. Several education sessions may be needed. Encourage other health professionals and relatives to discuss the topic with the patient as well.
- *Assessment*: Probe the patient to assess retention, understanding, and reasoning. In borderline or contentious cases employ a second opinion (often from a geropsychiatrist). The essential question is whether the patient can, in the clinician's judgment, understand the options that are available to him or her, and the consequences of the choice the patient is making.
- *Action*: Document the results of the assessment using observations and patient quotes. If the patient is incompetent, state how the substituted decision will be made e.g., medical decision in best interests, involvement of careers, case conference etc.

# Making financial decisions

Competent patients can make financial decisions.

## Power of attorney (POA)

A competent person, in this context called the "principal" or "grantor," can designate another, known as the "agent" or "attorney in fact," to act on behalf of the principal.

This is known as a *power of attorney (POA)*. If the principal dies or becomes incompetent, the POA generally becomes ineffective and the agent loses authority.

## Durable power of attorney (DPOA)

A *durable power of attorney (DPOA)* allows the grant of authority to continue even if the principal is incapacitated. A *springing* DPOA only takes effect when the principal becomes incompetent.

Patients, especially those with progressive cognitive impairment, should be encouraged, if their circumstances allow, to complete a DPOA for their financial affairs.

## Incompetent patients

Incompetent patients cannot name DPOAs. Circumstances may require an adversarial court proceeding to establish guardianship.

## Testamentary capacity

*Testamentary capacity* refers to the ability to make or change a will.

# Making medical decisions

Two cornerstone ethical principals guide medical decision-making. The first is that reverence for human beings must never be compromised; the second is that every person has a right to say, "Keep your hands off of me" (see Box 27.1). These two principles occasionally collide.

Far more commonly, difficulties arise in the care of a patient who has lost the ability to accept or to refuse a burdensome but potentially life-sustaining treatment.

### Glossary

Warning! None of the terms below has a universally accepted meaning. In general, there is a connotation that the decisions involve life-sustaining treatment (LST).

*Advanced directives:* Directives, especially when legally documented, given by a competent patient to guide medical care in a future when the patient has become incapacitated. These may be living will–type directives or designation of heath-care agents.

*Advanced care planning:* Plans made by (advance directives) or on behalf of (when capacity is already lost) patients in the event of future severe illness.

*Substitute decision makers (SDMs):* The SDM may be authorized to make medical decisions because he or she has been designated (health-care agent) or by default, because he or she is the logical (next of kin) person to help decide.

Jurisdictions vary greatly in how these SDMs are named and what authority is granted to them.

*Health-care agent:* Durable power of attorney for health care. A common term for a designated SDM.

*Surrogate/proxy:* There is no consensus in the meaning of these terms. In some states, *proxy* refers to a designated SDM and *surrogate* to a default SDM. In other states, the opposite is true. In some states, all SDMs are called by one of these names.

*Futile:* Operationalized, a physician calls a treatment "futile" when he or she plans to withhold that treatment despite a patient or family request that it be administered.

Legal and ethical definitions vary tremendously. In Texas a treatment is futile when a committee says it is. In Maryland, treatment is futile if "to a reasonable degree of medical certainty… [it] … will not prevent the impending death of the patient."

*Substituted judgment:* The SDM tries to convey what a patient would have wanted if the patient were still able to decide.

*Best interest:* The SDM decides what is best for the patient without appealing to a substituted judgment.

***Living will:*** A document where a patient with capacity specifies certain situations in which he or she would like to refuse LST. These directives are generally very limited. In more places, they are only enforced by statute if a "qualifying condition (QC)" is present. Terminal illness is the most common QC. Persistent vegetative state is a QC in about half of states. A few states have additional QCs such as advanced dementia.

***Health-care agent:*** The designation of a specific SDM. There are few or no restrictions on an agent's authority. In some states the distinction between a designated SDM and one who is acting by default is very important. In other states there is little difference. Some states assume the next of kin will act in ways that benefit the patient, whereas other states do not accept this trust.

## The standard paradigm
- Ask the patient.
- If the patient is incapacitated, seek previously expressed guidance (advanced directives).
  - Living will
  - Health-care agent
- If no advance directives are available seek the appropriate default SDM. (This may vary by jurisdiction, as above.)
  - Most states encourage default SDMs to decide on the basis of substituted judgment when possible.

---

### Box 27.1 Assessment of patient refusing a colectomy for cancer

Miss Joseph has told me she will not consent to a colectomy. She explains that in view of her age and lack of current symptoms she would rather not put herself through a major operation. She said, "I am 89 years old and I don't want to be put through all that." She understands that by refusing surgery she might be shortening her life and that she may become ill in the future as the tumor grows but feels that this is a "lesser evil" than an operation at the moment.

I believe she is making a competent decision and we have agreed to discuss it again in 2 weeks' time during an outpatient appointment after she has spoken to her family.

Dated 12.2.06 Signed

# Making social decisions

Patients with capacity are generally allowed to take risks. (Attempting to reach the summit of Mt. Everest carries a 1%–5% risk of death.)

Patients with marginal or uncertain capacity can be highly problematic. A "sliding scale" of capacity is generally applied; a person wishing to stay in a safe environment will not be scrutinized as closely as one who wishes to live in a risky environment.

State laws vary. If clear, imminent danger is present, some sort of "emergency petition" is usually available. If the situation is more chronically dangerous, some sort of Adult Protective Service is generally available. Many states only deploy this resource on behalf of incapacitated patients.

State laws vary in how they balance the difficult problems of freedom and safety when capacity is uncertain.

Guardianship is a court proceeding, usually cast as adversarial, where the "alleged disabled" patient is a "dependent," and the petitioner is a "plaintiff."

## Further reading

Lowe M, Kerridge IH, McPhee J, et al. (2000). A question of competence. *Age Ageing* **29**: 179–182.

## How to manage a patient insisting on returning home against advice

First assess whether the patient is competent.

- A competent patient should accept that they are at risk and reason that they prefer to take this risk rather than accept other accommodation.
- In borderline or contentious cases a second opinion, often from a geropsychiatrist, can be helpful.

If the patient is **competent**, they cannot be forced to abandon their home or accept outside help, although the health-care team and family can continue to negotiate and persuade.

- It is worth determining what motives lie behind the patient's insistence; sometimes misconceptions can be corrected.
- Patients will sometimes agree to a trial period of residential care or care package, and this often leads to long-term agreement.

When the patient is **incompetent**, there is a duty of care to ensure that the patient is not discharged to an environment where they will be at unreasonable risk (there is no such thing as a "safe" discharge, only a safer one).

- The team should still attempt to accommodate the patient's wishes.
- Disconnection or removal of dangerous items, placement of alarm systems, or regular visits by caregivers or aides, etc. may still allow a patient to return home.

Finally, be sure you record your competency assessment clearly, for example:

"Mr. King has been a patient of mine for over 2 years. He has a progressive dementing illness and concern has been expressed by his son and the aides that he is at risk to himself in continuing to live alone at home. He was admitted to the hospital on this occasion after a small house fire (he left an unattended pan on the stove). He has had three other admissions since Christmas with falls and accidents. Over the last 2 weeks I have had several discussions with him about why his family is concerned about him. The nurses, his son, and his home health aides have also had such discussions.

When I spoke to him today he was disoriented in person and place (believing he was in a police station and that I was a policeman). He expressed a wish to go home to be with his wife (who died 12 years ago) but could not tell me his address. He did not believe that there were any risks involved in going home and did not accept that there was a possibility of falling over again, saying 'I am a very strong man, you would be more likely to fall over than me.' When I discussed the fire he started talking about his war-time experiences and would not accept that there was a risk of fires in the future.

At present I believe that Mr. King is not competent to make a valid decision about his social circumstances. I have no reason to believe that his level of competency will improve with further education or time. A multidisciplinary case conference has been arranged for next week to discuss if it is practical to continue to support him in his own home or whether a residential long-term care placement should be sought."

Dated 12.2.06 Signed

# Cardiopulmonary resuscitation (CPR)

Most CPR is not, in fact, resuscitation or "a return to consciousness, vigor, life." "Successful" CPR is often defined as return of spontaneous circulation (ROSC). *Survival* is defined as survival to hospital discharge.

Characteristics of both the patient and the clinical circumstance affect the likelihood of success and survival with CPR. It is essentially impossible to know, for any individual patient, that a CPR has no chance of success. Beyond this, precise likelihoods probably would not help patients.

For the several thousand patients who died at Memorial Sloan Kettering from 2000 to 2005, over 80% had do not attempt resuscitation (DNAR) orders—also commonly referred to as do not resuscitate (DNR) orders. Most of there were written on the day of death.

Successful CPR is one of the most common causes of persistent vegetative state (along with traumatic brain injury).

CPR occupies a special place in medical ethics because
- Death is virtually certain if a CPR is withheld.
- It is an emergency, so consent is not required.
- It is technologic, dramatic, and, when shown on TV, often successful.

Given that death is certain without CPR, most patients and their SDMs are reluctant to forgo this chance at life.

DNAR orders may lead some providers to think that other forms of care, e.g., admission to intensive care units, should also be limited. Nothing in the DNAR order justifies this.

Both the American College of Surgeons (ACS) and the American Society of Anesthesiologists oppose the automatic suspension of DNAR orders during surgical procedures. The ACS suggests a "required reconsideration" of this order prior to anesthesia and surgery.

### Discussing a CPR with hospitalized patients or substitute decision-makers
- Begin by reassuring the patient or SDM that the questions you will ask are asked of all patients in the hospital or nursing homes. Emphasize, when true, that you have no special reason to believe that cardiac arrest is likely.
- Describe the decision that must be made if the patient suffers cardiac arrest. The choices are to undertake a CPR, or not to undertake a CPR and acknowledge that the patient has died a peaceful death.
- Many patients will be able to answer this question immediately, and most of them will want "everything" done.
- For patients who are unsure, describe the process, burdens, and general prognosis of a CPR in a fair way.
- Regardless of the decision, reassure your patient that all patients are asked this question. If it is true, tell the patient that you respect the decision.

# Elder abuse and neglect

Definitions of elder abuse and neglect are highly variable and imprecise. Some definitions in state law require that the older person must lack capacity to make decisions about the abusive relationship. In others, the older person must be vulnerable in any unspecified way. *Domestic abuse* is defined as mistreatment by someone in a familial or other special relationship with the older person that occurs in a domicile.

In 2002, the WHO proposed a broad definition: "a single or repeated act, or lack of appropriate action, occurring within any relationship where there is an expectation of trust, which causes harm or distress to an older person"

This definition potentially infantilizes older people; it is vague enough that older couples who argue vigorously are mutual abusers, for example, and any adult child who loses their temper with a parent over age 65 is abusive of that parent. The definition of *neglect* is similarly troubling, especially because charges of neglect are often made against those who have no legal duty to provide care to the older adult.

Most older people are fully responsible, participating members in interconnected human ecosystems. They love and are loved, harm and cause harm, support and are supported, some bully and are bullied, all to a greater or lesser extent. The threshold for when legal action should be considered is a very delicate question.

Both the U.S. Preventative Services Task Force in 2004 and the Canadian Task Force on the Periodic Health Examination in 1994 found no evidence that screening or case finding for elder mistreatment leads to any benefit. In fact, considerable harm can result when a physician reports a family member to legal authorities because of suspected abuse of an older person.

Advocacy groups work toward greater education about and recognition of elder abuse, and toward more vigorous reporting and treatment, without evidence of benefit. Despite the lack of a serviceable definition or evidence of benefit from screening, case finding, reporting, or treatment, many states have enacted statutes that establish mandatory reporting of even the suspicion of elder abuse.

In 2008 the American Medical Association (AMA) issued a report on elder mistreatment with nine recommendations. The eighth recommends that definitions and outcome measures be developed.

That said, clinicians must be sensitive to the possibility that a patient is being mistreated. Poverty, cognitive impairment, physical frailty and dependence, and, paradoxically, the accumulation of assets that might be bequeathed to descendants if not spent may make older people particularly vulnerable to abuse and neglect. Harm to vulnerable patients should be addressed vigorously, and selection among the many available tools should be made carefully.

Far more commonly, difficult choices in constrained circumstances are made imperfectly by and on behalf of vulnerable patients. Family members must often make the best of bad circumstances, and the fact that some of the family members are old is only one consideration.

Clinicians in these circumstances must balance their duty to their patients with their duty to follow laws of their state, however imperfect.

## Considerations in reporting elder abuse

- Know the relevant statutes. In particular:
  - How are abuse and neglect defined?
  - How strong is the duty to report?
  - What might the state's responses be to such a report?
- Is the patient so cognitively impaired as to be unable to judge the relationship or circumstance or to devise a plan for self-protection, such as leaving the relationship?
- Conversely, is the patient willingly engaged in the relationship or circumstance?
- Could the patient leave the relationship or circumstance independently?
- Is the patient worsening the situation in any way that might be modifiable?
- Are interventions available that are likely to improve the life of the patient? (One intervention could be a heightened level of scrutiny by a government agency.)

# Chapter 28

# Financing health care

**F. Michael Gloth, III**

# Overview

Before 1965, most seniors had inadequate health insurance coverage and catastrophic illness left many people severely impoverished. In 1965 the U.S. government enacted federal legislation to provide health insurance for the old, disabled, and poor. Today the Medicare and Medicaid programs that grew from that legislation cover the majority of healthcare expenditure for adults age 65 and over. In fact, Social Security and Medicare programs comprise over 40% of the U.S. federal budget.

Medicare is part of the Centers for Medicare and Medicaid Services (CMS). Eligible beneficiaries are individuals who (1) are over age 65, (2) are under age 65 with certain disabilities, and (3) have end-stage renal disease requiring dialysis or kidney transplant.

While originally designed to cover costs for hospitalization (Medicare Part A), Medicare has expanded to include physician office visits, house calls, hospice, and early post-hospital institutional care, among other services (Medicare Part B); specific insurance programs designed to provide comprehensive coverage (Medicare Part C); and prescriptions drug coverage (Medicare Part D). Note that Medicare does not include long-term nursing home care. Additional information about Medicare benefits is available at http://www.ssa.gov/pubs/10043.html.

Medicaid is a joint federal–state run program that provides health care and hospital insurance for low-income individuals. Eligibility differs by state. Medicaid typically covers nursing home long-term care for eligible seniors who meet financial qualifications.

In 2004, $1.5 trillion was spent for personal health care in the United States. About a third of that was spent by seniors 65 years of age and older. Hospitalization accounted for 37% of health-care expenditures by seniors. Another 20% went to physician and clinical services, 17% to nursing home care, 10% to prescription drug costs, and 4% to home health. Dental services, durable medical equipment, other nondurable medical products, and other personal health-care items each accounted for an additional 2%–3% of spending.

Table 28.1 shows the breakdown of health-care expenditures for seniors in the United States.

**Table 28.1** Sources of personal health-care financing for Medicare population, 2000

| Funding source | Percent funded |
|---|---|
| Medicare | 52.3 |
| Medicaid | 12.2 |
| Supplemental Medigap | 12.2 |
| Out of pocket | 19.4 |
| Other | 3.9 |

# Medicare benefits

### Medicare Part A: hospital insurance
- Financed through payroll taxes paid by an individual or spouse while working. A small percentage of individuals pay for this premium after retirement.
- After an individual pays the deductible, Medicare
  - Covers inpatient care in hospitals, including critical access hospitals, and skilled nursing facilities (not custodial or long-term care).
  - Covers hospice care and some home health care for beneficiaries that meet certain criteria.

### Medicare Part B: medical insurance
- Most individuals pay a monthly premium for Part B.
- After an individual pays the deductible, the benefit covers the following services:
  - Physicians' professional services and outpatient care
  - Portion of medical services that Part A does not cover, such as physical and occupational therapists, and home health care
  - Portion of some medical supplies when medically necessary

### Medicare Part C: Medicare advantage
- Eligible for those with Part A and B and includes the following:
  - Medicare managed care, preferred provider organizations (PPO), Medicare private fee-for-service (FFS) plans and Medicare specialty plans
  - Medigap supplemental insurance (see below) is unnecessary since benefits are typically covered under Medicare Advantage.

### Medicare Part D: prescription drug coverage
- Medicare prescription drug coverage is an insurance program available to all Medicare beneficiaries.
- Most individuals who are eligible choose to pay a monthly premium for this benefit, which started January 1, 2006.
- Beneficiaries choose a drug plan offered by one of a number of private companies offering this coverage. Beneficiaries then pay a monthly premium.
- If a beneficiary decides not to enroll in a drug plan when they are first eligible, they may join later, but pay a penalty.

### Medigap
- Supplemental insurance provided by private carriers that cover "gaps" in Medicare Part A and B benefits, i.e., deductible and co-pays not covered by Medicare which typically are the responsibility of the Medicare beneficiary.

## Program for all-inclusive care of the elderly (PACE)

This program is available in some locales whereby a health-care organization contracts with CMS and the state Medicaid agency to provide comprehensive health care services for nursing home–eligible individuals who remain at home and come to a daycare program during the week. Care is provided by an interdisciplinary team.

## Hospice

See Hospice section in Chapter 26, Palliative care and end of life.

# Medicaid

- This is available only to certain low-income individuals and families who fit into an eligibility group that is recognized by federal and state law.
- Medicaid is a state-administered program and each state sets its own guidelines regarding eligibility and services.
- Some states require the subscriber to pay a small part of the cost (co-payment) for some medical services.

There are special rules for those who live in nursing homes. Each state sets criteria for eligibility. Asset assessment is also somewhat detailed, with a limitation on transfers to beyond 5 years from the time of application for Medicaid (more information on this is available online at http://www.cms. hhs.gov/DeficitReductionAct/Downloads/TOAbackgrounder.pdf).

## Veterans Affairs (VA) system

Health-care benefit is available primarily to those who actively serviced in the U.S. Army, Navy, Marines, or Coast Guard.

Multiple health-care benefits are available in various settings (for more details go to http://www.va.gov/healtheligibility/coveredservices/).

### Home and community-based long-term care

- Community residential care
- Geriatric research education and clinical centers (GRECCs)
- Geriatric evaluation and management
- Geriatric primary care
- VA nursing home care
- Inpatient respite
- Contract community nursing home
- State Veteran Homes Program

# Physician billing

Physicians have the option of (1) participating in the Medicare FFS program, (2) not participating in the Medicare FFS program, or (3) entering into a private contract with older patients and forgoing payment by Medicare or Medigap insurance, i.e., opting out.

Physicians participating in Medicare FFS submit claims for professional fees to a Part B insurance carrier and agree to accept the Medicare fee for service, which is 80% of a pre-established allowed amount. The patient or the patient's secondary insurer (Medigap) is billed for the remaining 20% of the allowable fee.

Physicians who do not participate in the Medicare program can bill patients directly for no more than 15% above 95% of the Medicare allowed fee for service. A third option is to opt out of Medicare and bill patients directly. Physicians who opt out of Medicare agree not to re-enter the Medicare payment system for 2 years.

For more information regarding Medicare services and billing see the *Medicare Physician Guide: A Resource for Residents, Physicians and Other Health Care Professions* (2008), which can be downloaded from the Center for Medicare and Medicaid Services (CMS) Web site at http://www.cms.hhs.gov/.

# Dental and oral health

Janet Yellowitz

# Overview

Dental and oral diseases are not a normal consequence of aging. With the exception of subtle changes in tooth structure and reduced salivary reserve, the healthy aging mouth is not unusually prone to dental and oral problems. Nevertheless, many older adults are at increased risk for tooth and gum disease, oral cancer, and oral complications related to medications and comorbid illness. Furthermore, older adults tend to present with more advanced dental and oral pathology.

Various factors contribute to this:

• Increased prevalence of cognitive or physical impairments that limit brushing and flossing
• Presence of more dental restorations that are older and susceptible to decay
• Less oral pain with tooth and gum infection

As with younger adults, annual professional oral examinations are recommended for all, and regular assistance with oral hygiene is needed for those individuals requiring it.

# The older mouth

## Mouth
- Mucosa is thinner and more friable, rarely a functional problem.
- Tooth loss is not normal and fewer older adults are edentulous.
- Salivary glands do not produce less saliva, but causes of xerostomia are more frequent with increasing age.
- Bone resorption occurs in the mandible with osteoporosis. This is accelerated with periodontitis and progresses fast once teeth are lost, leading to a change in facial appearance.
- Orofacial muscle tone can also diminish, with consequent drooling.

## Mouth examination
Use gloves. Be systematic. Check the following:
- *Parotid glands* (enlarged in parotitis, alcoholism, CLL)
- *Temporomandibular joint* (arthritis causes crepitus, subluxation, pain). Dislocation can cause pain and an inability to close the mouth.
- *Soft tissues*: The tongue and floor of the mouth are the most common sites for oral cancer. Smokers and alcoholics have a greater risk of having oral cancer. Angular stomatitis
- *Salivation*
- *Teeth*: How many are missing, what is the condition of the teeth, gums and restorations how much pain or sensitivity is there? Caries are increased by poor brushing and low fluoride exposure, diet of soft sweet foods, xerostomia, poor-fitting dentures, and infrequent dentist visits.
- *Dentures*: Check for cleanliness, integrity, and fit. Friction from loose dentures may produce a fold of fibrous tissue at the junction of the gums and inner cheek (epulis fissuratum; see Plates 7a and 7b).

## Interventions
- Caregiver or nursing help with dental and mouth care is vital for anyone unable to help themselves.
- Dental checkups should continue every 6 months regardless of age or disability.
- Consider chlorhexidine mouthwash in addition to mouth care twice a day for patients with poor oral self-care, e.g., with stroke, dementia.
- Severe periodontal disease may require antibiotics (topical or systemic) and surgical debridement to arrest progress.
- Poor oral and dental health contributes to poor appetite, malnutrition and systemic diseases. The patient may require nutritional support in severe cases of malnutrition.
- Poor oral health is directly related to fevers and aspiration pneumonia.

## Taste
Olfactory function and, hence, taste discrimination decrease gradually with normal aging. Many medications can alter taste, and oral lichen planus is associated with a metallic taste.

## Facial pain

Dental and oral disease accounts for most cases. However, consider trigeminal neuralgia, temporal arteritis, parotitis, temporomandibular joint arthritis, radiation of angina pectoris, migraines, or subacute thyroiditis.

## Sore tongue

This can be a side effect of drugs, glossitis ($B_{12}$, iron, or folate deficiency), candida/thrush, especially with antibiotic or steroid use or in diabetes, or idiopathic "burning mouth syndrome."

## Parotitis

Acute bacterial parotitis is not uncommon in frail older patients who are not eating (e.g., postoperative). Low salivary flow (dehydration) and poor oral hygiene predispose to parotitis with mouth flora (staphylococci and anaerobes). Correct volume depletion and treat with intravenous antibiotics and chlorhexidine mouth rinses. Response to treatment is usually dramatic. If not, consider abscess formation or MRSA infection.

## Xerostomia

The perception of dry mouth is closely related to salivary flow. Saliva is needed for the following:
- *Taste*: it dissolves food to present to taste buds
- *Swallow*: it helps form food bolus
- *Protection* of teeth and mucosa: it contains antibacterials, buffers, and mucin. Rapid tooth decay is a risk of xerostomia.

Xerostomia is not a normal aging change and should always be investigated. Causes include the following:
- Drugs with anticholinergic side effects (e.g., tricyclic antidepressants, anti-Parkinson's agents).
- Sjögren's syndrome (an autoimmune destruction of salivary glands) can be primary or associated with other autoimmune conditions.
- Irradiation, salivary stones, tumors, siladenitis (viral or bacterial infections)
- Treatments depend on the cause; stop or decrease causative drugs, stimulate saliva with grapefruit juice or sugar-free sweets or mints, and promote frequent, careful mouth care. Keep the mouth moist with frequent sips of water. Artificial saliva can provide symptomatic relief for some patients but does not protect against caries.

## Oral manifestation of systemic diseases and drug reactions

There is a very long list including common and general diseases (e.g., oral candidiasis in immunosuppression) as well as rare and specific (e.g., oral lichen planus) ones. Remember that many drugs also affect the mouth, e.g., xerostomia (see above), tardive dyskinesia with antipsychotics, and gum hypertrophy with phenytoin.

## Systemic manifestation of dental diseases

Poor oral hygiene with dental or periodontal disease can cause septicemia, aspiration pneumonia or infective endocarditis. Poor dental health can contribute to poor nutrition.

# Diseases of the gingiva and teeth

### Periodontal disease

This includes gingivitis and periodontitis. Periodontal disease occurs when bacterial plaque is allowed to build up at the margin of the gingiva and base of the tooth. Chronic infection and inflammation results in loosening of the connective ligament anchoring the tooth to the bone, causing teeth to become loose. Gums are tender, appear shiny, swollen, bright red or red-purple, and bleed easily. Halitosis is common.

Calcification of plaque becomes visible, hard tartar (calculus) at the base of the teeth. Acute necrotizing ulcerative gingivitis (ANUG) occasionally develops, which is associated with stress, poor oral hygiene, and tobacco and alcohol use. This presents with fetid halitosis and sometimes systemic symptoms of fever and malaise.

Regular professional cleaning prevents disease, but surgery may be necessary to treat extensive periodontal disease. Meticulous home care is necessary after professional cleaning to limit further destruction. Bleeding and tenderness should resolve within 1 or 2 weeks of treatment. Possible complications include facial cellulitis, osteomyelitis, and, tooth loss.

### Dental caries

Tooth decay or caries result when normal oral flora convert food sugars into acids, which dissolve the hard tooth structure (enamel and cementum). It begins painlessly, but when not treated will eventually penetrate to the tooth pulp, which becomes infected. Pain results (after consuming sweet, hot, or cold foods or drinks) and ultimately the tooth is destroyed. Older adults are particularly susceptible to root caries and caries around existing restorations.

Treatment is dependent on the extent of the disease. For shallow decay not involving the pulp, removing the softened hard material and sealing the cavity suffices. For pulp infection and apical abscess, removal of the canal pulp (root canal therapy) and sterilizing and filling the canal with inert material are necessary. When the tooth is irreparably destroyed or very few functional teeth remain or in very frail patients, tooth extraction is sometimes the only practical treatment.

### Tooth abscess

Periapical (pulp) abscess (see Plate 8) follows bacterial infection of the tooth pulp, which contains the neurovascular supply of the tooth. This is due to either caries or trauma. It results in swelling at the apex of the tooth. Infection can spread to and destroy the bone around the infected tooth.

Severe pain, bitter taste, swollen glands, and fever may be present. Biting on the infected tooth will increase the pain. Pain may be minimal or absent in patients with diabetes mellitus or on steroids. Antibiotics are used for infection.

Warm salt-water rinses may be soothing. Over-the-counter pain relievers may reduce pain and fever. A root canal treatment and surgical drainage of the abscess may restore the tooth or it may need to be extracted. Prompt treatment usually cures the infection, but if left untreated it can lead to facial cellulitis, Ludwig's angina, or osteomyelitis of the jaw. It could also result in brain abscess, endocarditis, pneumonia, mediastinitis, and sepsis.

# Oral soft tissue diseases

### Leukoplakia and mixed erythroleukoplakia

White and white-red mixed plaques can be precancerous lesions (see Plate 9). They are often a response to chronic irritation (e.g., rough teeth, denture surface, or restorations) and from smoking or other tobacco use. Pipe users are at high risk, as are those who hold chewing tobacco or snuff in the mouth.

Leukoplakia and erythroleukoplakia usually appear on the tongue or the insides of the cheek. Patches may be white, gray, or red or mixed; they are usually slightly raised with a hardened surface. They may become rough in texture and sensitive to touch, heat, spicy foods, or other irritation. They usually develop slowly, over weeks to months.

Refer patient to a dentist for evaluation and biopsy lesions resembling leukoplakia and erythroplakia. The goal of treatment is to eliminate the lesion. Removal of the source of irritation may lead to disappearance, though surgical removal of the lesion may be necessary.

Approximately 3% of leukoplakia lesions develop cancerous changes. However, mixed erythroleukoplakia has a much higher likelihood of revealing cancer on biopsy.

### Oral cancer

Most cases are squamous cell carcinoma, which can spread rapidly (see Plate 10). Mean age of diagnosis is 63 years. Smoking and other tobacco use are associated with 70%–80% of oral cancer cases. Smoke and heat from cigarettes, cigars, and pipes irritate the mucous membranes of the mouth. Heavy alcohol use, old age, and prolonged sun exposure (i.e., lips) are other high-risk factors. Some cases begin as leukoplakia or mouth ulcers.

Oral cancer most commonly involves the lips or tongue, but also the floor of the mouth, cheek lining, and gingiva. It can appear red, white, or red and white (see Leukoplakia, above). It is usually painless at first but can be painful if it ulcerates or invades local nerves. Additional symptoms include pain with swallowing or swollen lymph nodes. An oral examination reveals a visible or palpable lesion of the lip, tongue, buccal mucosa, or lymph nodes. Dysarthria, chewing problems, or swallowing difficulties may develop.

Early biopsy is needed for all suspicious lesions.

#### Treatment

Treatment includes surgical excision, radiation therapy, and chemotherapy. Approximately 50% of people with oral cancer live more than 5 years after diagnosis and treatment. When detected early, the cure rate is nearly 75%. Most cases spread to the throat or neck.

Complications of radiation therapy include dry mouth and difficulty swallowing or metastasis of the cancer. Refer patient to a dentist for leukoplakia or for an ulcer that does not resolve within 2 weeks. Annual comprehensive oral examination is the recommended preventive approach.

## Oral candidiasis

This may manifest as oral thrush (removable white plaques on erythematous base), angular stomatitis (sore cracks in corner of the mouth), or, rarely, hyperplastic or atrophic forms (see Plate 11). It can be reversed when possible risk factors such as antibiotics steroids are removed or hyperglycemia and immunosuppression are corrected.

Use nystatin and have the patient rinse it around in the mouth for several minutes. In cases with painful swallowing or dysphagia (i.e., that might have esophageal involvement) and those who cannot comply with rinses, use oral fluconazole 50–100 mg for 7–14 days. Dentures should be kept out each day when possible and soaked in chlorhexidine during treatment.

## Mouth ulcers

Simple apthous ulcers and ulcers due to poorly fitting dentures should be treated with topical anti-inflammatory agents (salicylate gel or triamcinolone). Ulcers can occur as part or the first manifestation of systemic disease such as Beçhet's syndrome, leukemia, lymphoma, fungal infection, tuberculosis, or inflammatory bowel disease. Any oral lesion persisting more than 3 weeks merits referral and/or biopsy to exclude cancer, but most early-staged mouth cancers are painless.

## Lichen planus

This is an idiopathic disorder of the skin and mucous membranes, although it is associated with a large number of medications. Oral lesions may appear as white striae (see Plate 12) or occasionally lead to oral mucosal ulcerations or erosive gingivitis.

- It may be asymptomatic. However, it can also produce a metallic taste or painful, burning lesions.
- A preliminary diagnosis may be made on the basis of appearance of the lesion (see Plate 12). A biopsy of a mouth lesion can confirm the diagnosis.
- Mild symptoms may not require treatment. Antihistamines, lidocaine mouth washes, and topical, intralesional, or oral corticosteroids can reduce inflammation and suppress symptoms.
- Generally, lichen planus is not harmful and usually clears within 18 months.
- Long-standing mouth ulcers may develop into oral cancer.

## Further reading

Little JW, et al. (eds.) (2008). *Dental Management of the Medically Compromised Patient*, 7th ed. St. Louis: Mosby.

# The older driver

**Peter M. Abadir**
**Carlos Weiss**

# Key facts

- Older drivers constitute the fastest-growing segment of the driving population.
- In 2000, older adults constituted 13% of the total U.S. population but suffered 18% of all traffic fatalities.
- Car accidents are the leading cause of injury-related death for 65- to 74-year olds. They are the second cause after falls for 75- to 84-year-olds.
- While older drivers have the lowest collision rates per 100,000 of the U.S. population, when driving mileage is taken into account, the fatality rate for drivers 85 years and older is 9 times higher than the rate for drivers 25 to 69 years old.

New problems with driving can be the first sign of medical illness and should trigger a comprehensive evaluation. Among older drivers, accidents are usually caused by decline in more than one area of function, in contrast to younger drivers.

Older adults think of driving with a value that ranges from unimportant at the low end to being intertwined with a sense of self-worth and quality of life at the high end. This makes it important to do the following:

1. Affirm, when appropriate, that your primary responsibility is to your patient. This means that if the person places a very high value on driving you will help try to make it safe.
2. Clarify that your goal is to make an objective medical assessment, and to identify and treat medical conditions that lessen the ability to drive safely.
3. Acknowledge that you share a responsibility to society to prevent unnecessary accidents.

The most challenging situations occur with people who place a high value on driving yet have poor insight into poor driving performance. For information on the special case of a patient with dementia driving, see How to manage the driver who has dementia, in Chapter 9 (p. 195).

# Risk assessment

During patient encounters be alert for the following "red flags":

- Acute events: counsel prior to discharge for MI, stroke or brain injury, syncope or vertigo, seizures, surgery, or delirium
- Patient's or family member's concerns
- Chronic medical illness that may affect function
- Medical conditions with unpredictable or episodic events
- Medications, especially those affecting CNS or motor function (see next section, Examination)
- Review of systems can reveal symptoms or conditions that impair driving performance (e.g., weakness, dizziness, palpitations, joint pain or stiffness)
- New medication or change; new condition or change: address the effect on driving in assessment and plan for treatment

The following medications have a strong potential to affect the patient's driving performance:

- Anticholinergics
- Anticonvulsants
- Antidepressants
- Antiemetics
- Antihistamines
- Antihypertensives
- Antiparkinsonians
- Antipsychotics
- Benzodiazepenes and other sedatives or anxiolytics
- Muscle relaxants
- Narcotic analgesics
- Stimulants

*Source:* AMA Physician's Guide to Assessing and Counseling Older Drivers, used with permission.

**Always remember:** Physicians should warn patients about the effects of medications on driving and document that they did so.

## How to take a focused history to identify risky driving

| Ask the patient | Ask the family |
| --- | --- |
| 1. Have you noticed any change in your driving skills? | 1. Do you feel uncomfortable in any way driving with the patient? |
| 2. Do others honk at you or show signs of irritation? | 2. Have you noted any abnormal or unsafe driving behavior? |
| 3. Have you lost any confidence in your overall driving ability, leading you to drive less often or only in good weather? | 3. Has the patient had any recent crashes? |
| 4. Have you ever become lost while driving? | 4. Has the patient had near-misses that could be attributed to mental or physical decline? |
| 5. Have you ever forgotten where you were going? | 5. Has the patient received any tickets or traffic violations? |
| 6. Do you think that at present you are an unsafe driver? | 6. Are other drivers forced to drive defensively to accommodate the patient's errors in judgment? |
| 7. Have you had any car accidents in the last year? | 7. Have there been any occasions where the patient has gotten lost or experienced navigational confusion? |
| 8. Any minor fender-benders with other cars in parking lots? | 8. Does the person need many cues or directions from passengers? |
| 9. Have you received any traffic citations for speeding, going too slow, improper turns, failure to stop, etc.? | 9. Does the patient need a co-pilot to alert them of potentially hazardous events or conditions? |
| 10. Have others criticized your driving or refused to drive with you? | 10. Have others commented on the patient's unsafe driving? |

*Source:* The Dementia Network of Ottawa-Carleton and the Regional Geriatric Assessment Program of Ottawa-Carleton (2004). The Driving and Dementia Toolkit,

# Examination

Three key functions for safe driving are (1) vision, (2) cognition, and (3) motor function. Figure 30.1 shows a framework for evaluation of the older driver.

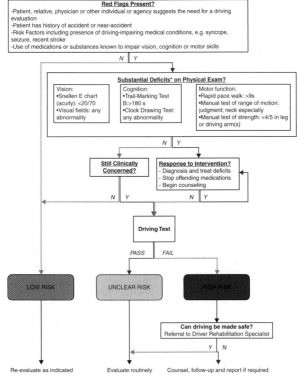

**Fig. 30.1** Suggested framework for evaluation of the older driver.
Exam branch points are based on observational data and expert opinion. Branch points and instructions are based on the *Physician's Guide to Assessing and Counseling Older Drivers*. Available at http://www.ama-assn.org/ama/pub/category/10791.html.

**Remember:** No single test predicts who will be involved in a motor vehicle accident. Clinical judgment that synthesizes findings from the history and exam is always needed and an on-road test of driving is sometimes needed.

# Driver rehabilitation programs

If the patient's functional deficits are not medically correctable, referral to driver rehabilitation specialists can help maximize driver safety. Driver rehabilitation specialists are often occupational therapists with additional training in driver rehabilitation.

Driver rehabilitation programs include three elements:

- Driver evaluation is conducted through clinical interview and assessment followed by on road assessment.
- Passenger vehicle evaluation assesses the client's vehicle in the context of the client's needs as a passenger. It also assists in the selection of adaptive equipment and provides guidance in the professional installation of this equipment.
- Treatment and intervention can include adaptive driving instruction or driver retraining, coordination of vehicle modifications, or recommendation of driving cessation.

**Remember:** Driver assessment and rehabilitation is expensive. Medicare and private insurance companies rarely pay for these services. To find a driver rehabilitation specialist in your area, review the Driver Rehabilitation Specialist Directory at http://www.driver-ed.org.

# Counseling and compensatory strategies

Enabling older drivers to stay on the road safely involves efforts to optimize their baseline health, functional abilities, and driving behaviors. Below is a list of possible compensatory strategies that can be used to maximize optimization of patient's driving behavior.

- Drive only familiar routes.
- Drive at an appropriate speed.
- Avoid night-time driving.
- Avoid distractions such as the radio.
- Avoid busy intersections.
- Don't drive with a distracting companion.
- Avoid expressways and freeways.
- Avoid rush hour traffic.

*Source:* The Dementia Network of Ottawa-Carleton and the Regional Geriatric Assessment Program of Ottawa-Carleton (2004). The Driving and Dementia Toolkit.

**Remember:** Compensatory strategies may not be enough and should be used after performing a full medical evaluation and deeming the patient safe to drive.

### How to tell your patient that he or she is unsafe to drive

In many situations an on-road test is necessary to make a decision about driving safety. When a clinical exam suggests driving is not safe:

- Discuss your concerns with the patient and caregivers before writing a letter and notifying others.
- Make safety the focus and provide alternatives to driving that maximize quality of life.
- Provide a letter explaining why you believe driving may be unsafe, as well as documenting your legal obligations (example is available in AMA Physician's Guide to Assessing and Counseling Older Drivers).
- Follow up with the patient and caregivers to assess for unwillingness to follow recommendations and establishment of alternative transportation.

# Legal and ethical responsibilities of the physician

Remember: In some states, physicians are required to report patients who have specific medical conditions (e.g., epilepsy, dementia) to their state Department of Motor Vehicles (DMV). In states where there are no laws authorizing physicians to report patients to the DMV, physicians must have patient consent to disclose medical information. Physicians should check with their own state's DMV regulations.

## Terms to know

### Reporting liability
Physicians have been held liable for civil damages caused by a patient's car crash when there was a clear failure to report an at-risk driver to the DMV prior to the incident.

### Immunity offered
Several states exempt physicians from liability for civil damages brought by the patient if the physician reported the patient to the DMV beforehand.

### Legal protection from breach of confidentiality
In states where there are no laws authorizing physicians to report patients to the DMV, physicians must have patient consent to disclose medical information. In these states, physicians who disclose medical information without patient consent may be held liable for breach of confidentiality. Nonetheless, this should not dissuade physicians from reporting when it is necessary and justified, as reporting may provide protection from liability for future civil damages.

Reporting requirements for your state:

_____

_____

_____

## Resources
- AMA Physician's Guide to Assessing and Counseling Older Drivers: http://ama-assn.org/ama/pub/category/10791.html
- When You Are Concerned: A Guide for Families, Friends and Caregivers Concerned about the Safety of an Older Driver: http://aging.state.ny.us/caring/concerned/handbook.pdf

## Further reading

Wang CC, Carr DB, for the Older Drivers Project (2004). Older driver safety: a report from the Older Drivers Project. *J Am Geriatr Soc* **52**:143–149.

# Preoperative evaluation

**Colleen Christmas**

## Overview

Advances in surgical, medical, and anesthetic techniques have expanded the surgical options for treating many diseases that are common in older adults. Currently, over half of all surgeries in the United States are performed on people over the age of 65, and the number of surgeries performed in older adults is expected to grow dramatically in the coming decade. Still, the majority of postoperative complications and deaths occur in the older age groups. Therefore, a cautious and comprehensive approach to the perioperative care of older adults is always warranted.

## Should this patient have surgery?

### Age, function, and physiology

Age alone should not be the sole determinant of whether to perform a surgical procedure. Most studies demonstrate that functional and physiological status is a more reliable predictor of adverse postoperative complications than chronological age.

### Likelihood of benefit

Understand the expected outcome of the planned surgery and consider what benefit the patient is expected to achieve. For example, surgery to repair an acute hip fracture is expected to restore ambulation or ability to weight bear and transfer for a patient who was functioning at this level before the trauma. However, a nursing home patient with severe dementia who does not weight bear may have little to gain from an operative repair. Healing in place may be a better option for this patient.

Clearly, all medical decisions involve considerations of the relative merits and risks of reasonable alternative approaches to treatments.

# Should this patient have surgery now?

### Emergent surgery

Surgical therapy for true emergencies (assuming that surgery is consistent with the patient's goals) must not be delayed. Less emergent, but still urgent conditions, such as repair of a hip fracture, should be not be delayed unnecessarily for preoperative testing that is unlikely to change management (e.g., echocardiogram for patient with benign murmur and no evidence of heart failure.)

In most cases, the sooner the patient can get back on their feet, the less deconditioning and the fewer complications they will experience.

### Less urgent surgery

One should search for and correct unstable medical conditions (e.g., recent myocardial infarction, active heart failure, severe anemia, uncontrolled hypertension, dehydration or electrolyte abnormalities, severe depression, and acute infection) before proceeding.

In some cases it is wise to delay surgery in order to allow the patient to undergo "prehab" to increase strength and fitness (e.g., before knee replacement). However, practice of delaying surgery for cancer treatments in order to give a patient time to gain weight has no scientific support.

# Preoperative medication review

Review all prescription and non-prescription medications during the preoperative assessment and ensure that each is indicated and effective. Most medications that are necessary for management of chronic conditions will be continued through surgery and the immediate perioperative period. Remember, however, that the risk of postoperative delirium increases with the number of medications used.

Review all chronic conditions and ensure that each is optimally managed (e.g., heart failure, COPD).

## Advice regarding specific medications

### Aspirin and antiplatelet drugs

Surgeons may prefer to stop these for some types of procedures (e.g., prostate and brain surgery) or where excessive bleeding is expected. For most surgeries stopping these medications is unnecessary.

When a coronary stent has been in place less than 6 months or there has been a myocardial infarction in the previous 3 months, it is preferable to delay surgery, if possible, rather than stop antiplatelets prematurely.

### Warfarin and injectable heparins

These agents should be held for most surgeries. Warfarin is usually held for 5 doses before the surgery and resumed the night after the procedure when used to prevent thrombosis in a patient with atrial fibrillation.

However "bridging heparin" therapy is indicated for specific circumstances: patients with artificial heart valves, particularly in the mitral position, recent embolic stroke, recent pulmonary embolus, or a known cardiac thrombus. IV heparin or subcutaneous low-molecular-weight heparin is started once the INR falls below the therapeutic range. The IV heparin or subcutaneous heparin is discontinued just before surgery and resumed immediately postoperatively.

The warfarin is restarted postoperatively and the heparin is continued until the INR is again therapeutic. Spinal epidural anesthesia is avoided in patients on heparin therapy.

### Benzodiazepines

These are best avoided in older patients. However, those who take these chronically are at risk for withdrawal symptoms and delirium if stopped. Therefore, continue benzodiazepines through surgery and the postoperative period.

### Insulin and oral hypoglycemics

Patients with type 1 DM need half of their regular dose of insulin the morning of surgery while receiving D5 NS infusion while NPO. Patients with type 2 DM need half or less of their usual hypoglycemic medications the day of surgery. This must be individualized on the basis of chronic dose and the anticipated duration of NPO.

Hypoglycemics are resumed once the patient is eating. Generally, this means giving half or less of morning oral hypoglycemics if only one meal will be missed or holding hypoglycemics altogether if two or more meals will be missed.

Metformin can cause lactic acidosis during times of severe systemic stress so should be discontinued the morning of surgery and is resumed when the patient is eating, afebrile, and hemodynamically stable.

### Acetylcholinesterase inhibitor

These include, e.g., donepezil, riaistigmine, and galantamine. They should be stopped if general anesthesia is planned, since these drugs can prolong the effects.

### Bisphosphonates

There is no urgency to resuming these. Hold until the patient is able to stay upright for 30 minutes after taking with a full glass of water.

### Estrogens

Because of their association with deep venous thrombosis, it is best to hold starting 4 weeks before the surgery and through the postoperative period until the patient is ambulatory.

### Seizure medications

These should be continued without interruption. If the patient will need to miss a dose or more from being NPO, seizure medications should be administered by intravenous infusion.

## Drugs to start or increase

### Infective endocarditis prophylaxis

The American Heart Association recommends antibiotic prophylaxis for specific cardiac conditions associated with the highest risk of infective endocarditis.[1] These conditions are (1) prosthetic cardiac valve and prosthetic material used to repair cardiac valve, (2) previous infective endocarditis, (3) congenital heart disease with specific conditions, and (4) cardiac transplantation recipients who develop valvulopathy. Note that for conditions such as aortic valve stenosis and mitral valve insufficiency, conditions that are common in older adults, antibiotic prophylaxis is no longer recommended.

For patients at highest risk, all dental procedures that involve manipulation of gingival tissue or the periapical region of the teeth or penetration of the oral mucosa should receive antibiotic prophylaxis. Antibiotic prophylaxis should also be provded for respiratory tract procedures with incision or biopsy of the respiratory mucosa.

Antibiotic prophylaxis may be indicated when there is incision of infected skin or bone. Antibiotic prophylaxis solely for genitourinary and gastrointestinal procedures is not recommended.

Perioperative antibiotics have been demonstrated to reduce postoperative wound infections associated with orthopedic and gastrointestinal procedures.

**1.** Wilson W, Taubert KA, Gewitz M, et al. (2007). Prevention of infective endocarditis. Guidelines from the American Heart Association. *Circulation* **116**:1736–1754.

*Prevention of venous thrombosis and pulmonary embolism*

Hospitalization and immobilization increases the risk for deep venous thrombosis (DVT) and pulmonary emboli, especially in high-risk patients (e.g., with obesity, cancer, previous DVT, age >65). DVT prophylaxis will be warranted according to the guidelines published by the American College of Chest Physicians.[2]

All geriatric patients are considered high risk, so they should receive DVT prophylaxis with either subcutaneous unfractionated heparin three times daily or low-molecular-weight heparin once daily. Mechanical devices may be added to this regimen for very high-risk patients or very high-risk surgeries.

*Beta-blocker therapy*

Patients taking beta-blocker for treatment of angina, arrhythmia, or hypertension or who are at high risk for myocardial ischemia should continue taking them through surgery. Unless contraindicated, beta-blocker therapy should be given preoperatively for those at high risk of myocardial ischemia who are undergoing vascular surgery and possibly for those undergoing intermediate-risk procedures (e.g., intra-abdominal surgery).

Prophylactic use of beta-blockers is not indicated in low-risk patients or low-risk procedures. Whether they should be used in patients with only one cardiac risk factor undergoing intermediate-risk surgeries or in patients with no risk factors undergoing a high-risk surgery is not known.

If the patient is not on a beta-blocker, it is ideal to start it several weeks in advance and target the heart rate to 60 bpm and systolic blood pressure >100 mmHg.

Whether aspirin, clonidine, or HMG co-A reductase inhibitors ("statin medications") should be initiated preoperatively to reduce cardiac risks is not well established. However, aspirin has been shown to reduce postoperative cardiac complications when starting within 24 hours after coronary artery bypass grafting (CABG) surgery.

If adrenal insufficiency is known or suspected, give IV hydrocortisone immediately preoperatively and continue for 24 hours postoperatively for minor surgery and 48 hours for major surgeries.

Drug allergies must be communicated to the surgeon and anesthesiologist.

---

2. For specific antibiotics and dosing instructions see The Johns Hopkins Antibiotic Guide at http://www.hopkins-abxguide.org/

# Further reading

1. Fleisher LA, Beckman JA, Brown KA, et al. (2007). ACC/AHA 2007 guidelines on perioperative cardiovascular evaluation and care for noncardiac surgery: a report of the American College of Cardiology/American Heart Association Task Force on Practice Guidelines. *J Am Coll Cardiol* **50**:e159–241.
2. Douketis JD, Berger PB, Dunn AS, et al. (2008). The perioperative management of antithrombotic therapy. American College of Chest Physicians Evidence-Based Clinical Practice Guidelines (8th edition). *Chest* **133** (6 Suppl):299S–339S.

# Reducing perioperative complications

In addition to measures taken for the preoperative medication review, aim to reduce risks of adverse pulmonary events, postoperative infections, deconditioning and pressure ulcers, and postoperative confusion.

## Pulmonary complications

These are most common in patients with underlying lung disease and with surgery closest to the thorax. Mobilize the patient early. To prevent destabilization of chronic obstructive lung disease, implement pulmonary toilet and use of inhaler therapies, and, if necessary, start perioperative steroid therapy.

Postoperative pneumonias are especially dangerous in this age group—recognize and treat them aggressively. Pneumonia is best prevented by deep breathing exercises (with or without incentive spirometry devices), early mobilization, controlling pain to enable deep coughing and clearing of secretions, and reducing risk of delirium, which can lead to aspiration. Perform a careful chest exam daily and obtain a chest X-ray for fever, cough, hypoxia, delirium, or other reason that would lead you to suspect pneumonia. Start appropriate antibiotics early when postoperative pneumonia is suspected.

Reduce aspiration risks by keeping the head of the bed elevated.

Prevent deep venous thrombosis and pulmonary embolism as discussed above (p. 742).

## Postoperative infections

These are reduced by appropriate use of preoperative prophylactic antibiotics if warranted. Remove Foley catheter and all unnecessary intravenous lines as soon as possible.

## Deconditioning and pressure ulcers

The key to prevention is early mobilization and time out of bed. Consult physical and occupational therapists for the patient who needs help with transfer and ADLs. Early attention to maintenance of strength, tone, and range of movement will pay dividends in recovery and reduce the risk of skin breakdown. Patients who are able to safely ambulate should be encouraged to do so.

IV lines act as tethers and inhibit mobility, which is another reason to remove them as soon as possible.

Patients at high risk for pressure ulcers need to be carefully positioned with pillows and pads (see Pressure injuries, Chapter 18, p. 521).

## Postoperative delirium

This prolongs hospitalization, increases the risk of falls and of aspiration in the hospital, delays rehabilitation, and may result in prolonged cognitive impairment. Preoperative review of medication (as noted above), ensuring hydration, anticipation and control of postoperative pain, a quiet room, and relaxing procedures to promote sleep (e.g., massage and soft music) and reorientation are recommended.

Avoid using sleep medications or sedatives (unless the patient habitually uses benzodiazepines). If delirium develops, see Delirium: treatment, in Chapter 9 (p. 206).

# Planning for postoperative care

Anticipate postoperative needs and discuss these with the patient, family, and/or caregiver during the preoperative evaluation. If a prolonged period of disability and rehabilitation is expected, work with the patient and family to plan for contingencies for family and social obligations. (Remember, many older patients are caregivers for a spouse or others.)

Engaging a social worker can be extremely helpful in these situations. It may also help the patient to understand when to reasonably expect transitions in their care, for example, from hospital to inpatient rehabilitation, if appropriate, and what the goals and focus at each stage of treatment will be.

Depending on the nature of the surgery, postoperative follow-up appointments and referrals needed after surgery may be scheduled at the time of the preoperative visit. In addition, education may be provided about ongoing risk factor modification that will be warranted after the surgery. In this way, the patient may be maximally prepared not only for the surgery but also for the events that will likely follow the surgery.

Finally, the preoperative evaluation may be an ideal opportunity to review and update advance directives and ensure that all appropriate documentation is completed.

# Chapter 32

# Preventive medicine

**Rachelle Gajadhar**
**Samuel C. Durso**

# Approach to the older adult

The aim of preventive care is to prevent or mitigate the experience of illness, functional decline, or premature death. These measures encompass a broad range of primary (e.g., immunization, exercise counseling, and warfarin for a patient with atrial fibrillation) and secondary (e.g., breast and colon cancer screening, lipid management in a patient after myocardial infarction) interventions.

Guidelines for implementing preventive care come from many sources with varying degrees of supporting evidence. Few have been tested in adults over age 75 or take into consideration comorbid conditions or functional health status.

Like other clinical decisions, recommendations for preventive care require knowledge of the individual patient and judgment in their application. This is especially true for those older patients who may already be burdened with functional impairments, medical illness, or complex medication regimens. As a result, physicians should exercise caution when recommending preventive guidelines to older adults that are developed for the general adult population.

Preventive measures that impose little burden or risk to patients, such as influenza vaccine, may benefit even the frailest patients and are recommended for nearly all older adults regardless of age or health status. However, procedures such as colorectal or breast cancer screening impose burdens and risks that are proportionally higher for frail older adults and are unlikely to benefit individuals with limited life expectancy.

In all cases, clinicians must consider the patient's preferences when making preventive care recommendation.

## Screening vs. diagnostic testing

When discussing preventive care with patients, it is important to distinguish between prevention (e.g., cancer screening in asymptomatic individuals) and diagnostic testing. This can be confusing to patients.

For example, it is important that a healthy older female with no personal or family history of breast cancer understand that her individual risk of breast cancer is low (10% lifetime cumulative risk) and that most abnormalities found by screening are likely to be benign. This is quite different than the consideration of mammography in an older woman with unexplained weight loss and axillary lymphadenopathy, or the decision to recommend bone densometry in a patient who has fractured his hip.

The following questions can help to frame the discussion of preventive care with patients.

• What are the patient's health-care experiences and preferences?

Patients who have had personal experience (e.g., a family member or themselves) with cancer, heart disease, or stroke may have strong opinions about the value of screening and preventive care.

• Does the person want to know if a problem exists and deal with it proactively, or do they prefer not to worry about the unknown?

Is this a person who will be very troubled by false-positive results? Does the patient have the cognitive capacity to understand complex choices that can result from screening or preventive care?

- Do the short-term risks outweigh the long-term benefit?

For example, is the patient frail and vulnerable to complications of the screening test (e.g., dehydration from preparation for colonoscopy) or from an additional test that might be necessary to resolve false-positive findings (e.g., angiography to evaluate findings from carotid ultrasound)?

- Is there comorbid illness that limits the benefit of detecting or preventing asymptomatic disease?

For example, screening for abdominal aortic aneurysm in a patient with severe COPD might impose such a limit.

- What is the impact of an intervention on absolute risk reduction of morbidity or mortality?

Remember that the relative risk reduction for an intervention may be impressive while the absolute risk reduction may be quite small (e.g., decrease in absolute risk from 2% to 1% over 5 years represents 50% relative risk reduction but only a 1% absolute risk reduction for that period). Some patients will understand and appreciate this type of information when making a decision regarding preventive care.

### Consider average life expectancy (ALE) rather than age alone

When considering preventive care recommendations, remember that older adults are a heterogeneous population and that health status is a better guide to average life expectancy (ALE) than age alone. Figure 32.1 illustrates this; note the wide distribution of ALE for different age cohorts of older women and men. The distribution correlates with functional status and comorbid illness.

For example, individuals in the top 25th percentile for ALE in each age cohort typically enjoy robust health: they have the ability to walk 2 miles or perform heavy gardening, have independence in higher-level functions such as managing personal finances and travel, and lack severe illness. In contrast, those in the lowest 25th percentile are usually dependent in one or more basic activities of daily living (e.g., bathing, dressing, feeding, transferring, etc.) or have an end-stage chronic illness such as oxygen-dependent COPD.

While physicians cannot precisely predict life expectancy for an individual patient, they can make a reasonable estimate of whether a patient is in an upper, middle, or lower quartile of ALE based on functional assessment and the presence or absence of end-stage illness. Physicians should keep this perspective in mind when considering the likelihood of future benefit balanced against risk for a given intervention such as colon or breast cancer screening, or long-term medication for reducing risk of complications from cardiovascular disease, diabetes mellitus, or osteoporosis.

*Example*
Consider two 70-year-old men. Mr. Smith has Parkinson's disease and needs assistance with transferring, bathing, and dressing. Mr. Jones is an avid gardener who can walk 2 miles easily. Mr. Smith is dependent in several ADLs and is probably in the lower quartile of ALE for his age (6.7 years). Mr. Jones exhibits robust health and is probably is in the upper quartile of ALE for his age (18 years).

The average time to benefit from colonoscopy for colorectal cancer screening is approximately 10 years. In addition to risks from the procedure, Mr. Smith is less likely to benefit from colonoscopy than Mr. Jones.

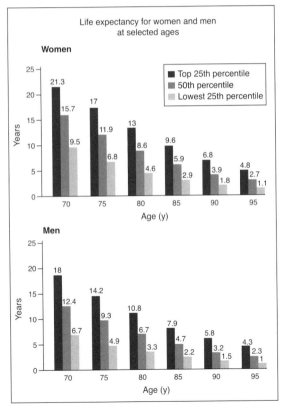

**Fig. 32.1** Life expectancy for women and men at selected ages. Adapted with permission from Walter LC, Covinsky KE (2001). Cancer screening in elderly patients: a framework for individualized decision making. *JAMA* **285**(21):2750–2756.

# Selected preventive care recommendations

Screening for function should be performed at the time of a new evaluation and at least annually thereafter (for the specific elements, see Chapter 3, Clinical assessment of older adults, p. 27). Recommendations for screening and evaluation of falls and unsafe driving are discussed in Chapters 5 and 30.

## Immunizations

### Influenza vaccination

Influenza is associated with 20,000–40,000 excess deaths each year. Older adults are disproportionately affected.

- Recommended for all patients over age 65
- Trivalent inactivated influenza vaccine (TIV)
- Given annually, optimally at beginning of flu season (October to mid-November)
  - Short-lived protection (4–5 months)
- Contraindicated in patients with egg allergy
- May be given concurrently with pneumococcal

### Pneumococcal vaccination

Protection wanes with age and efficacy is uncertain in debilitated older adults, but it is safe and inexpensive, so should be encouraged.

- 23–valence vaccine given at age 65
- Consider repeating every 5 years in those with chronic illness, including immunocompromised status.
- Contraindicated in those with history of allergy to vaccine

### Tetanus vaccination

Older adults who have never received the vaccine are at risk.

- If never vaccinated, administer 2 doses 1–2 months apart, followed by additional booster 6–12 months later
- If previously immunized, administer booster every 10 years
- Contraindicated if neurological or hypersensitivity reaction to previous dose

### Herpes zoster vaccination

Shingles is caused by reactivation of the varicella zoster infection. In the United States the incidence is approximately 0.5–1.0 million cases per year with an individual lifetime risk of 30%. The goal is to decrease shingles episodes and the sequelae, such as postherpetic neuralgia.

- Recommended for all adults >60 years, including those with prior history of herpes zoster infection
- Efficacy of the vaccine decreases with age
- Live attenuated vaccine is contraindicated in immunocompromised patients, including those on chronic steroids
- Requires storage at −20°C
- 0.65 mL dose subcutaneously in the deltoid region of the arm within 30 minutes of thawing the vaccine

## Cancer screening

### Colorectal cancer

- The U.S. Preventive Services Task Force (USPSTF) recommends screening using fecal occult blood testing, sigmoidoscopy, or colonoscopy between age 50 and 75.
- The USPSTF recommends against screening between ages 76 and 85 although individual considerations may justify it.

### Breast cancer

- The USPSTF recommends mammography every 1–2 years for women after age 40.
- The American Geriatrics Society recommends offering screening for women to age 85 who have good health and an estimated life expectancy of 5 or more years.

### Cervical cancer

- The USPSTF recommends against routine screening of women over age 65 who have had adequate screening with a normal Pap smear and are not at high risk for cervical cancer.
- Screening should be considered once in older women who are in good health and have not been previously screened.
- Older women without a cervix do not need a Pap smear.

### Prostate cancer

See Chapter 19, Genitourinary medicine (p. 529).

### Not recommended

Routine screening is not needed for lung, pancreatic, bladder, and ovarian cancer.

## Vascular disease

### Hypertension and lipid screening

The USPSTF recommends screening adults periodically for hypertension and lipid disorders. The value of screening for lipid disorders for the purpose of primary prevention is unclear in older adults. Individual circumstances must be weighed (e.g., presence of diabetes mellitus).

### Aspirin

The USPSTF recommends that physicians discuss the risks and benefits of aspirin therapy with adults who are at high risk for cardiovascular disease. Aspirin prophylaxis may not be justified in adults whose only risk factor for cardiovascular disease is advanced age, when balanced against the risk of gastritis, bleeding, or hemorrhagic stroke.

### Abdominal aortic aneurysm (AAA)

The USPSTF recommends one-time screening for AAA using ultrasonography for men ages 65–75 who have ever smoked. It should be recognized that screening men and repair of AAA that are ≥5.5 cm reduce AAA-related mortality but have not been shown to reduce all-cause mortality. The psychological stress of screening and monitoring small aneurysms and the risks of surgery must be considered on an individual basis.

*Not recommended*
The USPSTF does not recommend screening asymptomatic adults for carotid artery disease or peripheral vascular disease, and it does not recommend screening with electrocardiogram, exercise testing, or coronary artery calcium in adults at low risk of coronary artery disease.

## Miscellaneous
*Smoking and alcohol misuse*
The USPSTF recommends screening and counseling regarding tobacco use and alcohol misuse as well as appropriate interventions to assist patients with smoking cessation and reduction of alcohol misuse.

## Further reading
U.S. Preventive Services Task Force Recommendations: http://www.ahrq.gov/clinic/uspstfix.htm
Walter LC, Covinsky KE (2001). Cancer screening in elderly patients: a framework for individualized decision making. *JAMA* **285**(21):2750–2756.

# Appendix

# Barthel index

### Bowel status

| | |
|---|---|
| 0 | Incontinent |
| 1 | Occasional accident (once a week or less) |
| 2 | Continent |

### Bladder status

| | |
|---|---|
| 0 | Incontinent, or catheterized and unable to manage |
| 1 | Occasional accident (maximum once in 24 hours) |
| 2 | Continent (for more than 7 days) |

### Grooming

| | |
|---|---|
| 0 | Needs help with personal care (face, hands, teeth, shaving) |
| 1 | Independent (with equipment provided) |

### Toilet use

| | |
|---|---|
| 0 | Dependent |
| 1 | Can do some tasks, needs assistance |
| 2 | Independent (on/off, wiping, dressing) |

### Feeding

| | |
|---|---|
| 0 | Dependent |
| 1 | Can do about half, needs help with cutting, etc. |
| 2 | Independent (food within reach) |

### Transfers

| | |
|---|---|
| 0 | Unable (no sitting balance) |
| 1 | Major help (e.g., two people) |
| 2 | Minor help, able to sit (e.g., one person verbal or physical) |
| 3 | Independent |

### Mobility

| | |
|---|---|
| 0 | Immobile |
| 1 | Wheelchair independent |
| 2 | Able to walk with the help of one person |
| 3 | Independent (can use walking aids if necessary) |

### Dressing

| | |
|---|---|
| 0 | Unable |
| 1 | Can do about half unaided, needs some help |
| 2 | Independent |

### Stairs

| | |
|---|---|
| 0 | Unable |
| 1 | Needs some help (including stair lift) |
| 2 | Independent up and down |

### Bathing

| 0 | Dependent |
| 1 | Independent |

TOTAL POSSIBLE SCORE = 20

- Aim to record what the patient actually does in daily life, not what he or she can do (i.e., a poorly motivated but capable patient may score poorly).
- The score reflects the degree of independence from help provided by another person:
  - If supervision is required, the patient is not independent.
  - If aids and devices are used but no help is required, the patient is independent.
- Use the best available evidence, asking the patient or relatives, caregivers, nurses, and therapists, and using common sense. Observing the patient is helpful, but direct testing is not necessary.
- Middle categories imply that the patient supplies over 50% of the effort.
- It is useful to also ask about abilities before hospital admission or acute illness, and to compare both the total Barthel score and elements of it to determine the magnitude and nature of the setback.

# Geriatric depression scale

This scale is suitable as a screening test for depressive symptoms in the elderly. It is ideal for evaluating the clinical severity of depression and, thus, for monitoring treatment. It is easy to administer, needs no prior psychiatric knowledge, and has been well validated in many environments—home and clinical.

The original GDS was a 30-item questionnaire that was time consuming and challenging for some patients (and staff). Later versions retain only the most discriminating questions; their validity approaches that of the original form. The most common version in general geriatric practice is the 15-item questionnaire.

*Instructions*

Undertake the test orally. Ask the patient to reply indicating how they have felt over the past week. Obtain a clear "yes" or "no" reply. If necessary, repeat the question. Each depressive answer (bold) scores 1.

| | | |
|---|---|---|
| 1 | Are you basically satisfied with your life? | YES/**NO** |
| 2 | Have you dropped many of your activities and interests? | **YES**/NO |
| 3 | Do you feel that your life is empty? | **YES**/NO |
| 4 | Do you often get bored? | **YES**/NO |
| 5 | Are you in good spirits most of the time? | YES/**NO** |
| 6 | Are you afraid that something bad is going to happen to you? | **YES**/NO |
| 7 | Do you feel happy most of the time? | YES/**NO** |
| 8 | Do you often feel helpless? | **YES**/NO |
| 9 | Do you prefer to stay at home, rather than going out and doing new things? | **YES**/NO |
| 10 | Do you feel you have more problems with memory than most? | **YES**/NO |
| 11 | Do you think it is wonderful to be alive now? | YES/**NO** |
| 12 | Do you feel pretty worthless the way you are now? | **YES**/NO |
| 13 | Do you feel full of energy? | YES/**NO** |
| 14 | Do you feel that your situation is hopeless? | **YES**/NO |
| 15 | Do you think that most people are better off than you are? | **YES**/NO |

### Scoring intervals

| | |
|---|---|
| 0–4 | No depression |
| 5–10 | Mild depression |
| 11+ | Severe depression |

# Mini-cog and clock drawing

DATE_____ ID_____ AGE_____ GENDER M F LOCATION_____ TESTED BY_____

## MINI-COG ™

1) GET THE PATIENT'S ATTENTION, THEN SAY: "I am going to say three words that I want you to remember now and later. The words are

**Banana     Sunrise     Chair.**

Please say them for me now." (Give the patient 3 tries to repeat the words. If unable after 3 tries, go to next item.)

(Fold this page back at the TWO dotted lines BELOW to make a blank space and cover the memory words. Hand the patient a pencil/pen).

2) SAY ALL THE FOLLOWING PHRASES IN THE ORDER INDICATED: "Please draw a clock in the space below. Start by drawing a large circle." (When this is done, say) "Put all the numbers in the circle." (When done, say) "Now set the hands to show 11:10 (10 past 11)." If subject has not finished clock drawing in 3 minutes, discontinue and ask for recall items.

- - - - - - - - - - - - - - - - - - - - - - - - - - - - - - - - - - - - - - - - - - - - - - - - - - - - - - - - - - - - - -

3) SAY: "What were the three words I asked you to remember?"

(Score 1 point for each) 3-Item Recall Score ☐

Score the clock (see other side for instructions):      Normal clock      2 points
                                                         Abnormal clock   0 points      Clock Score ☐

**Total Score = 3-item recall plus clock score** ☐      *0, 1, or 2 possible impairment; 3, 4, or 5 suggests no impairment*

## CLOCK SCORING

### NORMAL CLOCK

A NORMAL CLOCK HAS ALL OF THE FOLLOWING ELEMENTS:
All numbers 1-12, each present only once, are present in the correct
order and direction (clockwise).
Two hands are present, one pointing to 11 and one pointing to
2.

ANY CLOCK MISSING ANY OF THESE ELEMENTS IS SCORED
ABNORMAL. REFUSAL TO DRAW A CLOCK IS SCORED
ABNORMAL.

SOME EXAMPLES OF ABNORMAL CLOCKS (THERE ARE MANY OTHER KINDS)

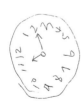

Abnormal Hands

Missing Number

# Glasgow coma score

The Glasgow coma scale (GCS) provides a framework with which to describe a patient's state in terms of three elements of responsiveness: eye opening, verbal, and motor.

The GCS is an artificial index obtained by adding scores for each of the three responses. The range of scores is 3 to 15, 3 being the worst, and 15 the best.

### Best eye response

| 4 | Spontaneous opening |
| 3 | Open to speech |
| 2 | Open to pain |
| 1 | No eye opening. |

### Best verbal response

| 5 | Orientated |
| 4 | Confused conversation |
| 3 | Inappropriate words |
| 2 | Incomprehensible sounds |
| 1 | None. |

### Best motor response

| 6 | Obey commands |
| 5 | Localize pain |
| 4 | Withdrawal from pain—pulls limb away |
| 3 | Abnormal flexion to pain (decorticate posture) |
| 2 | Extension to pain (decerebrate posture) |
| 1 | No motor response. |

Note that the term *GCS 11* has limited meaning. It is important to state the components of the GCS, e.g., E2V2M4 = GCS 8.

Broadly, a GCS of
≥13 suggests mild brain injury
9–12 suggest moderate injury
≤8 suggests severe brain injury (coma)

# Confusion assessment method

A positive test requires the presence of items 1 and 2, *and* 3 *or* 4.
   The positive likelihood ratio is 5.06 and negative likelihood ratio is 0.23.
1. *Acute onset and fluctuating course*. Evidence of acute change in mental status from baseline; behavior fluctuates during the day.
2. *Inattention*. Easily distracted, difficulty focusing attention and keeping track with conversation.
3. *Disorganized thinking*. Irrelevant conversation, unclear flow of ideas, unpredictable switching from subject to subject.
4. *Any mental state*, *other than alert*, *is abnormal*. Describe altered states as (a) vigilant, (b) drowsy, (c) difficult or unable to arouse.

## Further reading

Inouye SK, van Dyck CH, Alessi CA, Balkin S, Siegal AP, Horowitz RI (1990). Clarifying confusion. The Confusion Assessment Method. A new method for detection of delirium. *Ann Intern Med* **113**(12):941–948.

# Index